Palliative Surgery

Matthias W. Wichmann • Guy Maddern
Editors

Palliative Surgery

Springer

Editors
Matthias W. Wichmann, MD, FRACS
Department of General Surgery
Mount Gambier General Hospital
Flinders University—Rural
Medical School
Mount Gambier
SA, Australia

Guy Maddern, MBBS, PhD,
MS, MD, FRACS
Discipline of Surgery
The Queen Elizabeth Hospital
University of Adelaide
Woodville
SA, Australia

ISBN 978-3-642-53708-0 ISBN 978-3-642-53709-7 (eBook)
DOI 10.1007/978-3-642-53709-7
Springer Heidelberg New York Dordrecht London

Library of Congress Control Number: 2014933799

Printed on acid-free paper

Springer is part of Springer Science+Business Media (www.springer.com)

To my patients; to my family Juliane, Antoinette, Jakobus, and Evangelia; and to my parents Inga and Tonius. Thank you for all your help and support!

Matthias W. Wichmann, MD, FRACS

To my patients and their families.

Guy Maddern, MBBS, PhD, MS, MD, FRACS

Preface

The optimal care for patients suffering from terminal and end-stage disease due to malignancies or other conditions has gained significantly more attention by health-care professionals across all specialties. This is an important area for general surgeons – we always have performed procedures on terminally ill patients but rarely described it as "Palliative Surgery".

If we are already performing such surgery, why should we need to write a book about it? There are a number of excellent reasons to produce a book on this increasingly important subject.

The most important reason is perhaps our responsibility for such patients. During discussions with a colleague who is a palliative care physician, it became evident that surgeons are not keen to accept the responsibility for patients in their last weeks or even days of life. We might feel more comfortable with patients who have an excellent prognosis after our surgical efforts, and we might ignore the tremendous impact even a small improvement of quality of life can have for a palliative care patient. The idea for this book was born when another colleague could not find a surgeon who was willing to create a stoma for a patient dying from metastatic rectal cancer but was suffering from faecal vomiting due to his bowel obstruction.

This book encourages experienced as well as young surgeons to put their surgical skills and knowledge towards the symptomatic treatment of patients in their terminal phase of life. The book encourages us to assume the same responsibility for these patients as we are willing to take for those with a more positive prognosis.

A further important reason is the continuously increasing medical knowledge that can obscure the understanding on relevant research results. This book provides evidence – where it is available – to make our surgical treatment decisions reliable, reproducible and comparable. "Palliative Surgery" certainly is not to be placed at the end of the operating list to be done by the junior members of the surgical team. Surgical results must be of high quality, and research in this field of surgery must be encouraged. A surgical textbook can contribute to this research and will help make sound surgical treatment decisions.

The growing relevance of palliative surgery is not only a very significant development for surgeons but also for our patients: the end of curative surgery does not mean that there is no way of surgical intervention for improvement of quality of life. The surgeon who was involved with the care of an individual patient can and should stay involved even when the curative approach clearly has failed.

The growing need for surgical palliation has developed due to the increasing numbers of patients receiving palliative care as a consequence of our ageing population and the prolonged cancer survival as a result of improved treatment regimens.

Palliative care is usually provided within the setting of a multidisciplinary team, and a surgeon must be part of this team approach. Expert opinion of a general surgeon is needed to decide upon treatment options for a palliative care patient. It is therefore of importance to collect and analyse the available data on surgical treatment options for palliative patients in a consolidated reference textbook. This helps provide for sound judgement and reliable treatment planning for patients who are highly dependent on our help and guidance. Very often they are not fit for a second opinion or a trip to a different hospital to receive their care: this further increases our responsibility as care providers.

This book will help to improve surgical decision-making in palliative surgery, encourage surgeons to assume responsibility for palliative care patients and, most importantly, improve the care offered to these patients.

Mount Gambier, SA Matthias W. Wichmann, MD, FRACS
Woodville, SA Guy Maddern, MBBS, PhD, MS, MD, FRACS

Contents

Contributors

Markus Albertsmeier, MD Department of General, Visceral, Transplantation, Vascular and Thoracic Surgery, Ludwig Maximilians University, Munich, Germany

Martin K. Angele, MD, FACS Department of General, Visceral, Transplantation, Vascular and Thoracic Surgery, Ludwig Maximilians University, Munich, Germany

Oliver Ayres, MBBS, FRANZCR Benson Radiology, North Adelaide, SA, Australia

Department of Medical Imaging, Flinders Medical Centre, Bedford Park, SA, Australia

Giacomo Bovio, MD Metabolic-Nutritional Unit and Palliative Care Unit, Fondazione Salvatore Maugeri, Pavia, Italy

Nadine R. Caron, MD, MPH, FRCSC Department of Surgery and Northern Medical Program, University of British Columbia, Prince George, BC, Canada

Scott A. Carruthers, FRANZCR Department of Radiation Oncology, Royal Adelaide Hospital, Adelaide, SA, Australia

John Cartmill, MBBS, BSc(med), MM, FRACS Department of Surgery, Macquarie University Hospital, Australian School of Advanced Medicine, Macquarie University, North Ryde, NSW, Australia

Suzanne Chapman, RGN, MSc, BSc Department of Anaesthetics and Pain, The Royal Marsden NHS Foundation Trust, London, UK

Pierre-Alain Clavien, MD, PhD, FACS, FRCS Department of Surgery, Swiss Hepato-Pancreato-Biliary Center, University Hospital Zurich, Zurich, Switzerland

David C. Currow, MPH, BMed, FRACP Discipline of Palliative and Supportive Services, Repatriation General Hospital, Flinders University, Adelaide, SA, Australia

David J. David, MBBS, MD, FRCS, FRACS Australian Cranio-Facial Unit, David David Medical Services, Women and Children's Hospital, Royal Adelaide Hospital, North Adelaide, SA, Australia

Ashley Dennison, MD, FRCS Department of Hepatobiliary and Pancreatic Surgery, Leicester General Hospital, Leicester, UK

Paul Farquhar-Smith, MB BChir, MA, FRCA, PhD, FFPMRCA, FFICM Department of Anaesthetics and Pain, The Royal Marsden NHS Foundation Trust, London, UK

Marissa Ferguson, MBBS(hons), BmedSc Department of Anaesthesia and Pain Medicine, Peter MacCallum Cancer Centre, Melbourne, VIC, Australia

Jonathan G. Hiller, MBBS, FANZCA Department of Anaesthesia and Pain Medicine, Peter MacCallum Cancer Centre, Melbourne, VIC, Australia

Glyn G. Jamieson, MD, MD, MBBS, FRACS, FACS, FRCS Discipline of Surgery, Royal Adelaide Hospital, University of Adelaide, Adelaide, SA, Australia

Karl-Walter Jauch, MD, FACS Department of General, Visceral, Transplantation, Vascular and Thoracic Surgery, Ludwig Maximilians University, Munich, Germany

Nigel Jones, DPhil, FRACS, FFPMANZCA Department of Surgery, University of Adelaide, Adelaide, SA, Australia

Craig A. Jurisevic, MBBS, MS, FRACS Cardiothoracic Surgery Unit, Royal Adelaide Hospital, Adelaide, SA, Australia

Benjamin C. Knight, MBchB, FRCS Discipline of Surgery, Royal Adelaide Hospital, University of Adelaide, Adelaide, SA, Australia

Mickaël Lesurtel, MD, PhD Department of Surgery, Swiss Hepato-Pancreato-Biliary Center, University Hospital Zurich, Zurich, Switzerland

Guy Maddern, MBBS, PhD, MS, MD, FRACS Discipline of Surgery, The Queen Elizabeth Hospital, University of Adelaide, Woodville, SA, Australia

John Miller, MBBS, FRANZCOG CGO Department of Gynaecology, The Queen Elizabeth Hospital, Woodville, SA, Australia

Sheila Payne, BA, DipN, RN, PhD, C.Psychol Division of Health Research, International Observatory on End of Life Care, Lancaster University, Lancaster, Lancashire, UK

Jane L. Phillips, B.App.Sci(Nur), PhD School of Nursing and Sacred Heart Health Service, The University of Notre Dame Australia, Cunningham Centre for Palliative Care, St Vincent's Health Network, Darlinghurst, NSW, Australia

Nancy J. Preston, PhD, RGN Division of Health Research, International Observatory on End of Life Care, Lancaster University, Lancaster, Lancashire, UK

Timothy J. Price, MBBS, FRACP Department of Medical Oncology, The Queen Elizabeth Hospital and University of Adelaide, Adelaide, SA, Australia

Guy Rees, MBBS, FRCS, FRACS Department of Otolaryngology and Head and Neck Surgery, The Royal Adelaide Hospital, Adelaide, SA, Australia

Bernhard Riedel, MBChB, FCA, FANZCA, FASE, MMed, MBA, PhD Department of Anaesthesia and Pain Medicine, Peter MacCallum Cancer Center and University of Melbourne, Melbourne, VIC, Australia

Peter S. Savas, MBBS, BMedSci Department of Medical Oncology, The Queen Elizabeth Hospital, Woodville South, SA, Australia

Laurie Simard, MD, FRCSC Department of General Surgery, CHUS Hotel Dieu, Sherbrooke, QC, Canada

Dan Spernat, MBBS, MPH, MEd, AFRACMA, FRACS Department of Urology, The Queen Elizabeth Hospital, Woodville, SA, Australia

Sarah Thomasset, PhD, MRCS Department of Hepatobiliary and Pancreatic Surgery, Leicester General Hospital, Leicester, UK

Albert Tuca, MD, PhD Support and Palliative Care Unit, Medical Oncology, Hospital Clinic Barcelona, Barcelona, Spain

Frank Voyvodic, MBBS(Hons), FRANZCR Benson Radiology, North Adelaide, SA, Australia

Department of Medical Imaging, Flinders Medical Centre, Bedford Park, SA, Australia

Andrea Wirsching, MD Department of Surgery, Swiss Hepato-Pancreato-Biliary Center, University Hospital Zurich, Zurich, Switzerland

David C.A. Walsh, MBBS, FRACS Department of Surgery, The Queen Elizabeth Hospital, Adelaide, SA, Australia

Matthias W. Wichmann, MD, FRACS Department of General Surgery, Mount Gambier General Hospital, Flinders University—Rural Medical School, Mount Gambier, SA, Australia

Samuel Young, MBBS(Hons) Department of Orthopaedic Surgery, Royal Perth Hospital, Perth, WA, Australia

René Zellweger, FRACS, FACS Department of Orthopaedic Surgery, Royal Perth Hospital, Perth, WA, Australia

Part I

Palliative Surgery: Behind the Scenes

1 Surgery and Palliative Care: Is There Common Ground or Simply a Clash of Cultures?

David C. Currow and John Cartmill

Contents

The goal of clinical medicine is to improve or maintain the best possible health and well-being. An intervention is "palliative" when the primary aim is to optimise function or comfort without an expectation that the course of the illness will be changed. The philosophy of surgery is predicated on a localised, biomechanical intervention at a single point in time, often with an optimism focusing on what could be achieved. Conditions with potential surgical interventions that develop in advanced disease have widely varying manifestations and progression, making studies difficult, leading to greater reliance on clinical intuition for decision-making.

The person's premorbid level of function, and the likelihood that any intervention will help them to return to, or maintain, better function, becomes the measures for decisions when considering palliative interventions. Principles include:

- D*o no harm* as surgery is trauma and, in someone with progressive, irreversible cachexia, anything that accelerates his/her deterioration is likely to compound disease progression even when minimally invasive.
- Just because something *could* be done does not mean that it *should* be done.

1.1 Introduction

The goals of surgery and good palliative care are directly compatible, where shared clinical decision-making with a less-than-ideal evidence base requires close consultation between the

D.C. Currow, MPH, BMed, FRACP (✉)
Discipline of Palliative and Supportive Services, Repatriation General Hospital, Flinders University, Health Sciences Bldg, Daws Road, Daw Park, Adelaide 5041, SA, Australia
e-mail: david.currow@flinders.edu.au

J. Cartmill, MBBS, BSc(med), MM, FRACS
Department of Surgery, Macquarie University Hospital, Australian School of Advanced Medicine, Macquarie University, 2 Technology Place, 2109, North Ryde, NSW, Australia
e-mail: john.cartmill@mq.edu.au

M. Wichmann, G. Maddern (eds.), *Palliative Surgery*,
DOI 10.1007/978-3-642-53709-7_1, © Springer-Verlag Berlin Heidelberg 2014

disciplines. These decisions must be made with less certainty about outcomes and with greater regard for potential burdens because the risk/benefit ratio shifts rapidly at the end of life, and understanding this trajectory, above all else, is imperative to tailor such surgical care.

The goal of clinical medicine is to improve or maintain the best health and well-being possible. Many of the most striking advances in improving health outcomes in the last century have been driven by the ability of clinicians to safely deliver surgical interventions.

More recently, the advances in health outcomes have reflected decreasing mortality from many acute diseases, leaving instead an increasing and paradoxical legacy of chronic, complex diseases. Many of these diseases become progressive, leading eventually or contributing to death. The sum of these two changes across the second half of the twentieth century has fundamentally changed how we live and, subsequently, how we die. At the beginning of the twenty-first century, most people in our communities will have foreknowledge of their death as they are most likely to experience a chronic progressive disease. This growing cohort of patients (many of whom owe their survival to the success of acute medicine and surgery) challenge our institutions and models of care on many levels and to a large extent constitute the specialty of palliative care.

1.2 How Do Surgery and Palliative Care Fit Together?

Palliative care seeks to optimise comfort and function for people with advanced, progressive illness. Physical, social, existential, psychological and sexual dimensions of personhood are addressed. The goal of an intervention is "palliative" anytime that the primary aim of a clinician is to optimise function or comfort without the expectation that the course of the illness will be changed. The population under consideration are characterised by "frailty", irrespective of age. Much of the acute care that is offered has a palliative intent, with one recent census of hospital inpatients estimating that palliation was the goal of care for one third of all inpatients [1].

The philosophy of surgery on the other hand is predicated on a localised, biomechanical intervention: a blockage is stented or bypassed; a perforation is repaired; bleeding is stemmed; a cancer is excised. The whole patient and their context are considered and respected, but the therapy is localised in time and place – emphatic, targeted and often bold. For a surgeon, the well-being of the whole patient is improved by solving a discrete problem. The ability to perform a procedure and provide the immediate post-operative care safely has continued to improve rapidly. Surgery's advances have been enabled by quantitative methods of research and practice. Quantitative methods are at their finest in situations with some regularity and reproducibility: normal anatomy and tissue biomechanics, expectations of inflammation, healing and repair and a predictable natural history of well-understood and relatively common diseases. Conditions that develop subsequently are not so straightforward, and it becomes more difficult to predict outcomes once systemic disease is established with its widely varying manifestations and progression – once it is "off the rails".

Quantitative methods are less suited to the complexities of many of the palliative care problems that have a potential surgical intervention associated with them. Many competent researchers have looked at the problems of palliative care patients that might be amenable to surgery for consistency and patterns (signals within the noise) and have not found them. A Cochrane Review summarises them. So strong and embedded is the quantitative approach, however, that failures of the technique are seen to be failures of the researchers who have been bold enough to tackle these challenges – failures rather than an acknowledgment that many of these individual clinical problems reside in a realm of clinical experience beyond the quantitative, even when relatively large numbers of patients and their outcomes are aggregated, demanding instead a realm of "rule of thumb", based firmly on the basic principles of surgery and "surgical wisdom" (whatever that encompasses).

With a recurrence of cancer, for example, the anatomy is altered, the biomechanics of the tissue are different and the nutritional state is often already compromised. Such problems are multiplied if there are a number of sites of recurrence in the one person. Response to surgery is unpredictable, the risks are higher and the payoff can seem relatively poor. The systematic approaches on which we rely to build our practices may not provide the specific answers seen in other areas of surgery. This leads to a much greater reliance on narrative and intuition.

In parallel with the rapid advances in surgery and the clinical supports required before and after the operating suite that have developed in the last 50 years, palliative care developed as a counterculture to mainstream health services in reaction to:

- The perceived failure of the health system to acknowledge that people die
- That most deaths are *not* a failure of the clinicians involved in care nor the health systems that delivers care
- That people have specific conversations, goals and tasks that are important for them and their surviving families when death becomes the inevitable outcome of a particular condition

At its inception, this counterculture arguably ignored key opportunities for active intervention that might have improved the well-being of patients – because patients had been labelled "palliative". However, there have been fundamental shifts in attitude from both within and outside the specialty. Palliative care specialists are now more likely to actively embrace interventions that will optimise function or comfort in people likely to tolerate a procedure. Over the same period palliative care has proved its value to the extent that the interventional specialities are now more willing collaborators.

One of the challenges of collaboration between surgeons and palliative care physicians is their profound differences in focus and experience. Surgery usually encounters patients early in a disease with a discrete, localised mechanical problem, a problem with a surgical solution that is well practised, trusted and reliable. Palliative care encounters patients in much more general [global] terms. A surgeon considers the mobility of a tumour, for example, or the state of nutrition. A palliative care specialist, in the setting of metastatic cancer, considers the (often long) plateau phase where a person's overall condition (reflected in their level of function) is relatively stable, noting that once function starts to decline, the trajectory to death is rapid. In this setting, the major prognostic feature is overall well-being rather than the organs in which metastases appear, reflecting that advanced cancer is a systemic disease causing systemic decline. Increasing global frailty is the hallmark of death approaching.

There are few randomised controlled trials of surgical care compared to other ways of dealing with symptomatic problems, and the few studies that do exist often stratify on the basis of performance status. Those with poor performance status tend to be systematically excluded. The absence of research says a great deal about the complexity of the problem and how difficult it is to tease out strands of consistent experience that can be applied generally to clinical decision-making.

Where guidelines fail – and they fail often in the palliative care setting – the challenge becomes clinically dealing with uncertainty. Once such uncertainty is recognised because of a lack of applicable evidence, then there are ways to navigate the circumstances based on values, first principles and clinical experience. While acknowledging that some of the principles, aphorisms and rules of thumb are contradictory, some are presented here; some are surgical and some are palliative. Clinical experience, narrative evidence and intuition may be all the guidance that is available. First, *do no harm* is a good start. Surgery is trauma, not a magic wand, and we should never underestimate just how much worse an operation can make things for someone with established cachexia and no way of reversing the underlying disease state.

If a person is in a catabolic state, anything that accelerates his/her deterioration is likely to be irreversible. The trauma of surgery compounds the deterioration of the disease itself. The systemic well-being of the person is a key index of ability to withstand the catabolic insult of surgery, no matter how minimally invasive that surgical procedure may appear to be. People with established and progressive cachexia are unlikely to tolerate even the most straightforward procedure. Importantly, such cachexia is not limited to people with cancer but seen also in advanced AIDS, neurodegenerative diseases and end-stage organ failure. The ability to recover from surgery is going to be limited and arguably may hasten dying even if the surgery itself is deemed "a success". Minimally invasive techniques alter this balance between metabolic insult and benefit. Modern technologies (often minimally invasive) find niche applications in this area (stents, multiplex vascular access ports for isolated organ perfusion or transarterial embolisation, as examples).

The overall condition of the patient must be weighed against the proposed intervention in a multifactorial calculus that has little certainty. Systemically, what is the overall condition of the person? Where might this person be in their disease trajectory either with or without the intervention proposed? What has been the rate of (irreversible) systemic decline in the last week/month/quarter? Rapid decline without a reversible cause is likely to delineate a very short prognosis, while a slower decline is likely to indicate a longer prognosis. Ultimately, is this person otherwise going to tolerate this procedure and live long enough to recover from the effects of the procedure to enjoy the benefits offered?

Optimism underscores the surgical approach and where there is uncertainty there can be good surprises as well as sad ones; an obstruction can be benign but sadly even a benign obstruction in someone with widespread metastatic disease may be the harbinger of death, with or without surgery.

As an example, the surgical approach tailored to the person with advanced disease may include consciously seeking to:

- Make an incision to avoid tumour mass and come in close to adjacent loops of obstructed and collapsed bowel
- Use non-absorbable rather than a dissolving suture
- Bypass rather than attempting to resect a fistula

Should the patient be nursed on the surgical ward with its rigour and focus or stay where it might be quieter and enjoy his/her existing relationships with staff?

Within any health-care system, there will be additional layers of often confounding complexity to interpret and resolve: an operating room and staff must be available; does the surgeon have the emotional reserve or the time and energy to take the case on? To suggest that these factors may influence clinical decision-making is offensive to some clinicians; however, evidence suggests that logistics and even financial considerations do have a bearing on the care that is offered.

Conclusion

Ultimately, the goals of surgery and those of good palliative care are directly compatible. They belong in the realm of shared clinical decision-making where an evidence base may not be directly available and where the consequences of decision-making are profound. The decisions must be made with less certainty as to the outcome and with greater regard for potential burdens than one is used to as a surgeon.

Where there are no quantitative data to help the calculus of risk and benefit, uncertainty cannot be solved in prospect. Patterns may be discernible in retrospect, and as experience, however fragmented and heterogenous, accrues, such experience is audited with the expectation that at some point signals may emerge from the noise. Any data collection will be confounded by the development of new techniques as surgical and engineering imaginations innovate. It is complicated, it is changing and it is fuelled by an optimism of diversity, imagination and resilience. The advances of surgery in generating less morbidity and more predictable benefit that have been developed, especially in the last two decades, have opened opportunities for palliative interventions which, in carefully selected cases, offer demonstrable benefit. This "shifting ground" is to be welcomed in the palliative setting, tempered by profound and humble respect for the person who is dying and their family.

Just because something *can* be done does not mean that it *should* be done. As someone deteriorates systemically, the risk/benefit ratio starts to shift rapidly, and understanding this trajectory, above all else, is imperative to tailor surgical care to the individual as death approaches.

Reference

1. To THM, Greene AG, Agar MR, Currow DC. A point prevalence survey of hospital inpatients to define the proportion with palliation as the primary goal of care and the need for specialist palliative care. Intern Med J. 2011;41(5):430–3.

Models of Care in Palliative Medicine

2

David C. Currow and Jane L. Phillips

Contents

D.C. Currow, MPH, BMed, FRACP (✉)
Discipline of Palliative and Supportive Services, Repatriation General Hospital, Flinders University, Health Sciences Bldg, Daws Road, Daw Park, Adelaide 5041, SA, Australia
e-mail: david.currow@flinders.edu.au

J.L. Phillips, B.App.Sci(Nur), PhD
School of Nursing and Sacred Heart Health Service, The University of Notre Dame Australia, Cunningham Centre for Palliative Care, St Vincent's Health Network, Darlinghurst 2010, NSW, Australia
e-mail: jane.phillips@nd.edu.au, jphillips@stvincents.com.au

In resource-rich countries, chronic complex diseases have largely replaced acute causes of disability and death. There is now a need for every clinician to be able to take a *palliative approach*. This is defined as the ability to deal with key elements of clinical care for someone who has a progressive illness that is likely to lead to death and their caregivers. The key elements of a *palliative approach* are access; collaborative interdisciplinary team-based care; defining the goals of care; evaluating the "net effect" of any treatments or interventions addressing, where relevant, issues of withholding and withdrawing treatment; determining preferred place of care and, separately, the preferred place at the time of death; and managing care transitions.

For patients, there is evidence of improved symptom control, better met needs, better satisfaction with care and better quality of dying and improved comfort in the last 2 weeks of life. Having relinquished their roles, caregivers for people at the end of life who have used specialist palliative care services had better long-term survival and were better able to adjust to their changed circumstances. Specialist palliative care services are also associated with better met caregiver needs, improved satisfaction with care and less caregiver anxiety. For health systems, benefits include reduced inpatient stays, fewer presentations to the emergency department and reduced overall costs.

Patient-defined areas of importance include the ability to carry out one's affairs as the end-of-life approaches, resolving relationship issues and being involved in decision-making. Specialist

M. Wichmann, G. Maddern (eds.), *Palliative Surgery*,
DOI 10.1007/978-3-642-53709-7_2, © Springer-Verlag Berlin Heidelberg 2014

supportive and palliative care has services which are charged with providing team-based clinical care to people with the most complex end-of-life care needs and their families, as well as and consultative support for colleagues providing care where the patient or family have less complex needs. Ensuring all people have access to best palliative care is dependent upon an on going committment to ensuring that: there is adequate education at an undergraduate, postgraduate and post-registration level; and high-quality research that continues to refine the evidence base for clinical care that is offered; and health services are structured to optimally deliver these services.

2.1 Introduction

Palliative medicine grew out of a counterculture to perceptions in the 1950s and 1960s that the major causes of death and disability were all but addressed [1]. As such, death and dying were not areas that were receiving serious attention both academically and clinically. Palliative care was a reaction in many ways to the perception that death was a clinical "failure". Although much of our health system spends time concerned that death may be a consequence of poor care or iatrogenic, the vast majority of deaths are, or should now be, expected in clinical care, since mortality patterns have changed rapidly in the last century.

In resource-rich countries, chronic complex diseases have largely replaced acute causes of disability and death. This has meant that life expectancy has increased but, at the same time, the causes of death have shifted from maternal and child health, trauma, infection and acute cardiovascular diseases to chronic, progressive illnesses such as cancer, organ failure and neurodegenerative diseases. For example, rarely are young healthy people dying of community-acquired pneumonia and the rates of death from acute myocardial infarction in the fifth and sixth decade continue to decline. Such changes in the causes of death and disability have required a significant paradigm shift in the clinical care of people across the community. There is now a need for every clinician to be able to take a *palliative approach*. This is defined as the ability to deal with key elements of clinical care for someone who has a life-limiting illness as well as supporting their caregivers. A *palliative approach* is not limited by the physical setting in which care is delivered. Whether the person with the life-limiting illness is based at home, or in an institutional setting, quality palliative care can and should be delivered.

How does one define a patient where the intent should be palliative? Essentially, if a person has a progressive illness that is likely to lead to death, then a *palliative approach* should be taken. This in no way precludes the use of disease-modifying therapies. Indeed, a *palliative approach* should be taken in tandem with disease-modifying therapies, using both approaches to ensure that care is optimised for patients. Lynn et al. use the question "Would you be surprised to hear that this person had died in the next 12 months?" [2]. This question does not limit supportive and palliative care to the last 12 months of life, but does help to frame clinical thinking on the matter.

This chapter provides an overview of outcomes from quality research into the net effects of engaging palliative care, the palliative care needs of surgical patients and their caregivers, the models of care configured to address patients' palliative care needs and the key elements that clinicians need to consider when providing a *palliative approach*.

2.2 What Differences Do Hospice/Palliative Care Services Make?

Evidence from good quality health services research has been evolving over the last 30 years. This has been complemented by increasingly sophisticated population-based studies that help to identify key associations between the uptake of specialist palliative care services and outcomes for patients, for their caregivers and for the health system in which they are treated. This creates two levels of evidence – rigorous randomised trials and other interventional studies from which causality can be derived – and observational studies where only associations can be drawn. Data are available at patient, caregiver, service and health systems levels.

For patients, there is evidence of improved symptom control, better met needs, better satisfaction with care and better quality of dying and improved comfort in the last 2 weeks of life [3]. Both a randomised controlled trial (RCT) and a high-quality observational study have suggested that there may be survival benefit in late-stage disease with referral to palliative care [4, 5], although this may be that premature mortality was avoided in the hospice/palliative care group [6]. There appears to be benefit in better maintaining function in people with a multidisciplinary approach that includes specialists and primary clinical staff joining the patient and caregiver in at least one case conference [7]. Having controlled for major factors known to be associated with poor health in general, being a caregiver is a risk factor for poor health outcomes [8]. Having relinquished their roles, caregivers for people at the end of life who have used specialist palliative care services had better long-term survival and were better able to adjust to their changed circumstances [9, 10]. Specialist palliative care services are also associated with better met caregiver needs, improved satisfaction with care and less caregiver anxiety [3]. For health systems, benefits include reduced inpatient stays, fewer presentations to the emergency department and reduced overall costs [7, 11–13].

The World Health Organization has not only sought to define "palliative care" in ways that it has not done for other areas of clinical care but also set out the framework for service delivery [14]. The basic framework includes that:

- There should be early introduction of palliative care – that is, once there is recognition that this person's life is likely to be shortened as a result of this illness.
- Palliative care can and often should be provided in parallel with disease-modifying therapies.
- This requires careful and repeated assessment of the patient and their caregivers throughout the course of the life-limiting illness.

2.3 Needs and Priorities of Patients and Families

Patient-defined areas of importance include the ability to carry out one's affairs as the end-of-life approaches, resolving relationship issues and being involved in decision-making [15–17]. Without excellent physical symptom control, it is almost impossible to carry out these important end-of-life tasks [17]. Planning for one's death includes being part of discussing what is important at that time, ensuring that legacy issues are actively addressed (How does one want to be remembered? Are there unfinished projects?) and ensuring that one's wishes are known and are going to be respected while dying and once dead.

Being alert throughout the life-limiting illness is incredibly important to patients who are facing death. By contrast health professionals would often regard physical symptom control as more important than being cognitively intact [17]. Although a great deal of health policy is now advocating for home death, the place of care is actually far less important to patients if their family and friends are able to freely spend time with them and to support them. "Home death" as an outcome measure *per se* fails to reflect the complexities of care and the demands made of family and friends as they provide the bulk of that care.

2.4 Providing a Palliative Approach in the Surgical Setting

The speciality of supportive and palliative care has grown up charged with the responsibility of providing team-based clinical care to the people at the end of life with the most complex needs and their families and consultative support for colleagues providing care where the patient or family have less complex needs; ensuring that there is adequate education at an undergraduate, postgraduate and post-registration level; and ensuring that high-quality research is continuing to refine the evidence-base for clinical care that is offered and the way that health services are structured to deliver optimally these services.

In the developed world, the majority of deaths occur in acute care, and this trend is expected to increase in line with population ageing and changing patterns of caregiver availability. These secular trends in where care is provided, especially in the terminal phases of a life-limiting illness, vary widely from country to country depending on health and social system drivers. A small proportion of all acute care deaths will be managed by the patients' surgical team, with support from a specialist palliative care team, as required.

Despite the increase in the number of palliative care services within the acute care sector over the past two decades, in the USA these services are more likely to be based in larger hospitals, academic medical centres, not-for-profit hospitals and VA hospitals compared to other hospitals [18]. These consultative palliative care services are most frequently called upon to support the treating team with discussions about prognosis and goals of care, pursuing documentation of advance directives, discussion about foregoing specific treatments and/or diagnostic interventions, family and patient support, discharge planning and symptom management [19]. The input of hospital-based palliative care teams to patient's care has been shown to improve symptom control and quality of life, alleviate emotional burden and improve caregiver and patient satisfaction [3, 20, 21]. In the USA, palliative care provided to hospitalised patients with advanced disease has resulted in lower costs of care and less utilisation of intensive care compared to similar patients receiving usual care [22].

Following the high-profile randomised controlled trial (RCT) in the USA by Temel et al. [4] for people with advanced lung cancer where participants were randomised to either early referral to palliative care or to routine care, there is now increasing interest in encouraging earlier referral to specialist palliative care services [23], which is appropriate for people with more complex needs [24]. Simultaneously, the timely initiation of a *palliative approach* is appropriate for people whose care needs can be managed by their existing care team.

2.5 Key Elements of a Palliative Approach

The key elements of a *palliative approach* are access; collaborative interdisciplinary team-based care; defining the goals of care; evaluating the "net effect" of any treatments or interventions addressing, where relevant, issues of withholding and withdrawing treatment; determining preferred place of care and, separately, the preferred place at the time of death; and managing care transitions.

2.5.1 Access

Palliative care is not limited by diagnosis – people with cancer, AIDS, neurodegenerative diseases or end-stage organ failure are all going to benefit from a *palliative approach* and may require referral to specialist palliative care when the complexity of their needs exceeds the care offered by other disciplines including primary care or specialist surgery [25]. Likewise, palliative care is not limited by prognosis in the presence of a chronic, progressive life-limiting illness. The needs of patients and their caregivers should be the arbiter of the care that is offered in this setting. These needs include all of the domains that define each of us (physical, social, existential, sexual, emotional, financial and logistical). The aim of care is to optimise function and comfort in each of these domains having been adequately assessed, minimise dependence and determine each caregiver's willingness and ability to provide care and support. This approach enables the implementation of systematic care planning based upon a multifaceted assessment of the patients and their caregivers' support needs.

2.5.2 Collaborative Interdisciplinary Team-Based Care

Given the breadth of issues faced by people at the end of life, there is a need for true interdisciplinary care. Every team member brings a combination of skills: those inherent in any fellow human, those of a health professional and those of the specific discipline in which the person has been trained. As noted, a number of skills need to be shared at the level of a health professional (a *palliative approach*) and those that are dealt with at specialist level (*specialist palliative care*). Configuring the interdisciplinary team to the patients' needs requires consideration.

A key clinician has to take responsibility for overseeing care and optimising its coordination. In many health systems this may be the general practitioner/family physician or the primary specialist charged with that care. Patients benefit from having the input of all of the disciplines that can add to the quality of their clinical care. Other specialist medical teams with skills related to the underlying life-limiting illness and any co-morbid conditions are crucial to optimise the care of anything that will predictably improve the control of the disease and to help in decisions about rationalising medications and contributing to discussions on the changing goals of care.

Nurses' proximity to patients and their caregivers enable them to identify people who would benefit from a *palliative approach* and to advocate for this approach to care. Nurse practitioners and nurse specialists have key roles including management of medications/medication compliance, overall evaluation of the patient in the setting of their caregivers and community more broadly and comprehensive evaluation of the health of the person. The expertise of a range of other specialist nurses is often required to manage surgical patient's complex wounds, continence and stomas.

In the light of widespread polypharmacy that increases as death approaches, the pharmacist's role is of critical importance [26]. Not only are medications for long-term co-morbidities continued, but medications for symptom control are added. This needs ongoing review and rationalisation with the emphasis on medications whose continuation will deliver a demonstrable benefit to the patient.

As people are living longer with non-communicable diseases, there is a need to optimise their level of physical functioning in a setting where physical decline is an almost universal experience. Physical and occupational therapists are central to achieving this outcome [27]. Better maintaining function is a pivotal patient-centred goal of care.

The practical issues of facing death (ensuring that wills and powers of attorney are all in place, financial support) are also a central concern of many patients. Social workers have a key role in helping to ensure these issues are addressed. Counselling skills for patient and their families are another key part of the role.

For people who are exploring existential questions for the first time or in new ways, for people who may not have a faith community or where their faith community is not meeting his/her needs, contact with pastoral care can be helpful. These are often difficult issues and, at times, frightening conversations. Often people's world views and belief systems are challenged by news of their impending death.

Art therapists and music therapists can help in exploring ways of expressing difficult-to-articulate issues. By using a variety of media people may be able to create a legacy as an important part of their end-of-life work [28].

Oral historians help to capture particular aspects of life, some of which may not have been discussed or require a particular perspective. It is also a rich legacy that many people want to leave for their families.

2.5.3 Defining the Goals of Care

Above all, patients expect that clinicians are going to be honest in discussing issues about end-of-life care, are competent to raise these issues and will do so in a timely manner. This requires excellent communication skills by clinicians and a level of candour that balances hope (an incredibly plastic concept that sees people shift what they hope for, which at times may be for better moments as opposed to better days) and honesty. Above all else, patients will value honesty in this setting in a way that can optimise care and allow them the time to arrange their affairs as they would wish [15].

2.5.4 Evaluating the "Net Effect" of Treatment

A *palliative approach* requires integrating evidence-based palliative non-pharmacological and pharmacological interventions tailored to specific disease conditions and symptoms. However, interventions (whether they are pharmacological, surgical or psychological) need to be evaluated for their "net effect". This means that both the benefits and the burdens of any interventions need to be carefully, prospectively evaluated. Anything less than this is likely to limit the ability of clinicians to provide quality care predictably and limit the ability to tailor interventions to individuals who are most likely to benefit from them.

There should be a focus on optimising the management of the life-limiting illness. Again, this needs to be in the context of the net clinical effect (benefit and burdens). Treating with low odds of benefit and high risk of toxicity is unlikely to be of net benefit for most patients late in the course of most life-limiting illnesses. Interventions need to predictably improve this person's well-being in order to be justified.

While in developed countries approximately one in three people referred to palliative care services are under the age of 65, many people referred to palliative care are elderly, which means that an increasing number of co-morbid illnesses will be encountered and also have to be managed actively. In this setting, the goals of care in treating the co-morbid illness need to be clear. For example, many patients are continued on anti-hypertensive medications long after they have lost weight, have become normotensive and indeed may now have iatrogenic postural hypotension. In managing type II diabetes with increasing cachexia, weight loss and anorexia, an early decision needs to be made in order to avoid fatal or life-threatening hypoglycaemia. It is crucial that we better understand the role of other long-term interventions such as the use of "statins". If the number needed to treat (NNT) requires hundreds of people to be treated for several years in order to avoid one particular event, continuing those medications late into the course of a life-limiting illness is probably going to be counterproductive more often than not. The balance between benefit and an increasing likelihood of toxicity as frailty becomes prominent needs to be considered carefully.

2.5.5 Addressing Issues of Withholding and Withdrawing Treatment

The clinical decisions surrounding withdrawing and withholding treatment towards the end of life are particularly challenging when many of the life-sustaining interventions, such as renal dialysis and implantable defibrillators, are initiated earlier in the person's illness with the goal of managing symptoms and prolonging life [29]. If the reality of needing to withdraw treatment at some stage has not previously been discussed with the patient and his/her family, then these conversations take on a new urgency and often become more challenging as the patient's condition deteriorates and these interventions become progressively more burdensome. Clarifying and renegotiating the goals of care with the patient and family is crucial as it allows them to plan accordingly, limits their exposure to unnecessary and potentially distressing care [30] and ensures that the interdisciplinary team is clear on the intent(s) of treatment. Reviewing and clarifying the goals of care with the patient and their caregivers is something that clinicians should actively initiate. In the future, with technological and pharmaceutical advances, it is likely that health professionals will be faced with these clinical dilemmas on a more frequent basis.

2.5.6 Determining Preferred Place of Care and Place of Death

There is an often expressed view that people with life-limiting illnesses would most like to be cared for at home. Certainly in surveys of well members of the community, there is a preference that home is where people would like to be if they have a life-limiting illness. However, this should not be translated into a policy that home is where care must be, especially in the terminal phases (last hours or days of life) of a life-limiting illness. Indeed, many people would actively choose an inpatient setting as the place they would like to die even if they had expressed a wish that the majority of their care were to be provided in the community setting. People's preferences for where care should be may also change over time [31].

Central to this is the need to have an able and willing caregiver [32]. It seems that clinicians assume that a person will happily take on the caregiving role, and rarely do we ask if they are willing or able to do so. Yet, the strongest predictor of care at home and subsequent death at home is the presence of a caregiver who is prepared to take on the role. If there are disagreements between the person dying and the caregiver, it is ultimately the caregiver who makes the greatest impact on where care will be. Recent data suggest that having taken on a caregiver role, there are an identifiable group of people who would not take on such a role again [33].

2.5.7 Managing Care Transitions

A rapid change in the palliative patient's clinical status and or caregiver circumstances often necessitates transitions between hospitals, subacute and post-acute nursing facilities, the patient's home, primary and specialty care offices and long-term care facilities. A rapid change may also include, at times, an improvement in their condition where people may wish to make the most of "windows of opportunity" to return home from an inpatient unit while they still can. Coordination and continuity of care between different locations or levels of care within the same location are a priority for palliative patients and their families. Patients and caregivers may lack knowledge of what services are available and how to access them [34]. Navigating the transition from inpatient to community-based care requires intensive effort and coordination to put management plans and caregiver support in place. Current information about the patient's goals, preferences and clinical status along with a comprehensive plan of care needs to accompany the transfer of the patient across care settings. Specifically planning for patient's and caregivers' responses to clinical scenarios that may occur for this patient is a key role for health professionals when caring for someone in the community. For example, if systemic sepsis from a urinary tract infection has precipitated two admissions to hospital in the last 7 weeks, then contingency planning for the next episode is crucial.

2.6 Minimal Palliative Care Competencies Required by All Health Professionals

In a recent Australian process, a survey sought views from specialist palliative care providers, generalists and educators nationally [35]. There was widespread agreement that there were four competencies required by all clinical staff in order to be able to provide a *palliative approach*. These include:

- Basic principles of palliative care including understanding disease trajectories (with and without disease-modifying treatment) and the net effects (burdens and benefits) of any clinical intervention
- Good communication skills
- Excellent assessment skills not limited to physical well-being, but also to the social, emotional and existential problems that people frequently face in these circumstances
- Optimising the comfort and function of the person and their caregivers in each of the domains outlined in the third competency

2.7 Summary

The heterogeneity of the palliative care population requires collaboration across care teams, with a focus on a *palliative approach* for the majority of people and referral to specialist palliative care services for a smaller number of people based on needs rather than diagnosis nor prognosis. Such a system-based approach delivers benefits to patients, their caregivers and the health system in which care is delivered. Existing evidence reinforces the importance of shared communication, skill enhancement and clarifying goals of care through advanced care planning.

References

1. Clark D. From margins to centre: a review of the history of palliative care in cancer. Lancet Oncol. 2007;8(5):430–8.
2. Lunney JR, Lynn J, Foley DJ, Lipson S, Guralnik JM. Patterns of functional decline at the end of life. JAMA. 2003;289(18):2387–92.
3. Currow DC, Wheeler JL, Abernethy AP. International perspective: outcomes of palliative oncology. Semin Oncol. 2011;38(3):343–50.
4. Temel JS, Greer JA, Muzikansky A, Gallagher ER, Admane S, Jackson VA, et al. Early palliative care for patients with metastatic non-small-cell lung cancer. N Engl J Med. 2010;363(8):733–42.
5. Pyenson B, Connor S, Fitch K, Kinzbrunner B. Medicare cost in matched hospice and non-hospice cohorts. J Pain Symptom Manage. 2004;28(3):200–10.
6. Currow DC, Foley K, Zafar SY, Wheeler JL, Abernethy AP. The need for a re-evaluation of best supportive care studies reported to date. Br J Cancer. 2011;104(3):390–1.
7. Abernethy AP, Currow DC, Shelby-James T, Rowett D, May F, Samsa GP, et al. Delivery strategies to optimize resource utilization and performance status for patients with advanced life-limiting illness: results from the "Palliative Care Trial" [ISRCTN81117481]. J Pain Symptom Manage. 2013;45(3):488–505.
8. Schulz R, Beach SR. Caregiving as a risk factor for mortality: the Caregiver Health Effects Study. JAMA. 1999;282(23):2215–9.
9. Christakis NA, Iwashyna TJ. The health impact of health care on families: a matched cohort study of hospice use by decedents and mortality outcomes in surviving, widowed spouses. Soc Sci Med. 2003; 57(3):465–75.
10. Abernethy AP, Currow DC, Fazekas BS, Luszcz MA, Wheeler JL, Kuchibhatla M. Specialized palliative care services are associated with improved short- and long-term caregiver outcomes. Support Care Cancer. 2008;16(6):585–97.
11. Connor SR, Pyenson B, Fitch K, Spence C, Iwasaki K. Comparing hospice and nonhospice patient survival among patients who die within a three-year window. J Pain Symptom Manage. 2007;33(3):238–46.
12. Costantini M, Higginson IJ, Boni L, Orengo MA, Garrone E, Henriquet F, et al. Effect of a palliative home care team on hospital admissions among patients with advanced cancer. Palliat Med. 2003; 17(4):315–21.
13. Brumley RD, Enguidanos S, Cherin DA. Effectiveness of a home-based palliative care program for end-of-life. J Palliat Med. 2003;6(5):715–24.
14. World Health Organisation. WHO definition of palliative care. 2003. Retrieved 16 January 2014, from http://www.who.int/cancer/palliative/definition/en/
15. McCaffrey N, Currow DC, Eckermann S. Measuring impacts of value to patients is crucial when evaluating palliative care. J Pain Symptom Manage. 2009;37(6): e7–9.
16. Singer PA, Martin DK, Kelner M. Quality end-of-life care: patients' perspectives. JAMA. 1999;281(2): 163–8.
17. Steinhauser KE, Christakis NA, Clipp EC, McNeilly M, McIntyre L, Tulsky JA. Factors considered important at the end of life by patients, family, physicians, and other care providers. JAMA. 2000; 284(19):2476–82.
18. Morrison RS, Maroney-Galin C, Kralovec PD, Meier DE. The growth of palliative care programs in United States hospitals. J Palliat Med. 2005;8(6): 1127–34.
19. Manfredi PL, Morrison RS, Morris J, Goldhirsch SL, Carter JM, Meier DE. Palliative care consultations: how do they impact the care of hospitalized patients? J Pain Symptom Manage. 2000;20(3):166–73.
20. Hanks GW, Robbins M, Sharp D, Forbes K, Done K, Peters TJ, et al. The imPaCT study: a randomised controlled trial to evaluate a hospital palliative care team. Br J Cancer. 2002;87(7):733–9.
21. Higginson IJ, Finlay IG, Goodwin DM, Hood K, Edwards AGK, Cook A, et al. Is there evidence that palliative care teams alter end-of-life experiences of patients and their caregivers? J Pain Symptom Manage. 2003;25(2):150–68.
22. Penrod JD, Deb P, Dellenbaugh C, Burgess Jr JF, Zhu CW, Christiansen CL, et al. Hospital-based palliative care consultation: effects on hospital cost. J Palliat Med. 2010;13(8):973–9.
23. Meier DE, Brawley OW. Palliative care and the quality of life. J Clin Oncol. 2011;29(20):2750–2.
24. Waller A, Girgis A, Davidson P, Newton P, Lecathelinais C, Macdonald P, et al. Facilitating needs based support and palliative care for people with chronic heart failure: preliminary evidence for the acceptability, inter-rater reliability, and validity of a needs assessment tool. J Pain Symptom Manage. 2013;45(5):912–25.
25. Waller A, Girgis A, Johnson C, Mitchell G, Yates P, Kristjanson L, et al. Facilitating needs based cancer care for people with a chronic disease: evaluation of an intervention using a multi-centre interrupted time series design. BMC Palliat Care. 2010;9:2.
26. Currow DC, Stevenson JP, Abernethy AP, Plummer J, Shelby-James TM. Prescribing in palliative care as death approaches. J Am Geriatr Soc. 2007;55(4): 590–5.

27. Taylor K, Currow D. A prospective study of patient identified unmet activity of daily living needs among cancer patients at a comprehensive cancer care center. Aust Occup Ther J. 2003;50:79–85.
28. Bradt J, Dileo C. Music therapy for end-of-life care. Cochrane Database Syst Rev 2010;(1):CD007169.
29. Beattie J. A discussion document for health professionals: implantable cardioverter defibrillators in patients who are reaching the end of life. London: British Heart Foundation; 2009.
30. Hillman K. Vital Signs: stories from intensive care. Sydney: University of New South Wales Press; 2009.
31. Agar M, Currow DC, Shelby-James TM, Plummer J, Sanderson C, Abernethy AP. Preference for place of care and place of death in palliative care: are these different questions? Palliat Med. 2008;22(7): 787–95.
32. Grande G, Ewing G. Death at home unlikely if informal carers prefer otherwise: implications for policy. Palliat Med. 2008;22(8):971–2.
33. Currow DC, Burns C, Agar M, Phillips J, McCaffrey N, Abernethy AP. Palliative caregivers who would not take on the caring role again. J Pain Symptom Manage. 2011;41(4):661–72.
34. Burns CM, Dixon T, Smith WT, Craft PS. Patients with advanced cancer and family caregivers' knowledge of health and community services: a longitudinal study. Health Soc Care Community. 2004; 12(6):488–503.
35. Hegarty M, Currow D, Parker D, Turnbull B, Devery K, Canning DF, et al. Palliative care in undergraduate curricula: results of a national scoping study. Focus Health Prof Educ. 2010;12(2):97–109.

Psychosocial and Ethical Aspects 3

Sheila Payne and Nancy J. Preston

Contents

S. Payne, BA, DipN, RN, PhD, C.Psychol (✉)
N.J. Preston, PhD, RGN
Division of Health Research, International Observatory on End of Life Care, Lancaster University, Lancaster, Lancashire LA1 4YG, UK
e-mail: s.a.payne@lancaster.ac.uk; n.j.preston@lancaster.ac.uk

This chapter reflects on some of the realities of providing psychosocial care and the ethical dilemmas that are raised in the context of very sick and dying patients who require palliative surgery. We start by defining psychological, social and spiritual care and then highlight the evidence for integrating these elements of care in palliative surgery. We address the important topic of communication, information exchange, decision-making and ethical choices that are relevant to all types of surgical practice but especially when cure is not the likely or intended outcome. The objective of the chapter is to demonstrate how individual differences in appraisals of stress lead to a variety of coping responses. We also present an overview of psychological issues associated with cancer-related pain management, psychological and psychosexual consequences of palliative surgery and the psychological effects of cancer or surgically induced changes.

3.1 Introduction

Most patients with cancer will have been treated with surgery following diagnosis, and for some this will have required extensive and potentially mutilating procedures [1]. While the majority of surgical interventions for cancer are designed to cure the disease, a large number of operations are undertaken with non-curative (palliative) intent such as tumour de-bulking procedures, insertions of stents and those designed to improve cosmetic

M. Wichmann, G. Maddern (eds.), *Palliative Surgery*,
DOI 10.1007/978-3-642-53709-7_3, © Springer-Verlag Berlin Heidelberg 2014

appearance or remove distressing fungating wounds. There have been exciting developments in surgery where improvements in health technologies and diagnostics have resulted in less invasive procedures, more use of localised resections and improvements in functional outcomes, aided by better rehabilitation. These innovations are likely to benefit those with advanced disease. Globally, the majority of patients who are diagnosed with cancer have advanced disease which is no longer amenable to curative treatment. This means that they are likely to experience distress from pain and other symptoms and psychosocial concerns [2].

For anyone facing surgery, either elective or emergency, there is likely to be heightened anxiety about the outcomes of the procedure and fear about pain and disability and potential complications. The normal trade-off for the patient undergoing surgery is that the short-term pain and distress are balanced by long-term benefits, especially the potential of cure. Clearly in patients approaching the final stage of life, there needs to be careful consideration of this balance to prevent futile and expensive procedures that extend hospital stays and have little impact on quality or duration of life [3]. Yet a recently published review indicates there is little research on the preferences of patients or the impact on quality of life of palliative surgery [1].

This chapter focuses on psychosocial and ethical issues in palliative surgery. We start by defining psychological and social care and then highlight the key ethical issues which will underpin the following sections. We start by addressing the important topic of communication, information exchange, decision-making and ethical choices that are relevant to all types of surgical practice but especially when cure is not the likely or intended outcome. Further sections address individual differences in stress and coping, the psychological issues associated with pain related to surgery, psychological and psychosexual consequences of palliative surgery and the psychological effects of cancer or surgically induced changes.

3.2 What Do We Mean by Psychosocial Care in Palliative Care?

The principles of palliative care have long stressed the interrelationship between four domains of care: physical, psychological, social and spiritual which are acknowledged in the World Health Organization definition [4]. More recent accounts expand this definition to also include structure and processes of care, cultural aspects of care, end-of-life care and ethical and legal aspects of care [5]. Psychosocial care refers to enhancing the psychological, emotional, social, spiritual and existential well-being of patients and their families, not merely identity and treating psychopathology [6]. Psychological care refers to managing emotional and cognitive changes which may or may not be linked to the disease process. Social care encompasses the social functioning of the patient, their relationships and meaningful roles such as participation in employment, education and leisure and financial and environmental situations [7]. Spiritual care may include meaning making and existential and religious beliefs and practices that are important to patients.

3.3 Communication, Information, Informed Consent, Decision-Making and Ethical Considerations in Palliative Surgery

As in all aspects of medicine, the ability to communicate with patients and their families effectively and compassionately is the foundation of psychosocial care. This is especially important when surgeons are required to explain complex procedures where patients need to make decisions about surgery compared to nonsurgical interventions. For example, in prostate cancer treatment options include watchful waiting, radical prostatectomy, radiation therapy and hormonal therapy [8]. The side effects (including urinary incontinence and erectile dysfunction) of a radical prostatectomy are known to be debilitating and life altering for the patient and their partner [8].

In the United Kingdom (UK), for example, services are expected to carry out a *Holistic Needs Assessment* for people with cancer which includes identifying the psychosocial and spiritual needs of the patient across the care pathway, from diagnosis and treatment and into survivorship or end-of-life care [9]. Similarly in the USA the National Quality Forum includes psychosocial, spiritual, religious and existential aspects of care in their quality framework for palliative care [10].

In the UK, the National Institute for Clinical Excellence (NICE) [11] guidance for adults with cancer recommended a four-tiered model of psychological assessment, support and intervention based upon the complexity of the needs of patients and the expertise of professionals involved. This indicated that all health professional should have the expertise to offer basic psychological care, recognise distress and make appropriate referrals, while more complex assessment and psychotherapeutic interventions required the skills of psychologists or psychiatrists. Much psychological morbidity goes unrecognised and therefore untreated because clinicians are reluctant to question people directly about their feelings and patients fail to report their concerns because they fear wasting professional's time, are afraid that they may be construed as ungrateful or "weak willed" or do not believe that surgeons are interested in their psychological state [6]. Asking patients explicitly if they are depressed or anxious should become part of routine surgical follow-up. However, evidence suggests that surgeons are unlikely to have received adequate training in palliative care, pain management or psychosocial care [1].

3.4 Individual Differences in Stress and Coping

One of the main problems in the way psychological care is often construed is to emphasise the abnormal or pathological ways to respond. Relatively little attention is focused on the way that the majority of people affected by cancer manage to contain their distress, carry on with their everyday lives and maintain good relationships with those around them. These are remarkable achievements and only recently have psychologists started to study what is now called "positive psychology". Little is known about the individual differences that predict who will manage difficult challenges associated with palliative surgery and who will be overwhelmed by the experience of cancer and late-stage disease.

One seminal model of stress and coping is based on the notion that patients make primary appraisals of phenomena to determine if they are construed as threatening, followed by secondary appraisals to examine the resources at their disposal to deal with the stressor [12]. It is important to recognise that people have intrinsic (e.g. their personality, life experiences, education) and extrinsic (e.g. family, community, religion, money) resources. These different ways to cope with threat tend to be categorised as problem-focused and emotion-focused coping. The former is more action oriented and may involve seeking information and mobilising resources to seek solutions to a challenge, while the latter tends to emphasise dealing with distressing emotions such as anxiety or anger, by, for example, learning to relax or distract oneself, and tends to be regarded as a more passive response. No one type of coping style is better, as different responses are suitable in different situations or stages of illness. For example, immediately after surgery it may be more helpful if patients can learn to relax and rest, while later they may require an active engagement with rehabilitation. Arguably most people with cancer are very resilient and cope well with the challenges facing them. But when external stressors exceed their capacity to adapt, either because the stressors are so overwhelming or because there are concurrent problems, then psychological distress, depression and anxiety can happen to anyone.

This model has been adapted by Stroebe and Schut [13] to account for the stress and coping associated with bereavement (called the "dual process" model). It may help to account for differences between people in their responses to loss, especially gender differences.

Psychological research shows that some people have personalities that are better able to deal with difficult and challenging situations such as "hardiness" [14]. There are three key characteristics in hardiness: commitment (active involvement in life), control (a belief in the ability to influence life events) and challenge (a stance that regards change as normal and not threatening). People with these attributes are more likely to be optimistic, deal better with stressful situations and engage in healthy behaviours. More recently research has focused on resilience as a protective characteristic following bereavement [15] and in end-of-life care [16].

3.5 Psychological Issues in the Experience of Pain Associated with Surgery and Its Management

Cancer-related pain is defined as the pain experienced by adults and children with cancer in which the pain is due to the tumour itself, to cancer therapy or to associated problems. There is overwhelming evidence that cancer-related pain is common with more than 90 % of patients reporting suffering from pain in the final year of life. Inadequate pain management results in significant psychological consequences such as anxiety, fear, anger, depression and sleep disturbance, which all impact upon recovery from surgery and reduced quality of life. Access to effective pain medication is an essential requisite to palliative surgery, including painful and invasive investigatory procedures. In the early days of palliative care, Cecily Saunders introduced the concept of "total pain" and called for rigorous assessment and treatment of the four domains (as highlighted previously) [17]. In the mid-1980s the World Health Organization introduced a three-step approach (called the pain ladder) to titrate analgesia to pain experiences [18]. Despite some criticism, these remain a cornerstone of effective pain management. Recent clinical guidelines from the European Association for Palliative Care make recommendations on using opioids effectively to manage cancer pain [19]. However, there remain many structural, procedural and educational barriers to ensuring adequate, affordable and timely access to pain medication with huge disparity in morphine consumption across the world [20]. There is evidence that knowledge about how to manage cancer-related pain and other common symptoms near the end of life is poor in many surgeons [1].

3.6 Psychosocial Aspects of Patient and Family Relationships, Including Psychosexual Aspects

Family carers are important companions in the final phase of life and offer vital support to patients that enable them to make choices about the nature and place of death [21, 22]. A recent population-based study in the UK indicates that being single, widowed or divorced (i.e. lacking a family carer) is an important predictor for dying in a hospital [23]. In the context of palliative surgery, family members may have an influential role in helping patients understand the information on treatment options and in considering the risks of complications, morbidity and mortality associated with surgical procedures and weighing them in relation to potential benefits. However, families are often enthusiastic to seek further treatment, both to do their "best" and to be seen not to be giving up on patients. They may underestimate the degree of suffering associated with the surgery. This may mean that they encourage patients to contemplate futile or risky procedures. Alternatively, family members are known to experience vicarious suffering in witnessing the pain and distress of the patient [21, 22].

3.7 Psychosocial Aspects of Palliative Surgery

When patients present with advanced disease, their surgery is often palliative and an example of this would be ovarian cancer. However, subsequent minor surgical procedures may then be required such as drainage of ascites (paracentesis). Malignant ascites is the build-up of large volumes of fluid (about 5 l) in the peritoneal cavity resulting in a large distended abdomen producing abdominal discomfort, difficulty mobilising and fatigue. For many patients, particularly with ovarian cancer, this is the first visible manifestation of their cancer and is a profoundly negative experience [24].

Treatment for ascites is commonly by intermittent drainage using an external cannula inserted at the hospital or treatment centre, often requiring an inpatient admission. Palliative care physicians are less likely to use drainage than their medical or surgical colleagues as they see it as too invasive [25]. Patients generally tolerate drainage well and welcome the relief it brings. However, there is an increased drive to use permanent drainage catheters which can be left in place and the fluid drained as required at home. Patients do not always welcome their use, and in a study by O'Neil and colleagues [26], 16 out of 40 patients turned down the permanent catheter preferring to attend hospital for drainage as required. A small study of just four patients showed that patients found the idea of the permanent drain distasteful, but most of them decided it was worthwhile [27].

Another similar area to consider is the use of ureteric stents to bypass uropathy [28]. While they may improve renal function, research has shown that ureteral stents interfere with patient's daily activities and resulted in a reduced quality of life in 80 % of cases [29]. Perhaps patients need to decide whether the stents are worthwhile or would other less invasive forms of management be preferred, even if this might reduce survival. Indeed, we often fail to assess patients' preference about treatment in research studies, instead measuring symptoms on pre-existing scales. Hence, for even relatively minor surgical procedures such as the choice of ascetic drain, the patient needs to be counselled and consulted before a decision is made; otherwise, they can have psychologically negative impacts upon them.

3.8 Conclusions and Recommendations

In conclusion, this chapter has reviewed the evidence for psychosocial support in patients facing palliative surgery. It has offered working definitions to guide readers and provided a framework for understanding psychological care. It has considered the impact of changing patterns and styles of communication and information provision on the expectations of patients and their engagement in decision-making. Finally, there is recognition that surgeons generally receive little training in palliative care and often do not know how to present and discuss complex palliative treatment choices with patients and families. The implications for recognising individual differences in approaches to stress and coping means that what is perceived as stressful or overwhelming is not merely external factors but an interaction between the person, their internal (psychological) and external (social, financial and cultural) resources. Future policies while being steadfast in their determination to ensure the delivery of high-quality palliative care, and where necessary palliative surgery to patients and their family carers, need to address priorities of service provision and financial support and expand the engagement of surgeons in the multidisciplinary team. The next 10 years will provide many opportunities for the development of better research about patients' preferences for palliative surgery, for crossing or blurring of boundaries between palliative and curative surgical care and for advancing a stronger recognition of a partnership between surgeons and specialist palliative care professionals. Roy [30] highlights the ambiguities inherent in palliative care situations, where differences, contradictions and tensions are balanced with desire for unity, harmony, love and compassion; this is the essence of psychosocial care.

References

1. Mols A, Reiter-Theil S, Oertli D, Viehl CT. Palliative surgery in cancer patients: what do we know about it? Eur J Palliat Care. 2013;20(1):9–13.
2. Kaasa S, Payne S, Sjogren P. Challenges related to palliative care. Lancet Oncol. 2011;12:925–7.

3. Easson AM, Lee F, Brasel K, Krouse RS. Clinical research for surgeons in palliative care: challenges and opportunities. J Am Coll Surg. 2003;196(1): 141–51.
4. Sepulveda C, Marlin A, Yoshida T, Ullrich A. Palliative care: the world health organization's global perspective. J Pain Symptom Manage. 2002;24:91–6.
5. Wittenberg-Lyles E, Goldsmith J, Ferrell B, Ragan SL. Communication in palliative nursing. New York: Oxford University Press; 2013.
6. Lloyd Williams M, editor. Psychosocial issues in palliative care. 2nd ed. Oxford: Oxford University Press; 2008.
7. Altilio T, Otis-Green S, editors. Oxford textbook of palliative social work. New York: Oxford University Press; 2011.
8. Wittmann D, Northouse L, Foley S, Gilbert S, Wood JRDP, Ballon R, Montie JE. The psychosocial aspects of sexual recovery after prostate cancer treatment. Int J Impot Res. 2009;21:99–106.
9. National Cancer Action Team. Holistic needs assessment for people with cancer. London: National Cancer Action Team; 2011. Available from: http://ncat.nhs.uk/sites/default/files/HNA_practical%20guide_web.pdf.
10. National Quality Forum. A national framework and preferred practice for palliative and hospice care quality. Washington DC: National Quality Forum; 2006. Available from: http://www.qualityforum.org/Publications/2006/12/A_National_Framework_and_Preferred_Practices_for_Palliative_and_Hospice_Care_Quality.aspx.
11. National Institute for Clinical Excellence. Supportive and palliative care guidance for adults with cancer. London: National Institute for Clinical Excellence; 2004.
12. Lazarus RS, Folkman S. Stress, appraisal and coping. New York: Springer; 1984.
13. Stroebe M, Schut H. The dual process model of coping with bereavement: rationale and description. Death Stud. 1999;23:197–224.
14. Kobasa SC. Stressful life events, personality and health: an inquiry into hardiness. J Pers Soc Psychol. 1979;37:1–11.
15. Bonanno G, Moskowitz J, Tedlie J. Resilience to loss in bereaved spouses, bereaved parents, and bereaved gay men. J Pers Soc Psychol. 2005;88:827–43.
16. Monroe B, Oliviere D, editors. Resilience in palliative care – achievement in adversity. Oxford: Oxford University Press; 2007.
17. Clark D. "Total pain", disciplinary power and the body in the work of Cicely Saunders 1958–67. Soc Sci Med. 1999;49(6):727–36.
18. World Health Organisation analgesic ladder for cancer pain relief. http://www.who.int/cancer/palliative/painladder/en/. Accessed online on 23 July 2012.
19. Caraceni A, Hanks G, Kaasa S, et al. Use of opioid analgesics in the treatment of cancer pain: evidence-based recommendations from the EAPC. Lancet Oncol. 2012;13:e58–68.
20. Global State of Pain Treatment. http://www.hrw.org/reports/2011/06/01/global-state-pain-treatment-0. Accessed 4 Apr 2012.
21. Payne S. EAPC task force on family carers white paper on improving support for family carers in palliative care: part 1. Eur J Palliat Care. 2010;17(5):238–45.
22. Payne S. EAPC task force on family carers white paper on improving support for family carers in palliative care: part 2. Eur J Palliat Care. 2010;17(6):286–90.
23. Gao W, Ho YK, Verne J, Glickman M, Higginson I. Changing patterns in place of cancer death in England: a population-based study. PLOS Med. 2013;10(3): e1001410.
24. Preston N. A review of the management of malignant ascites. Eur J Palliat Care. 2005;12(2):57–60.
25. Macdonald R, Kirwan J, Roberts S, Gray D, Allsopp L, Green J. Ovarian cancer and ascites: a questionnaire on current management in the United kingdom. J Palliat Med. 2006;9:1264–70.
26. O'Neill MJ, Weissleder R, et al. Tunneled peritoneal catheter placement under sonographic and fluoroscopic guidance in the palliative treatment of malignant ascites. AJR Am J Roentgenol. 2001;177(3):615–8.
27. Day R, Mitchell T, Keen A, Perkins P. The experiences of patients with ascites secondary to cancer: a qualitative study. Palliat Med. 2013;27(8):739–46.
28. Joshi HB, Stainthorpe A, Macdonagh RP, Keeley FX, Timoney AG. Indwelling ureteral stents: evaluation of symptoms, quality of life and utility. J Urol. 2003; 169(30):1065–9.
29. Lapitan MCM, Buckley BS. Impact of palliative urinary diversion by percutaneous nephrostomy drainage and ureteral stenting among patients with advanced cervical cancer and obstructive uropathy: a prospective cohort. J Obstet Gynaecol Res. 2011;37(8):1061–70.
30. Roy DJ. Ambiguity in palliative care? (editorial). J Palliat Care. 2009;25(4):243–4.

Part II

Palliative Surgery: The Framework

Anaesthetic Considerations

4

Marissa Ferguson, Jonathan G. Hiller,
and Bernhard Riedel

Contents

M. Ferguson, MBBS(hons), BmedSc
J.G. Hiller, MBBS, FANZCA
Department of Anaesthesia and Pain Medicine,
Peter MacCallum Cancer Centre,
Melbourne 8006, VIC, Australia
e-mail: marissa.ferguson@gmail.com;
jonathan.hiller@petermac.org

B. Riedel, MBChB, FCA, FANZCA, FASE, MMed,
MBA, PhD (✉)
Department of Anaesthesia and Pain Medicine,
Peter MacCallum Cancer Center and University
of Melbourne, Melbourne 8006, VIC, Australia
e-mail: bernhard.riedel@petermac.org

The provision of high-quality surgical palliative care requires a coordinated team approach, and in this context anaesthetists are valuable members of the perioperative palliative care team. In particular, the relief of suffering and distressing symptoms has been a core component of anaesthesia practice since its inception. Anaesthetists possess valuable skills important to the provision of perioperative care for patients

M. Wichmann, G. Maddern (eds.), *Palliative Surgery*,
DOI 10.1007/978-3-642-53709-7_4, © Springer-Verlag Berlin Heidelberg 2014

undergoing palliative surgery. These include the ability to provide effective analgesia; to relieve symptoms of nausea, anxiety, and dyspnoea; and to stabilize perioperative physiological derangements in this vulnerable patient population. This chapter will review the core principles underlying effective perioperative management for patients undergoing palliative surgical procedures, with a focus on perioperative pathophysiological considerations, effective intraoperative management and perioperative symptom control.

4.1 Introduction

4.1.1 Definition

Palliative care is a unique discipline of medicine which has evolved as "an approach that improves the quality of life of patients and their families facing the problems associated with life-threatening illness, through the prevention and relief of suffering", as defined by the World Health Organization [1].

The core principles of palliative care are [1, 2]:

- Effective treatment of pain and other symptoms
- Striving to increase quality of life
- Incorporation of a biopsychosocial approach
- Formation of support networks for patients and families
- Respect for patient rights, including self-determination
- A team-based and patient-centred approach

Surgical palliative care is based on similar principles encompassing "the treatment of suffering and the promotion of quality of life for patients who are seriously or terminally ill under surgical care [3]". Palliative surgical procedures are defined as those "used with the primary intention of improving quality of life or relieving symptoms caused by advanced disease [3]". Although palliative surgery may prolong survival, there is a consensus that the primary goal of palliative procedures should be improved quality of life and reduced suffering [4–6].

Table 4.1 Indications and examples of common palliative surgical procedures

Indication	Example
Pain control	Tumour debulking/cytoreduction
	Pathological fracture fixation
	Neural plexus ablation
	Relief of visceral obstruction
Management of dyspnoea	Tracheostomy
	Endobronchial stenting, laser procedures
	Drainage of pericardial or pleural effusions
Management of abdominal and urogenital symptoms	Relief of obstructive symptoms:
	Stoma, stent, or bowel resection for obstruction
	Oesophageal stent/dilatation for dysphagia
	Percutaneous gastrostomy or jejunostomy tube insertion
	Biliary stent or operative bypass
	Nephrostomy/ureteric stenting
	Perforation or fistula repair
	Ascitic drainage (LeVeen/Denver shunt)
	Control of gastrointestinal bleeding
Management of neurological symptoms	Spinal decompression or stabilization
	Management of intracranial bleeding
	Resection of intracranial metastases
	Ventriculoperitoneal shunt
Palliative procedures for non-malignant conditions	Lung volume reduction surgery (chronic obstructive pulmonary disease)
	Porto-systemic shunt procedures (hepatic failure)

4.1.2 Incidence and Types of Palliative Surgical Operations

Patients with advanced cancer represent the largest group requiring palliative care services. Palliative surgical procedures account for 6–13 % of all surgical oncology procedures [4, 7]. However, surgical palliative care may also be beneficial for patients with non-malignant conditions including those with chronic organ failure (cardiac, respiratory, renal, and hepatic failure), neurodegenerative diseases, acquired immunodeficiency syndrome (AIDS), as well as post-transplant and critical care patients – all of whom share distressing symptoms and life-threatening illnesses [3].

Patients with terminal illness may experience a range of symptoms depending on the underlying disease pathophysiology and the biopsychosocial context. Pain, dyspnoea, nausea, depression, and fatigue are all reported by patients with both malignant and non-malignant terminal illnesses [8]. Importantly, some symptoms are more amenable to surgical palliation than others. In particular, anorexia, fatigue, and depression all have a devastating impact upon quality of life, but are difficult to relieve through surgical intervention [9].

Palliative procedures may involve a range of interventions, including open surgery, laparoscopic surgery, endoscopy, interventional radiology, brachytherapy, radio-frequency ablation, and intraoperative radiotherapy or chemotherapy administration (Table 4.1). Less invasive operative approaches such as laparoscopy and endoscopy are associated with lower rates of perioperative morbidity [10]. Endoscopic procedures account for approximately 30 % of all palliative surgical procedures in this high-risk patient population [4]. Of patients receiving palliative surgery for malignant disease, 50 % will also receive adjuvant chemotherapy and 20 % adjuvant radiotherapy [4]. (Neo)adjuvant therapies are an important consideration as they contribute to an increased risk of postoperative complications and further symptom burden.

4.1.3 Challenges Associated with Palliative Surgery

Patients undergoing palliative procedures represent a high-risk population. Due to recent advances in medical therapies, overall life expectancy is greater, and many terminal illnesses which would have previously had a short natural history now have a more chronic time-course [3]. This prolongation in life expectancy may be accompanied with a significant symptom burden. As a result, palliative surgical procedures are more often being performed in an elderly population with limited physiological reserve.

The patient receiving palliative surgery is at high risk of complications due to comorbidities, organ impairment, and surgical risks. Hence, palliative surgical procedures carry a risk of shortening remaining life and worsening quality of life [11]. For example, the 30-day morbidity and mortality rates after palliative surgery for advanced malignancy range from 21–29 % and 5–12 %, respectively [4, 7, 12, 13]. Overall, perioperative surgical morbidity occurs in approximately 40 % of patients undergoing palliative surgery [4, 13]. This is particularly significant given that major postoperative complications significantly reduce the chance of effective symptom palliation [4]. Additional challenges accompany the provision of anaesthesia for urgent or emergency procedures; these account for approximately 20 % of palliative surgical procedures [4]. Emergency procedures allow little opportunity for preoperative optimization for patients who are often acutely and systemically unwell. As a result, urgent operations are associated with increased risk – a 30-day mortality of up to 28 % for patients with disseminated malignancy [12].

Despite these risks, patients may experience significant benefits from palliative procedures, with observation studies demonstrating that 80–90 % of patients undergoing palliative surgery experience symptom improvement or resolution [4, 13]. However, approximately 25 % of patients experience symptom recurrence, and up to 30 % develop new symptoms requiring further treatment [4]. Furthermore, symptomatic improvement may not equate to improved postoperative quality of life [14]. As a result, careful patient selection and clear indications for palliative surgery are important to minimize risk maximize quality of life improvement [5]. Despite this, there is little evidence comparing the efficacy of surgical and medical palliative care or indications to guide patient selection [10, 15].

4.2 Preoperative Assessment

4.2.1 General Principles of Preoperative Assessment

Individualized patient care is of particular importance in palliative care [16], as outcomes relating to symptom relief and quality of life are necessarily subjective. In order to maximize the potential for a successful outcome, it is important to know the patient's goals, values, and concerns relating to the upcoming procedure. Effective communication is therefore an essential component to ensuring that the patient's specific goals are met [5]. Patient decisions may be influenced by their understanding of the disease process and beliefs about expected survival [10], as well as spiritual or religious beliefs, personal values, and external influences such as family wishes. In addition to a patient-centred approach, a multidisciplinary team approach is particularly important in the perioperative management of patients undergoing palliative surgery. This involves collaboration with the patient and their next of kin/carers, surgeons, nursing staff, pastoral care, social workers and other allied health staff including physiotherapy, dieticians, speech therapists, occupational therapists, and pharmacists.

4.2.2 Risk Assessment and Minimization

Assessing perioperative risk is a complex process, but is particularly important in the palliative surgical population due to the high rates of postoperative morbidity and mortality previously discussed. Risk assessment involves integrating the risks related to the palliative surgical procedure, the underlying pathology necessitating surgery, the patient's comorbidities, as well as the patient's overall functional status and physiological reserve. Patients presenting for palliative surgery often have multisystem organ impairment, and a thorough history and examination is essential, with consideration for focused investigations. However, the relative benefit from the results of an investigation must be balanced with the discomfort, delay, and inconvenience of performing additional testing.

The surgical risk associated with palliative procedures varies from low-risk (e.g. percutaneous gastrostomy tube insertion [17]) to high-risk procedures such as resection of large tumour masses which may be associated with significant physiological derangements [18]. Accurate information about prognosis and the risk of surgical morbidity and mortality is important for decision-making around palliative surgery. Recent work has been done to improve prognostication using data from the American College of Surgeons National Surgical Quality Improvement Program to create a nomogram predicting 30-day morbidity and mortality after surgery for disseminated malignancy [12].

The risk related to the patient's functional status varies greatly from the relatively young and systemically well patient with locally invasive disease to the physiologically unstable patient with an acute complication of metastatic disease in the context of multiple medical comorbidities. Specific risk factors associated with morbidity and mortality after palliative surgery for advanced malignancy include advanced age, impaired performance/functional status, impaired renal and respiratory function, ascites, hypoalbuminaemia, and abnormal white cell count [4, 12]. Postoperative cardiorespiratory risk can be objectively assessed using validated scoring tools such as the Lee Revised Cardiac Risk Index [19] as well as more recently developed tools to predict respiratory complications postoperatively [20, 21].

Following on from a thorough risk assessment is the implementation of strategies to reduce risk to be discussed next. In the situation where risk is believed to outweigh possible benefits of palliative surgery, some difficult questions must be considered, including "Has the least invasive therapy been trialed first?" and "Should this operation be done for this patient at this time? [10]"

4.2.3 Formulation of a Patient-Centred Perioperative Management Plan

Core components of the perioperative management plan include:

1. Optimize function preoperatively.
2. Maximize the potential for symptom relief and comfort.
3. Minimize the risks of perioperative complications.

The perioperative management plan should be formulated in collaboration with the patient and their family/carers as well as the perioperative surgical and allied health team. The plan should focus on effectively addressing the symptoms most concerning to the patient while minimizing the risk of perioperative complications. This includes discussing the available options regarding anaesthetic technique and the risks and benefits specific to that patient as well as exploring current symptoms and specific concerns relating to the upcoming surgery.

Therapies to optimize the patient's preoperative physiological status should be implemented based on issues identified in the preoperative assessment. These include correction of electrolyte and coagulation abnormalities, optimization of oxygen-carrying capacity (e.g. haematinic supplementation such as preoperative iron infusion), optimization of organ function (e.g. optimal medical therapy for cardiac failure), as well as nutritional supplementation and "prehabilitation" exercise programmes where appropriate. Here, a multidisciplinary team approach is particularly important, and expert input from specialist physicians and allied health colleagues is valuable in ensuring optimal patient care.

Finally, the patient should be counseled in order to provide a reasonable expectation of how their symptoms may change in the perioperative period as well as formulation of a plan for perioperative symptom control. The preoperative consultation should also clarify the patient's wishes about various life-sustaining and life-prolonging interventions specific to the perioperative period – this will be discussed further under Ethics section later in this chapter.

4.3 Perioperative Pathophysiological Considerations in Palliative Surgery

Patients undergoing palliative surgery are susceptible to the pathophysiological changes associated with their underlying malignant disease. The malignant process and the effects of treatment often have complex effects which may impact upon every organ system. In advanced disease, knowledge of tumour biology is important in predicting likely complications; this guides strategies that minimize risk and can effectively control symptoms.

Table 4.2 Pathophysiological effects of malignancy

1. Direct effects of the primary malignancy
2. Secondary effects due to metastatic disease
3. Systemic effects
4. Iatrogenic or treatment-related effects

Table 4.2 summarizes the major mechanisms underlying the pathophysiological effects of malignancy; these may also apply to other non-malignant life-limiting illnesses. Primary and secondary (metastatic) tumour effects may result in bleeding, infection, compression, obstruction, and destruction of organ structure and function. These effects often translate into symptoms of pain, functional impairment, and reduced quality of life. Systemic effects include paraneoplastic syndromes, as well as pathophysiological changes of malignant cachexia, systemic inflammatory activation, coagulation abnormalities, and endothelial dysfunction.

4.3.1 Alterations in Anatomy and Physiology

The anaesthetic implications relating to alterations in anatomical integrity and physiological function of the major organ systems of patients presenting for palliative surgery are discussed next.

4.3.1.1 Airway

Patients presenting for palliative surgery often have risk factors predicting difficulty airway management additional to standard predictors of difficult intubation [22]. The direct anatomical effects of advanced oropharyngeal, laryngeal, oesophageal, and thoracic malignant mass lesions may make intubation and ventilation difficult (or even impossible) via standard techniques. Prior radiotherapy may also contribute to difficult direct laryngoscopy due to restricted neck extension, limited mouth opening, and fibrosis of the tongue and submandibular tissues [23]. Furthermore, patients presenting for palliative surgery may have reduced physiological reserve to tolerate hypoxaemia if any difficulty in securing the airway is encountered.

4.3.1.2 Respiratory System

Patients undergoing palliative surgery often have reduced cardiorespiratory reserve with dyspnoea and hypoxaemia often being multifactorial in origin. Shunt and ventilation-perfusion mismatch may arise from pulmonary parenchymal invasion, infection, bronchial obstruction with collapse of distal lung units, pneumothorax, and pleural effusion. Impaired diffusion of oxygen across the alveolar membrane may be due to chemotherapy- or radiation-induced pulmonary fibrosis, pulmonary oedema, or lymphomatosis carcinomatosa. Pulmonary embolic phenomena, resulting from either venous thromboembolism or tumour embolism, may lead to significant dead space fraction, lung infarction, and associated haemodynamic instability due to excessive right ventricular afterload. Finally, the not infrequent occurrence of a bronchopleural fistula in the setting of palliative surgery represents a particular challenge to the anaesthetist [24, 25].

4.3.1.3 Cardiovascular System

Reduced cardiovascular reserve may be related to primary cardiac failure, direct cardiac involvement by tumour, pericardial effusion, systemic comorbidities, or toxicity related to chemoradiotherapy. Note that myocardial and intracavity involvement by cancer metastases may not result in symptoms experienced by the patient [26]. Vascular effects of malignancy and related comorbidities include arterial insufficiency related to radiotherapy, great vessel venous obstruction, and venous thromboembolism; all of these may have implications for central venous and arterial cannulation.

4.3.1.4 Neurological

Mass lesions in the central nervous system may cause focal weakness, seizures, visual loss, and aphasia (supratentorial lesions) or cerebellar symptoms (infratentorial lesions). Other central nervous system pathology encountered in the palliative setting includes spinal cord compression due to tumour invasion or pathological vertebral fracture, leptomeningeal disease, as well as neurodegenerative conditions. Peripheral neuropathy may be related to chemotherapy or radiotherapy or may be due to direct nerve infiltration or compression by tumour. In addition, encephalopathy may result from renal or hepatic failure or as a result of exogenous agents including analgesic metabolites and chemotherapeutic agents.

4.3.1.5 Gastrointestinal

Nausea is a frequent symptom in the palliative care setting. In particular, fasting status may be compromised due to mechanical obstruction from gastrointestinal mass lesions as well as impaired gastrointestinal motility due to high-dose opioids and electrolyte derangement. Hepatic impairment may occur as a result of tumour infiltration, previous resection, or iatrogenic toxicity, and this has significant pharmacologic implications for the perioperative period, discussed later in this chapter.

4.3.1.6 Renal

Renal impairment may be multifactorial in the patient presenting for palliative surgery. Prerenal causes include hypovolaemia and cardiac failure. Direct nephrotoxicity may result from drug toxicity, tumour lysis syndrome, or long-term effects of other chronic comorbidities such as diabetes mellitus and hypertension. Post-renal impairment may result from mechanical obstruction due to malignant disease. The implications of renal disease in the perioperative period are extensive, including electrolyte and acid–base abnormalities, volume overload, and impaired drug elimination.

4.3.1.7 Paraneoplastic Syndromes

Paraneoplastic syndromes may result from a number of mechanisms, including tumour secretion of peptides and autoimmune reactions resulting from sensitization to tumour antigens with subsequent cross-reactivity. Common tumours associated with paraneoplastic syndromes are summarized in Table 4.3 [27]. Eaton-Lambert

Table 4.3 Paraneoplastic syndromes associated with malignancy

Syndrome	Associated malignancies
Endocrine	
Syndrome of inappropriate antidiuretic hormone production	Small cell lung cancer (most common)
	Mesothelioma
	Urinary tract malignancies
	Ewing sarcoma
	Thymoma
	Lymphoma
Hypercalcaemia (Secretion of PTH or PTHrP[a])	Breast cancer
	Multiple myeloma
	Renal cell carcinoma
	Squamous cell lung cancer
Cushing's syndrome	Small cell lung cancer
	Bronchial carcinoid
Hypoglycaemia	Insulinoma
	Sarcoma
Neurologic	
Eaton-Lambert myaesthenia	Small cell lung cancer
Limbic encephalitis	Small cell lung cancer
	Germ cell tumours
	Breast cancer
Paraneoplastic cerebellar degeneration	Small cell lung cancer
	Hodgkin's lymphoma
	Breast cancer
Autonomic neuropathy	Small cell lung cancer
Myaesthenia gravis	Thymoma
Other	
Dermatomyositis	Multiple: ovarian, breast, lung, colorectal, and prostate cancers; non-Hodgkin's lymphoma
Hypertrophic pulmonary osteoarthropathy	Intrathoracic malignancies

Modified with permission from Pelosof and Gerber [27]
[a]*PTH* parathyroid hormone, *PTHrP* parathyroid hormone-related protein

syndrome has particular relevance in the peri-operative period as patients are sensitive to both depolarising and non-depolarising muscle relaxants. This is due to reduced acetylcholine release as a result of antibodies to presynaptic voltage-gated calcium channels [28].

4.3.1.8 Endocrine

A primary malignancy may cause significant endocrine organ destruction and alteration in function due to previous resection or paraneoplastic effects. These effects can impact on thyroid, adrenal, pancreatic and pituitary function. Furthermore, patients presenting for palliative surgery may be receiving exogenous glucocorticoid therapy and hence consideration should be given for stress-dose supplementation of corticosteroids. Hypercalcaemia is relatively common in malignant disease and may be due to humoral mechanisms (parathyroid hormone-related protein) or direct mobilization associated with bony spread of disease from breast carcinoma metastases or multiple myeloma [29].

4.3.1.9 Immunological and Haematological

Anaemia is common in patients receiving palliative care, occurring in approximately 70 % of patients [30], and may contribute to symptoms of fatigue and dyspnoea. Pathophysiological mechanisms involved include blood loss, haemolysis, and impaired erythropoiesis. Erythrocyte production may be impaired due to inappropriately low erythropoietin levels from renal disease, haematinic deficiency [30], or bone marrow suppression resulting from either the iatrogenic effects of chemoradiotherapy or direct marrow invasion by tumour cells. Thrombocytopenia may occur due to impaired production and release of platelets, the effects of chemoradiotherapy or splenic sequestration [29]. Leukopenia is also commonly encountered due to malignant bone marrow infiltration or as a result of chemotherapy. Alternatively, leukocytosis may be present in association with infection or haematological malignancy, and thrombocytosis may occur in the setting of systemic inflammation. In addition, malignancy is associated with a prothrombotic state, and patients are at an increased risk of venous thromboembolism in the perioperative period [31].

Tumour lysis syndrome is a potentially fatal condition which may occur on initiation of anticancer therapy in patients with haematological malignancies (most commonly high-grade lymphomas or acute lymphoblastic leukaemia) as well as in patients with solid organ malignancies involving high tumour burden, rapidly proliferative disease, or tumours that are very sensitive to cytotoxic chemotherapy [32]. Tumour lysis may also uncommonly occur spontaneously and, in rare circumstances, may be inadvertently precipitated perioperatively by corticosteroid administration or even by surgery itself [33]. The resultant massive lysis of tumour cells is a medical emergency causing hyperkalaemia, hyperuricaemia, hyperphosphataemia, and acute renal failure.

Patients undergoing palliative surgery may be immunocompromised from bone marrow infiltration, infection from human immunodeficiency virus, as well as immunosuppressant medications (chemotherapeutic agents, corticosteroids, post-transplant immunosuppressant medication). As a result, the palliative surgical population is at increased risk for disseminated opportunistic infection and impaired wound healing.

Finally, malignant cachexia is a complex pathophysiological phenomenon related to both malnutrition as well as the biological effects of malignancy and organ failure (including humoral and inflammatory mediators). It culminates in profound loss of muscle and adipose mass [34] and has significant implications for drug dosing and distribution as discussed next.

4.3.2 Anaesthetic Implications of Chemotherapy and Radiotherapy

Patients undergoing palliative surgery have often received multiple treatment cycles of chemotherapy or radiotherapy. The toxic effects of these therapies may occur acutely or subacutely or may be delayed many years.

4.3.2.1 Chemotherapy

Important considerations related to chemotherapy in the perioperative period include recognition of delayed organ toxicity due to previous cycles of chemotherapy, detection of acute toxicities related to recent chemotherapy for symptom palliation, as well as planning for possible perioperative chemotherapy administration. Chemotherapy may be used intraoperatively in conjunction with cytoreduction to reduce pain and to treat or prevent intestinal obstruction resulting from abdominal and peritoneal tumours. An example is hyperthermic intraperitoneal chemotherapy (HIPEC) for pseudomyxoma peritonei. Commonly used chemotherapeutic agents used in this setting include intraperitoneal mitomycin C, cisplatin, and oxaliplatin, combined with intravenous 5-fluorouracil [35].

Treatment-related toxicities common to most chemotherapeutic agents include fatigue, anorexia, nausea and vomiting, mucositis, and varying degrees of myelosuppression and immunosuppression [36]. Table 4.4 summarizes the organ-related toxicities commonly associated with chemotherapeutic agents. The effects of chemotherapeutic agents on organ toxicity are complex and are often difficult to attribute to a single agent given the frequent use of combination chemotherapy agents. Furthermore, there are numerous new anticancer drugs emerging each year (often with novel mechanisms of action), and the toxicity profiles of these new agents may only become clear with ongoing post-marketing toxicity reporting.

Several chemotherapeutic agents have particular significance to the anaesthetist. In particular, bleomycin is associated with a life-long risk of pulmonary fibrosis. A high inspired oxygen fraction perioperatively has been implicated in triggering a potentially fatal outcome in patients with bleomycin-induced pulmonary fibrosis [42]. Other risk factors for bleomycin pulmonary toxicity include total dose, advanced age, and renal impairment [43, 44]. Pulmonary toxicity associated with bleomycin is thought to result from low levels of the deactivating enzyme "bleomycin hydrolase" in the lung, with resultant free radical generation leading to cellular damage and inflammatory injury in the lung epithelium and endothelium [43]. Limiting the fractional inspired oxygen concentration less than 0.3 is recommended [43]. To improve oxygenation without the use of supplemental oxygen, strategies such as the optimal use of positive end-expiratory pressure, recruitment manoeuvres, and avoidance of fluid overload are useful in this setting [36].

In addition, cardiac toxicity related to prior chemotherapy is important to recognize preoperatively as the haemodynamic effects of anaesthesia can unmask or lead to decompensation of previously unrecognized or asymptomatic cardiac toxicity [40]. Specific risk factors for chemotherapy-induced cardiac toxicity include advanced age and comorbid cardiovascular disease [37].

4.3.2.2 Radiotherapy

Radiotherapy is a common modality for both treatment and palliation of malignancies. Multiple organ systems may be affected from radiotherapy, and this depends on the field of irradiation and dose administered; the toxic effects of chemotherapy may be additive. Patients undergoing palliative surgery may have delayed complications from previous radiotherapy or may be suffering from acute toxicities of palliative radiotherapy, which may occasionally necessitate surgical intervention. Table 4.5 summarizes the major organ toxicities associated with radiotherapy.

The fibrotic effects of radiotherapy on tissues have numerous perioperative implications including increasing the risk of difficult intubation and the difficulty performing a tracheostomy as well as contributing to difficult surgical dissection related to adhesion formation. Furthermore,

Table 4.4 Common organ toxicities associated with chemotherapeutic agents

Organ system	Toxicity	Causative agents
Cardiovascular [36, 37]	Cardiac failure	Anthracyclines (doxorubicin, idarubicin, danorubicin, epirubicin)
		Trastuzumab
		Cyclophosphamide (high dose), ifosfamide
		In combination with anthracyclines: paclitaxel, bevacizumab
	Myocardial ischaemia	Cisplatin, fluorouracil, vinca alkaloids
	Arrhythmias	Paclitaxel, ifosfamide, rituximab, cisplatin, anthracyclines
	Pericarditis/myocarditis	Cyclophosphamide
Respiratory [36, 38]	Pneumonitis/pulmonary fibrosis	Bleomycin
		Other: methotrexate, busulfan, carmustine, mitomycin, cyclophosphamide, cytarabine
Renal [36, 39]	Nephrotoxicity	Cisplatin (and other platinum-based agents)
		Other: ifosfamide, nitrosoureas, mitomycin, azacitidine, methotrexate
	Haemorrhagic cystitis	Cyclophosphamide, ifosfamide
Hepatic [40, 41]	Variable toxicity:	Methotrexate, 6-mercaptopurine, tamoxifen, irinotecan, imatinib, L-asparaginase, flutamide
	Hepatocellular injury, cholestasis, fibrosis, veno-occlusive disease	Rare case reports of fatal cholestatic hepatotoxicity: gemcitabine, oxaliplatin, azathioprine
		Many other agents may cause idiosyncratic liver injury or transient derangements in liver enzymes
Neurological [36, 40]	Encephalopathy	Ifosfamide, methotrexate (high dose)
	Autonomic neuropathy	Vincristine
	Peripheral neuropathy	Vincristine, paclitaxel, oxaliplatin, cisplatin

Table 4.5 Adverse effects associated with radiotherapy

Organ system	Effects
Cardiovascular [36, 37]	Pericardial disease (most common)
	Valvular disease
	Myocardial damage
	Coronary artery disease
	Carotid artery disease
	Peripheral vascular disease
Respiratory [45]	Radiation pneumonitis (acute)
	Pulmonary fibrosis (delayed)
Airway [46]	Soft tissue fibrosis, restricted neck mobility
	Trismus
Gastrointestinal [46]	Oesophagitis (acute), oesophageal stricture (delayed)
	Gastritis
	Enteritis
	Adhesion formation
	Hepatic injury

wound healing in the radiotherapy field is often impaired.

4.3.3 Alterations in Pharmacology and Anaesthetic Implications

There are complex interactions between patient comorbidities, preoperative medication therapy, anaesthetic drug administration, as well as surgical stress in the perioperative period.

4.3.3.1 Pharmacokinetics

Absorption

Gastrointestinal absorption of orally administered medications may be reduced and unreliable in the perioperative period due to delayed gastric emptying related to high-dose opioids, mechanical bowel obstruction, ileus, and mucosal oedema. In addition, absorption of medication delivered in a transdermal formulation may be reduced in the cachectic patient with limited subcutaneous adipose tissue.

Distribution

Patients undergoing palliative surgery are often malnourished with reductions in body fat and lean body mass. Furthermore, alterations in fluid and drug distribution may occur due to cardiovascular and renal impairment, while chronic illness may lead to hypoalbuminaemia. These factors can have significant implications for drugs which are highly protein bound and can result in large variations in a drug's steady state plasma concentrations. Drug doses must be adjusted for reduced body weight in the cachectic patient. All of these factors must be considered and are relevant for drug prescription to avoid underdosing or toxicity.

Metabolism and Elimination

Reduced hepatic and renal function may contribute to drug and active metabolite accumulation, with resultant toxic effects. In renal impairment, the opioid metabolites norpethidine and morphine-3-glucuronide have been described to cause signs of neurotoxicity such as myoclonus and seizures (although this association has more recently been challenged [47]).

4.3.3.2 Pharmacodynamics

Drug-Drug Interactions

Our understanding of the interactions of chemotherapeutic drugs with anaesthetic agents is predominantly based on the results of in vitro findings [48]. There are reports that patients receiving neoadjuvant methotrexate may be at increased risk of adverse effects from nitrous oxide exposure due to potential synergistic negative effects on folate metabolism. MTX inhibits dihydrofolate reductase, and nitrous oxide inhibits methionine synthetase, which converts methyltetrahydrofolate to tetrahydrofolate as part of a cofactor reaction [48].

Drug-Receptor Interactions

Drug-receptor interactions may affect intraoperative physiological responses to anaesthetic drugs as well as having implications for perioperative analgesia. For example, antihypertensive agents may need dose reduction, particularly for patients with cardiac and autonomic nervous system dysfunction. In addition, patients taking high-dose opioids may have significant drug tolerance; perioperative analgesia can be particularly challenging for this patient group.

Pharmacodynamic Effects in the Context of Altered Physiology

There may be pronounced cardiovascular changes in response to both general and neuraxial anaesthesia in elderly patients and those with cardiac and autonomic dysfunction. Several conditions have particular significance in patients undergoing palliative surgery. For example, neuromuscular blocking agents have a prolonged duration of action in patients with neuromuscular disease or prolonged immobility. In patients with carcinoid syndrome, a life-threatening carcinoid crisis may be precipitated by drugs used in the perioperative period such as adrenergic agonists and any drug that induces histamine release, e.g. atracurium.

4.4 Intraoperative Management

The general principles of intraoperative management for palliative surgery include:

- Choosing the safest anaesthetic technique, with an emphasis on relief of symptoms and preservation of dignity
- Preservation of normal physiology
- Employment of strategies to reduce perioperative complications

4.4.1 General Anaesthesia

4.4.1.1 Airway Management

While the standard principles of anaesthesia apply to approaching the airway of a patient receiving palliative surgery, added challenges can arise. Difficulty may be encountered if a patient is unable to lie flat due to dyspnoea or stridor resulting from upper airway malignancies. Induction techniques chosen in these circumstances include inhalational induction of volatile anaesthetic agents or an awake fibreoptic intubation. These techniques are limited in the acutely decompensating patient or in the case of upper airway bleeding (such as friable laryngopharyngeal or tracheal tumours). Effective communication with a head and neck surgeon in clinical attendance is critical. Elective or semi-urgent tracheostomy performed under local anaesthetic can be safely and swiftly performed in the hands of an experienced surgeon and is well tolerated by the patient.

4.4.1.2 Respiratory

Under anaesthesia, ventilation strategies that emphasize lung protection are important in patients at risk of lung injury. Such strategies include use of low tidal volumes (6 ml/kg) and low peak airway pressures and the use of positive end-expiratory pressure to maintain oxygenation [49]. The avoidance of high intraoperative inspiratory oxygen concentrations is important not only for the prevention of postoperative atelectasis, but is particularly relevant for the prevention of pulmonary toxicity in those patients with a history of bleomycin exposure.

Patients who are at high risk for respiratory failure postoperatively may benefit from "bridging" non-invasive respiratory support in a postoperative high-dependency unit environment. This has been shown in high-risk patients to decrease the risk of patients requiring re-intubation in the intensive care setting [49–51]

4.4.1.3 Cannulation

Establishing venous access in patients requiring sedation or general anaesthesia may be challenging amongst a patient group who have often had recurrent or prolonged hospitalizations, received multiple cycles of chemotherapy, may be thrombocytopenic (with associated limb ecchymosis) or have had axillary lymph node removal. Furthermore, if superior vena caval obstruction is present and not amenable to stenting preoperatively, then upper limb venous return may be impaired, and lower limb vein cannulation should be considered [52].

In patients requiring intermediate to long-term venous access, a peripherally inserted central catheter or central venous catheter (CVC) may be useful to avoid repeated attempts at peripheral venous cannulation. A low threshold for the use of ultrasound guidance for the insertion of central venous catheters should be employed. The placement of a CVC may be particularly difficult in an unwell patient receiving palliative surgery due to the high incidence of thrombocytopenia, anatomical variation, venous stenosis, and thrombosis from previous cannulation and the inability to lie flat [29]. In addition to the reliability of central venous access, a CVC provides multiple forms of intravenous access for the delivery of perioperative vasoactive infusions and a mechanism for postoperative blood sampling and delivery of parenteral nutrition. Consideration should always be given to a patient's specific requests or refusal for such a device.

4.4.1.4 Cardiovascular Support and Fluid Management

Patients receiving palliative surgical procedures are at risk for cardiovascular instability. Additional to the perioperative risks associated with age-related disease (hypertension, ischaemic heart disease, diabetes mellitus) are those arising from the frequent comorbidities of a patient receiving palliative surgery including dilated cardiomyopathy, chemotherapy-induced cardiomyopathy, pulmonary fluid overload, and pulmonary hypertension. A patient receiving palliative surgery is at risk for perioperative arrhythmia arising from electrolyte disturbance (particularly, hyperchloraemic metabolic acidosis, hypokalemia, and hypomagnesaemia), fluid overload, sepsis, hyperpyrexia, and drug toxicity. Due to the reduced physiological reserves of these patients, including the potential for impaired renal and cardiac function and a tendency to fluid overload (peripheral and pulmonary oedema), fluid prescription strategies in the perioperative period should be judicious.

4.4.1.5 Intraoperative Medication

The anaesthetic adage of the approach to medication delivery for the elderly "go low and go slow" can equally be applied to the patient receiving anaesthesia for palliative surgery. In general, the pharmacodynamic and pharmacokinetic fragility of these compromised patients is such that overdosage of intraoperative opioids and anaesthetic agents is common [53]. For this reason, anaesthetic techniques should be characterized by the use of non-sedating multimodal analgesia techniques, avoidance of long-acting benzodiazepines, and the employment of depth of anaesthesia monitoring to minimize anaesthesia overdose. Choice of muscle relaxant, where necessary, should be made with mindfulness to the drug's mechanism of metabolism (preferably organ-independent). Case reports exist of hyperkalaemic arrest due to the use of suxamethonium in patients who have experienced prolonged periods of immobility [54]. Due to the increased risk of cardiovascular instability during anaesthesia or sedation for palliative surgery, the immediate availability of vasoconstrictors and drugs of resuscitation is prudent.

4.4.2 Regional Anaesthesia

The use of regional anaesthesia and postoperative analgesic regimens incorporating local anaesthesia infusions are useful to assist in avoiding sedating opioid-based analgesia. The advantages of neuraxial-based analgesic techniques (intrathecal and epidural injection) must be balanced with the risks of neuraxial intervention. Patients may develop a hypocoagulable clotting state from thrombocytopenia, chronic low-dose thromboprophylaxis prescription, and impairment of platelet clotting function from chronic disease; an increased risk of spinal haematoma exists in these patients when neuraxial anaesthesia or analgesia is attempted. Caution must be placed in the use of local anaesthetic infusions due to the risk of toxicity from impaired local anaesthesia metabolism and excretion in patients with cardiac, hepatic, and renal disease.

4.4.3 Other Intraoperative Considerations

4.4.3.1 Monitoring

The relevant institutional or national guidelines regarding standards of monitoring apply for any sedation or anaesthetic procedure; however, a heightened level of awareness is relevant to the patient receiving palliative surgery. Because of the elevated risk of perioperative cardiorespiratory complications in patients with multiple comorbidities and decreased functional reserve, consideration should be given to more invasive monitoring, weighing this carefully against potential discomfort to the patient and the risk of complications. The insertion of an arterial cannula for invasive blood pressure monitoring is a quick, relatively painless, cost-efficient, and reliable intervention that can provide the anaesthetist and perioperative clinician with immediate information on a patient's cardiovascular stability and blood gas composition – it is highly recommended. Of increased importance in the patient with reduced physiological reserve is monitoring of temperature, neuromuscular activity (nerve stimulator), and depth of anaesthesia.

4.4.3.2 Blood Product and Transfusion Management

Patients undergoing palliative surgery have specific risk factors increasing their likelihood of requiring blood product transfusion in the perioperative period. For most procedures and surgery, increased intrinsic clotting capacity is required compared with what may be acceptable on the ward. Acceptable coagulation parameters are important for prolonged operations involving debulking of large vascular tumours and organ resection, but also for brief interventions to manage tumours of the airway and bronchial tree which may be particularly friable and prone to bleeding (e.g. bronchoscopy and laser resection). This includes attention to optimizing acid-base status, avoidance of hypothermia, and prevention of coagulopathy. Attention to adequate platelet count (>50 × 10 [9]/l), correction of inadequacies in clotting function, and appropriate avoidance of preoperative anticoagulants are vital in the care of a debilitated patient receiving palliative surgery.

Preoperative anaemia is common amongst patients with chronic illness undergoing palliative surgery, and preoperative optimization of haematinic status should be considered where possible. As with any blood product, the administration of red cells to increase a patient's oxygen-carrying capacity is a decision that must be made between the patient and clinicians after determining and balancing the risks and benefits of transfusion when compared with alternatives. For the immunocompromised patient, it is appropriate to use irradiated blood products for a patient at risk of graft-versus-host disease [55].

4.4.3.3 Infection Control

Patients receiving palliative procedures are often significantly immunocompromised and are at particular risk of opportunistic and wound infections. This risk is heightened for procedures involving the insertion of medium- to long-term foreign objects including venous access devices, stents, and implants. For this reason, strict attention to hygienic work practice and adherence to antibiotic prophylaxis based on local institutional guidelines are essential. The single most effective measure for the reduction in transmission of bacterial contamination is an effective hand hygiene practice before and after any procedure or contact with an immunocompromised patient [56]. Due to their lengthy exposure to the hospital system, patients receiving palliative surgery have a high frequency of colonization with multiresistant organisms such as vancomycin-resistant Enterococcus and multi-resistant *Staphylococcus aureus* [57]. Perioperative clinicians have a responsibility to limit the institutional spread of these organisms following interaction with immunocompromised patients.

4.5 Specific Clinical Presentations and Challenges

4.5.1 Cardiothoracic Procedures

Palliative cardiothoracic procedures commonly include drainage of pleural and pericardial effusions as well as interventions to relieve tracheobronchial obstruction. Anaesthetic considerations include lung isolation for thoracotomy or thoracoscopy, prevention of hypoxaemia and ventilator-induced lung injury, and the maintenance of haemodynamic stability, particularly in patients with pericardial tamponade and those undergoing drainage of large-volume pleural effusions.

Endobronchial stenting and/or lasering may provide significant symptomatic relief of dyspnoea [58]. Depending on the degree of intervention required and anatomical location of the lesion, this may involve a brief bronchoscopic intervention or may involve several hours of treatment, potentially with multiple airway interventions if both rigid and flexible bronchoscopes are employed. For these procedures, general anaesthesia is usually required although awake techniques have been described [59, 60]. Total intravenous anaesthesia and muscle relaxation is required if rigid bronchoscopy is used. Specific risks include the potential for airway fires with laser use, airway trauma causing pneumothorax and/or pneumomediastinum, airway obstruction related to stent misplacement or migration, or airway oedema and bleeding [52]. Airway bleeding related to laser or manual tumour debulking may be significant, particularly if underlying vessels are inadvertently damaged. In addition, patients may be at increased risk of awareness due to the stimulating nature of airway interventions and a shared airway in an often frail patient population, and depth of anaesthesia monitoring should be considered [52]. Despite these risks, the mortality rate in the first week postoperatively following endobronchial stenting of airway tumours may be as low as 0.4 % [58].

4.5.2 Abdominal Surgical Procedures

Palliative abdominal surgical procedures may involve major operations such as pelvic exenteration, debulking procedures, and HIPEC in selected patients. These procedures are often associated with significant perioperative physiological stress, including large fluid shifts and the potential for significant blood loss. In addition, postoperative pain may be significant, and epidural analgesia should be considered. HIPEC involves administration of intraperitoneal chemotherapeutic agents heated to 40–43 °C (with the aim of increased tissue penetration at hyperthermic temperatures) in conjunction with cytoreductive surgery. The technique is used to increase success of curative surgery or prolong disease-free survival, but may be used in the palliative setting for patients with locally advanced peritoneal malignancy and symptomatic burden from ascites or other pressure effects. This may be performed laparoscopically or as an open procedure and results in several important pathophysiological effects including systemic temperature changes, increased oxygen consumption, significant third-space fluid losses and potential coagulopathy as well as the potential adverse effects related to the chemotherapeutic agents used [35].

4.5.3 Other

Brachytherapy is the "implantation of radioactive sources in or near tumors" [61]. Common indications in the palliative setting include treatment of inoperable or recurrent local disease involving breast, bronchial, and pelvic malignancies [62]. The patient population undergoing brachytherapy is often at high risk of perioperative events due to advanced age and comorbidities – in one study, over 30 % of patients were of American Society of Anaesthetists grade III or IV [61]. Essential elements of anaesthesia for brachytherapy are analgesia and immobility. Regional or neuraxial techniques are often favoured for pelvic brachytherapy [60, 61]. Challenges in providing anaesthesia for brachytherapy include the unpredictable and potentially long duration of procedure, remote location, and a period of remote access to patient during high-dose-rate radiation delivery [62].

4.6 Postoperative Care

4.6.1 Postoperative Destination

Following a palliative procedure requiring anaesthesia or sedation, the patient must be recovered in an environment appropriate for postoperative care. In an operating theatre, this is usually the postoperative care unit. However, because many palliative procedures are being performed for symptom control, more and more of these procedures are being performed "off-the-floor" and in specialist, remote areas of the hospital.

These areas include the radiology, respiratory, gastroenterology, and haematology departments. This presents a potentially hazardous situation where, for convenience and efficiency, standards of recovery care may be compromised unknowingly by ward staff not familiar with the added risks posed by the postoperative care of the frail or sick patient. Examples include inadequate amount and duration of monitoring as well as the failure to recognize the over-sedated patient [63].

Appropriate ongoing care in a surgical ward environment will be the standard of postoperative care for patients in most institutions. Consideration must be given to the experience of the ward staff (surgical versus medical) appropriate to the circumstances of the patient when approaching the discharge destination of the patient from the recovery area. Patients receiving palliative surgery can be considered higher risk due to the frequency of concurrent comorbidities that make them prone to hypoxia, prolonged hypotension, oliguria, dysrhythmia, surgical bleeding, and over-sedation. For high-risk patients, the availability of a high dependency or intensive care for postoperative recovery is dependent on the wishes of the patient and bed availability. Given the expense of this resource and the increasing awareness that the majority of postoperative complications are observed in the first 12–24 h following surgery, "overnight recovery" units have been developed. These units are characterized by increased nursing resources, the availability of rapid escalation of care as needed, and an expected discharge to ward of 24 h. In the future, this model is likely to be the most effective means for cost-efficient prevention and management of postoperative complications in patients thought to be at risk [64].

4.6.2 Analgesia

4.6.2.1 General Principles

Postoperative analgesia for patients undergoing palliative procedures may be particularly challenging due to the presence of pre-existing chronic pain. In this situation, the perioperative clinician must be prepared for an exaggerated postoperative pain response and analgesic requirements. In addition, some palliative procedures will carry a risk for development of persistent postsurgical pain. The approach to any patient with pain always begins with prompt attendance, conduct of a thorough history and examination, and subsequent formulation of a mechanism-based assessment and plan. An appreciation by the perioperative clinician of the significance of different pathological processes causing pain in the postoperative patient will assist with the construction of an appropriate analgesia plan. Specialist pain management or palliative care teams, where available, should be consulted.

4.6.2.2 Postoperative Pain

The International Association for the Study of Pain (IASP) have defined pain as "an unpleasant sensory and emotional experience associated with actual or potential tissue damage, or described in terms of such damage" [65]. The importance of pain in the postoperative period is such that it has become known as the "fifth vital sign".

Acute pain, such as that in the postoperative period, has been defined as "pain of recent onset and probable limited duration. It usually has an identifiable temporal and causal relationship to injury or disease" [66]. By the nature of its temporal association with surgical injury, pain experienced by patients following palliative procedures tends to be nociceptive (somatic or visceral) and associated with actual tissue damage sensed and transmitted by peripheral nociceptors. In contrast, neuropathic pain can be defined as "pain arising as a direct consequence or a lesion or disease affecting the somatosensory system" [66] and, in general, can be thought of as relating to damage to neural structures [67]. The damage induces functional and structural changes in afferent nociceptive pathways leading to a dysaesthesia experienced by the patient. The role of neuropathic pain in postoperative pain is underestimated and is a key risk factor in the development of chronic pain; persistent postsurgical pain can exist in up to 50 % of patients following a high-risk procedure [68]. Multiple risk factors often exist for the development of neuropathic and subsequent chronic pain in the palliative surgical patient. These include preoperative pain or anxiety, perioperative chemoradiotherapy and procedures involving iatrogenic nerve injury (thoracotomy, lumbosacral pelvic dissection, amputation, and repeat surgery).

4.6.2.3 Management of Postoperative Pain

Beyond the scope of this chapter, comprehensive postoperative analgesia should incorporate components of preoperative preparation (patient education, planning), pre-emptive analgesia (generally paracetamol, anti-inflammatory agents, and neuropathic analgesics), and intraoperative analgesics (for physiological stability) that are ultimately aimed at managing predicted postoperative analgesia requirements. A postoperative analgesic plan is always required.

The World Health Organization's Pain Relief Ladder emphasizes the use of non-pharmacologic and basic analgesic (paracetamol, cyclo-oxygenase inhibitors, tramadol) prior to the introduction of strong opioids for the management of pain [69]. Severe postoperative nociceptive pain invariably requires oral (oxycodone, morphine, hydromorphone) or intravenous opioid (morphine, oxycodone, fentanyl, hydromorphone) best prescribed "as required" or on a "patient-controlled" basis. Where possible, the enteral route is preferred for patient tolerance and minimization of side effects [70].

Identification of the underlying pathological basis (neuropathic or nociceptive) for a patient's pain is important. For example, the use of cyclo-oxygenase inhibitors and opioids is of particular benefit for the management of nociceptive pain. A distinct neuropathic component to a patient's report of pain is better managed with gabapentanoid agents, tricyclic antidepressants, clonidine, systemic lignocaine infusion, and NMDA receptor antagonists such as ketamine. Many of these agents have been administered preventatively with success in at-risk patients undergoing high-risk surgery.

The role of regional or neuraxial analgesia in the patient undergoing a palliative procedure is largely dependent on the severity of anticipated postoperative pain. Where possible, local anaesthetic catheter infusions are an excellent form of postoperative analgesia with few side effects and are particularly useful in the opioid-tolerant patient. Comparisons between epidural- and intravenous-based analgesic regimens have been extensively studied. In general, there is agreement that for particularly painful procedures (e.g. thoracotomy), postoperative epidural-based analgesia reduces pain on rest and movement with fewer side effects of sedation and nausea [71]. The avoidance of sedating opioids is of particular benefit to the patient receiving palliative surgery. The results of a large prospective trial examining the impact of epidural (versus morphine)-based postoperative opioid analgesia highlighted a benefit of epidural-based analgesia in those patients with pre-existing lung disease, but also the difficulties in obtaining and maintaining epidural analgesia in the postoperative period [72].

4.6.3 Non-pain Symptom Management

Symptoms other than pain may account for a significant burden of illness, including physical symptoms of dyspnoea, nausea/vomiting, fatigue, and sedation. These symptoms have been extensively studied in the outpatient palliative care setting; there is less evidence to guide management specific to the palliative surgical setting. When assessing the individual patient, it is important to have an understanding of the biopsychosocial context in which the symptoms are occurring and to assess the resulting impact of each symptom in terms of distress suffered and effect on quality of life [73].

Dyspnoea is "a subjective sensation of breathlessness" [74]. Due to the subjective nature of dyspnoea, it can be difficult to assess, as objective signs of respiratory distress often do not correlate with the degree of symptomatic distress experienced by the individual [75]. Management includes treatment of the underlying cause as well as medical therapy to reduce the severity of symptoms, including morphine, supplemental oxygen, benzodiazepines, and non-pharmacologic methods such as fans and relaxation techniques [75].

Nausea and vomiting are common amongst patients with terminal illnesses including those with cancer, organ failure, and other conditions such as Parkinson's disease and AIDS. These symptoms may be increased in the postoperative period as a result of anaesthetic and analgesic adverse drug effects, direct surgical manipulation of the gastrointestinal tract, and the systemic inflammatory response associated with surgery. Perioperative management includes employing a low threshold for intraoperative administration of prophylactic antiemetic medication, appropriate prescribing of antiemetic agents in the immediate postoperative period, as well as prevention and management of contributing factors such as constipation.

Fatigue and sedation can be distressing to patients due to reduced ability for social interaction with loved ones; this accounts for a significant reduction in quality of life. Other symptoms which may be distressing include hiccoughs, constipation, oedema, and delirium/confusion. Constipation is particularly common in the postoperative period and is exacerbated by opioid medications, immobility, and electrolyte abnormalities.

4.6.4 Psychosocial and Spiritual

Patients with life-limiting illness commonly experience symptoms of depression and anxiety; these symptoms may be exacerbated in the perioperative period. Furthermore, feelings associated with a loss of hope, meaning, and integrity can compound alterations in mood [73]. Psychological distress may contribute to pain in the perioperative period, and consideration of alternative therapies such as music therapy, relaxation techniques, attentional techniques, and massage therapy may be beneficial [70].

4.6.5 Prevention of Complications

The avoidance of postoperative complications is an important consideration in surgical palliation where the goal is improved quality of life and reduced symptom burden. This is because the occurrence of a major postoperative complication has been shown to significantly reduce the chance of symptom improvement after palliative surgery [4]. See Table 4.6.

Table 4.6 Common postoperative complications and methods of risk reduction

Complication	Preventive measures
Wound complications	Antibiotic prophylaxis
Dehiscence, infection, fistula formation	Nutritional optimization
Respiratory failure	Chest physiotherapy
	Consideration of extubation to non-invasive ventilation in high-risk cases
Venous thrombosis	Mechanical thromboprophylaxis (e.g. calf compressors, compression stockings)
	Pharmacologic thromboprophylaxis
Pressure ulcers	Early mobilization
	Strict pressure care
Cardiac complications	Minimize physiological stress (e.g. avoidance of tachycardia, hypertension, and hypotension)
	Optimize oxygen delivery
Gastrointestinal ulceration	Pharmacologic stress ulcer prophylaxis where appropriate

4.7 Ethical Considerations: "Do Not Resuscitate" Orders in the Perioperative Period

Providing perioperative care for patients with "do not resuscitate" (DNR) orders in place preoperatively raises a number of complex and challenging ethical issues. Discussions with patients and their families regarding perioperative resuscitation orders requires adept communication (as well as thorough documentation) [76]. Throughout these discussions it is important to demonstrate respect for the individual patient's dignity, values, and goals, as well as showing compassion and empathy and understanding of the reasons underlying their wishes.

4.7.1 Ethical Principles

Core principles in medical ethics include [77]:

- Autonomy in informed decision-making
- Justice
- Beneficence
- Non-maleficence

A particular ethical dilemma specific to the perioperative care of a patient receiving palliative surgery is that of the validity of "do not resuscitate" (DNR) orders. The right to refuse resuscitation arises from the ethical principle of patient autonomy [78], and automatic suspension of DNR orders in the perioperative period may violate this right [76]. This has the potential to create further distress and suffering in a particularly vulnerable patient group.

The concept of "required reconsideration" [79] has been suggested as an alternative to automatic suspension of DNR orders (or automatic continuation of DNR orders). This involves reconsidering whether cardiopulmonary resuscitation would be appropriate as well as considering whether limited specific resuscitative measures would be acceptable to the individual patient in the perioperative period.

4.7.2 Suggested Approach to the Patient with an Existing "Do Not Resuscitate" Order in the Perioperative Period

The discussion regarding a patient's resuscitation wishes in the perioperative period may be difficult for both the anaesthetist and the patient for a number of reasons. The anaesthetist often has no prior therapeutic relationship with the patient, and the anaesthetist assessing the patient in a preadmission clinic often will not be the treating anaesthetist on the day of surgery. Finally, addressing resuscitation wishes on the day of surgery or in an emergency setting can be confronting for patients who often need time to reflect of their goals and values with their family. The American Society of Anesthesiologists Committee of Ethics has produced guidelines that act as a framework to guide discussion and decision making regarding DNR orders in the perioperative period [76]. The discussion should involve the patient, surgeon, physician, anaesthetist, and the next of kin where appropriate.

4.7.2.1 What Orders Are Currently in Place?

Although seemingly obvious, resuscitation wishes of patients often are not known by the treating doctor. For example, the SUPPORT study demonstrated that amongst patients who were hospitalized with life-limiting illnesses, less than 50 % of doctors were aware of their patients' resuscitation wishes [80].

4.7.2.2 What Are the Patient's Goals and Values?

An understanding of a patient's goals and values that underpin their resuscitation wishes is crucial in order to formulate an appropriate perioperative plan. Active listening in a non-judgmental and empathetic fashion is paramount in order to facilitate this discussion. Furthermore, it is important to discuss the existing resuscitation order in the context of the specific procedure planned and relating this back to the patient's underlying values.

4.7.2.3 Consider Clarifying and/or Revising the DNR Order, Keeping in Mind That Resuscitation Is Not "All or Nothing"

In discussing whether to reconsider or continue do not resuscitate orders in the perioperative period, it is important to explain to a patient what "resuscitation" involves. In particular, certain interventions which are often standard components of anaesthesia (such as endotracheal intubation, supported ventilation, and the use of vasopressors) may be viewed as resuscitation in the nonoperative setting [76]. Furthermore, the discussion should address possible modifications in DNR orders to allow treatment of reversible complications during surgery [76]. This is particularly relevant if the procedure may improve the patient's quality of life or reduce the distress of their symptoms (e.g. relieving dyspnoea via drainage of pneumothorax complicating CVC insertion).

Two approaches have been described which can be used to clarify a DNR order: (1) "Procedure-directed limitations" [76], whereby the specific resuscitative measures acceptable to a patient are explicitly stated preoperatively, or (2) "Goal-directed limitations" [76], whereby the patient delegates decision-making to the treating team while in accordance with the patient's goals and values.

If a procedure-directed approach is taken, the exact therapies which are acceptable to the patient need to be explicitly stated and documented [78]. Decisions regarding the specific interventions, which are acceptable to the individual patient, should be consistent with their overall goals and values. Specific therapies, which should be discussed, include cardiopulmonary resuscitation, defibrillation, intubation and ventilation, vasopressor use, blood product administration, care escalation, renal replacement therapy, antibiotic therapy, fluid therapy, and parenteral nutrition. An advantage of this approach is that the patient's wishes are explicitly documented. However, discussing a variety of technical interventions may be overwhelming for a patient and difficult to understand. Goal-directed limitations for resuscitation [76] places great responsibility on the anaesthetist and surgeon. Consultation with the patient's next of kin is essential [78]. An advantage of this approach is that the doctrine allows for a less regimented approach to patient care, allowing clinicians to act in the best interests of their patients in a variety of often unpredictable clinical circumstances.

4.7.3 The Postoperative Period

If the preoperative DNR order is modified, there should be a plan for when it is to be reinstituted in its original form postoperatively [76].

4.7.4 Dealing with Conflict Regarding Perioperative DNR Orders

The responsibility of providing anaesthesia for patients with DNR orders or treatment-limiting orders can be confronting for the anaesthetist, whose ultimate goal is usually to ensure that the patient survives the operation.

In cases of medical objection, whereby the physician believes that proceeding with an intervention with the patient refusing specific therapies would compromise safety or be inconsistent with accepted standards of care, then ethical board review of the case may be appropriate [76, 78]. In cases of moral objection, whereby the anaesthetist is unable to accept a patient's wishes regarding perioperative DNR orders, attempts should be made to find an alternative anaesthetist. However, if an alternative anaesthetist is not available, then experts agree that there are no ethical grounds for refusing to proceed [76, 78], and the anaesthetist should follow the patient's directives as best as possible to prevent further suffering [76].

Conclusion

Palliative surgery offers the opportunity to affect a positive and meaningful impact upon patients' quality of life. Beyond the focus of surgery, it is of great importance to provide high-quality perioperative care that considers a patient's symptoms and wishes in these frequently challenging and complex clinical situations. Pathophysiological changes specific to the patient receiving palliative surgery emphasize the importance of careful history taking, examination, and clinical decision-making. The complexity of many palliative procedures, as well as the frequency comorbidities in this patient population, underscores the importance of open and honest dialogue between patient, anaesthetist, and surgeon to attain the best possible outcomes for patients.

References

1. World Health Organization. Palliative care. Switzerland: World Health Organization; 2007.
2. American College of Surgeons Committee on Ethics and Surgical Palliative Care Task Force. Statement of principles of palliative care. Bull Am Coll Surg. 2005;90(8):34–5.
3. Dunn GP. Surgical palliative care: recent trends and developments. Anesthesiol Clin. 2012;30(1):13–28.

4. Miner TJ, Brennan MF, Jaques DP. A prospective, symptom related, outcomes analysis of 1022 palliative procedures for advanced cancer. Ann Surg. 2004;240(4):719–26.
5. Miner TJ. Communication as a core skill of palliative surgical care. Anesthesiol Clin. 2012;30(1):47–58.
6. McCahill LE, Krouse R, Chu D, Juarez G, Uman GC, Ferrell B, et al. Indications and use of palliative surgery – results of Society of Surgical Survey. Ann Surg Oncol. 2002;9(1):104–12.
7. Krouse RS, Nelson RA, Farrell BR, Grube B, Juarez G, Wagman LD, et al. Surgical palliation at a cancer center: incidence and outcomes. Arch Surg. 2001;136(7):773–8.
8. Solano JP, Gomes B, Higginson IJ. A comparison of symptom prevalence in far advanced cancer, AIDS, heart disease, chronic obstructive pulmonary disease and renal disease. J Pain Symptom Manage. 2006;31(1):58–69.
9. Cady B, Easson A, Aboulafia AJ, Ferson PF. Part 1: surgical palliation of advanced illness–what's new, what's helpful. J Am Coll Surg. 2005;200(1):115–27.
10. Workgroup SPC. Office of promoting excellence in end-of-life care: Surgeon's Palliative Care Workgroup report from the field. J Am Coll Surg. 2003;197(4):661–86.
11. Dunn GP. Palliative surgical outcomes: are we looking through a keyhole? Ann Surg Oncol. 2012;19(12):3637–8.
12. Tseng WH, Yang X, Wang H, Martinez SR, Chen SL, Meyers FJ, et al. Nomogram to predict risk of 30-day morbidity and mortality for patients with disseminated malignancy undergoing surgical intervention. Ann Surg. 2011;254(2):333–8.
13. McCahill LE, Smith DD, Borneman T, Juarez G, Cullinane C, Chu DZ, et al. A prospective evaluation of palliative outcomes for surgery of advanced malignancies. Ann Surg Oncol. 2003;10(6):654–63.
14. Podnos YD, Juarez G, Pameijer C, Choi K, Ferrell BR, Wagman LD. Impact of surgical palliation on quality of life in patients with advanced malignancy: results of the decisions and outcomes in palliative surgery (DOPS) trial. Ann Surg Oncol. 2007;14(2):922–8.
15. Badgwell B, Krouse R, Cormier J, Guevara C, Klimberg VS, Ferrell B. Frequent and early death limits quality of life assessment in patients with advanced malignancies evaluated for palliative surgical intervention. Ann Surg Oncol. 2012;19(12):3651–8.
16. Thomay AA, Jaques DP, Miner TJ. Surgical palliation: getting back to our roots. Surg Clin North Am. 2009;89(1):27–41.
17. Gutt CN, Held S, Paolucci V, Encke A. Experiences with percutaneous endoscopic gastrostomy. World J Surg. 1996;20(8):1106–8.
18. Young-Spint M, Guner YS, Meyers FJ, Schneider P, Khatri VP. Radical palliative surgery: new limits to pursue. Pediatr Surg Int. 2009;25(10):917–21.
19. Lee TH, Marcantonio ER, Mangione CM, Thomas EJ, Polanczyk C, Cook EF, et al. Derivation and prospective validation of a simple index for prediction of cardiac risk of major noncardiac surgery. Circulation. 1999;100:1043–9.
20. Arozullah AM, Daley J, Henderson WG, Khuri SF. Multifactorial risk index for predicting postoperative respiratory failure in men after major noncardiac surgery. The National Veterans Administration Surgical Quality Improvement Program. Ann Surg. 2000;232(2):242–53.
21. Canet J, Gallart L, Gomar C, Paluzie G, Vallès J, Castillo J, et al. Prediction of postoperative pulmonary complications in a population-based surgical cohort. Anesthesiology. 2010;113(6):1338–50.
22. el-Ganzouri AR, McCarthy RJ, Tuman KJ, Tanck EN, Ivankovich AD. Preoperative airway assessment: predictive value of a multivariate risk index. Anesth Analg. 1996;82(6):1197–204.
23. Iseli TA, Iseli CE, Golden JB, Jones VL, Boudreaux AM, Boyce JR, et al. Outcomes of intubation in difficult airways due to head and neck pathology. Ear Nose Throat J. 2012;91(3):E1–5.
24. Shekar K, Foot C, Fraser J, Ziegenfuss M, Hopkins P, Windsor M. Bronchopleural fistula: an update for intensivists. J Crit Care. 2010;25(1):47–55.
25. Konstantinov IE, Saxena P. Independent lung ventilation in the postoperative management of large bronchopleural fistula. J Thorac Cardiovasc Surg. 2010;139(2):e21–2.
26. Reynen K, Köckeritz U, Strasser RH. Metastases to the heart. Ann Oncol. 2004;15(3):375–81.
27. Pelosof LC, Gerber DE. Paraneoplastic syndromes: an approach to diagnosis and treatment. Mayo Clin Proc. 2010;85(9):838–54.
28. Small S, Ali HH, Lennon VA, Brown RHJ, Carr DB, de Armendi A. Anesthesia for an unsuspected Lambert-Eaton myasthenic syndrome with autoantibodies and occult small cell lung carcinoma. Anesthesiology. 1992;76(1):142–5.
29. Arain MR, Buggy DJ. Anaesthesia for cancer patients. Curr Opin Anaesthesiol. 2007;20(3):247–53.
30. Dunn A, Carter J, Carter H. Anemia at the end of life: prevalence, significance, and causes in patients receiving palliative care. J Pain Symptom Manage. 2003;26(6):1132–9.
31. Falanga A, Russo LV, Verzeroli C. Mechanisms of thrombosis in cancer. Thromb Res. 2013;131 Suppl 1:S59–62.
32. Mughal TI, Ejaz AA, Foringer JR, Coiffier B. An integrated clinical approach for the identification, prevention, and treatment of tumor lysis syndrome. Cancer Treat Rev. 2010;36(2):164–76.
33. Lee MH, Cheng KI, Jang RC, Hsu JH, Dai ZK, Wu JR. Tumour lysis syndrome developing during an operation. Anaesthesia. 2007;62(1):85–7.
34. MacDonald N, Easson AM, Mazurak VC, Dunn GP, Baracos VE. Understanding and managing cancer cachexia. J Am Coll Surg. 2003;197(1):143–61.
35. Raspe C, Piso P, Wiesenack C, Bucher M. Anesthetic management in patients undergoing hyperthermic chemotherapy. Curr Opin Anaesthesiol. 2012;25(3):348–55.

36. Allan N, Siller C, Breen A. Anaesthetic implications of chemotherapy. Contin Educ Anaesth Crit Care Pain. 2012;12(2):52–6.
37. Yeh ET, Tong AT, Lenihan DJ, Yusuf SW, Swafford J, Champion C, et al. Cardiovascular complications of cancer therapy: diagnosis, pathogenesis, and management. Circulation. 2004;109(25):3122–31.
38. Meadors M, Floyd J, Perry MC. Pulmonary toxicity of chemotherapy. Semin Oncol. 2006;33(1):98–105.
39. de Jonge MJ, Verweij J. Renal toxicities of chemotherapy. Semin Oncol. 2006;33(1):68–73.
40. Huettemann E, Sakka SG. Anaesthesia and anti-cancer chemotherapeutic drugs. Curr Opin Anaesthesiol. 2005;18(3):307–14.
41. Floyd J, Mirza I, Sachs B, Perry MC. Hepatotoxicity of chemotherapy. Semin Oncol. 2006;33(1):50–67.
42. Goldiner PL, Carlon GC, Cvitkovic E, Schweizer O, Howland WS. Factors influencing postoperative morbidity and mortality in patients treated with bleomycin. Br Med J. 1978;24(1):1664–7.
43. Froudarakis M, Hatzimichael E, Kyriazopoulou L, Lagos K, Pappas P, Tzakos AG, et al. Revisiting bleomycin from pathophysiology to safe clinical use. Crit Rev Oncol Hematol. 2013;87(1):90–100.
44. O'Sullivan JM, Huddart RA, Norman AR, Nicholls J, Dearnaley DP, Horwich A. Predicting the risk of bleomycin lung toxicity in patients with germ-cell tumours. Ann Oncol. 2003;14(1):91–6.
45. Merrill WW. Radiation-induced lung injury. In: Kavanagh B, Hollingsworth H, editors. UpToDate. Waltham: UpToDate; 2013.
46. Galloway T, Amdur RJ. Management of late complications of head and neck cancer and its treatment. In: Basow DS, editor. UpToDate. Waltham, MA: UpToDate; 2013.
47. McCann S, Yaksh TL, von Gunten CF. Correlation between myoclonus and the 3-glucuronide metabolites in patients treated with morphine or hydromorphone: a pilot study. J Opioid Manag. 2010;6(2):87–94.
48. Zaniboni A, Prabhu S, Audisio RA. Chemotherapy and anaesthetic drugs: too little is known. Lancet Oncol. 2005;6(3):176–81.
49. Mols G, Priebe HJ, Guttmann J. Alveolar recruitment in acute lung injury. Br J Anaesth. 2006;96(2): 156–66.
50. Ferrer M, Valencia M, Nicolas JM, Bernadich O, Badia JR, Torres A. Early noninvasive ventilation averts extubation failure in patients at risk: a randomized trial. Am J Respir Crit Care Med. 2006;173(2): 164–70.
51. Nava S, Gregoretti C, Fanfulla F, Squadrone E, Grassi M, Carlucci A, et al. Noninvasive ventilation to prevent respiratory failure after extubation in high-risk patients. Crit Care Med. 2005;33(11):2465–70.
52. Nethercott D, Strang T, Krysiak P. Airway stents: anaesthetic implications Contin Educ Anaesth Crit Care Pain. 2010;10(2):53–8.
53. Mercadante S. Intravenous patient-controlled analgesia and management of pain in post-surgical elderly with cancer. Surg Oncol. 2010;19(3):173–7.
54. Racca F, Mongini T, Wolfler A, Vianello A, Cutrera R, Del Sorbo L, et al. Recommendations for anesthesia and perioperative management of patients with neuromuscular disorders. Minerva Anestesiol. 2013;79(4):419–33.
55. Australian Red Cross Blood Service. Blood component information: a circular of information. Melbourne, Australia: Australian Red Cross Blood Service; 2012.
56. Ferguson JK. Preventing healthcare-associated infection: risks, healthcare systems and behaviour. Intern Med J. 2009;39(9):574–81.
57. Denkinger CM, Grant AD, Denkinger M, Gautam S, D'Agata EM. Increased multi-drug resistance among the elderly on admission to the hospital – a 12-year surveillance study. Arch Gerontol Geriatr. 2013;56(1):227–30.
58. Cavaliere S, Venuta F, Foccoli P, Toninelli C, La Face B. Endoscopic treatment of malignant airway obstructions in 2,008 patients. Chest. 2006;110(6):1536–42.
59. Profili S, Manca A, Feo CF, Padua G, Ortu R, Canalis GC, et al. Palliative airway stenting performed under radiological guidance and local anesthesia. Cardiovasc Intervent Radiol. 2007;30(1):74–8.
60. Coolen D, Slabbynck H, Galdermans D, Van Schaardenburg C, Mortelmans LL. Insertion of a self-expandable endotracheal metal stent using topical anaesthesia and a fibreoptic bronchoscope: a comfortable way to offer palliation. Thorax. 1994;49(1):87–8.
61. Benrath J, Kozek-Langenecker S, Hüpfl M, Lierz P, Gustorff B. Anaesthesia for brachytherapy–51/2 yr of experience in 1622 procedures. Br J Anaesth. 2006;96(2):195–200.
62. Roessler B, Six LM, Gustorff B. Anaesthesia for brachytherapy. Curr Opin Anaesthesiol. 2008;21(4): 514–8.
63. Bryson EO, Sejpal D. Anesthesia in remote locations: radiology and beyond, international anesthesiology clinics: gastroenterology: endoscopy, colonoscopy, and ERCP. Int Anesthesiol Clin. 2009;47(2):69–80.
64. Reed H. The development of an extended care facility in the recovery unit: the post-anaesthesia care unit. J Perioper Pract. 2011;21(6):210–4.
65. IASP Task Force on Taxonomy. In: Merskey H, Bogduk N, editors. Classification of chronic pain. Seattle: IASP Press; 1994.
66. Taskforce on Acute Pain. In: Ready BL, Edwards WT, editors. Management of acute pain: a practical guide. Seattle: IASP Press; 1992.
67. Loeser JD, Treede RD. The Kyoto protocol of IASP basic pain terminology. Pain. 2008;137(3):473–7.
68. Kehlet H, Jensen TS, Woolf CJ. Persistent post-surgical pain: risk factors and prevention. Lancet. 2006;367(9522):1618–25.
69. World Health Organization. Cancer pain relief: with a guide to opioid availability. Geneva: WHO; 1996.
70. APM: SE Working Group of the Australian and New Zealand College of Anaesthetists and Faculty of Pain Medicine. Acute Pain Management: Scientific Evidence. In: Macintyre PE, Schug SA, Scott DA,

Visser EJ, Walker SM, editors. Melbourne: ANZCA & FPM; 2010.
71. Wu CL, Cohen SR, Richman JM, Rowlingson AJ, Courpas GE, Cheung K, et al. Efficacy of postoperative patient-controlled and continuous infusion epidural analgesia versus intravenous patient-controlled analgesia with opioids: a meta-analysis. Anesthesiology. 2005;103(5):1079–88.
72. Rigg JR, Jamrozik K, Myles PS, Silbert BS, Peyton PJ, Parsons RW, et al. Epidural anaesthesia and analgesia and outcome of major surgery: a randomised trial. Lancet. 2002;359(9314):1276–82.
73. Dunn GP. Patient assessment in palliative care: How to see the "big picture" and what to do when "there is no more we can do". J Am Coll Surg. 2001;193(5):565–73.
74. Dunn GP, Milch RA. Is this a bad day, or one of the last days? How to recognize and respond to approaching demise. J Am Coll Surg. 2002;195(6): 879–87.
75. Mosenthal AC, Lee KF. Management of dyspnea at the end of life: relief for patients and surgeons. J Am Coll Surg. 2002;194(3):377–86.
76. American Society of Anesthesiologists Committee of Ethics. Ethical guidelines for the anesthesia care of patients with do-not-resuscitate orders or other directives that limit treatment. Park Ridge, Illinois: American Society of Anesthesiologists; 2008.
77. Beauchamp TL, Childress JF. Principles of biomedical ethics. Oxford, United Kingdom: Oxford University Press; 2012.
78. Scott TH, Gavrin JR. Palliative surgery in the do-not-resuscitate patient: ethics and practical suggestions for management. Anesthesiol Clin. 2012;30(1): 1–12.
79. Rothenberg DM. Informed refusal - DNR orders in the patient undergoing anesthesia and surgery at the end-of-life. In: Van Norman GA, Jackson S, Rosenbaum SH, Palmer SK, editors. Clinical ethics in anesthesiology. New York: Cambridge University Press; 2011.
80. The SUPPORT, Investigators P. A controlled trial to improve care for seriously ill hospitalized patients. The study to understand prognoses and preferences for outcomes and risks of treatments (SUPPORT). JAMA. 1995;274(20):1591–8.

Pain Management

5

Suzanne Chapman and Paul Farquhar-Smith

Contents

The principles of management of pain after palliative surgery are essentially the same as after any type of surgery. However, there are certain aspects for patients undergoing palliative surgery that need increased vigilance. Patients are often taking opioids for moderate to severe pain ("strong" opioids) which requires careful assessment and a detailed perioperative management plan, providing analgesia but minimising risk of withdrawal, uncontrolled pain and overdose. Multimodal analgesia should be utilised in an opioid-reducing strategy. It is imperative that pain and possible adverse perioperative sequelae should not compromise a quick recovery to allow the patient to have high-quality end-of-life care. Neuraxial blockade, continuous peripheral nerve block techniques and other analgesic adjuvants should be considered. Patient-controlled analgesia offers the flexibility in opioid delivery to adapt to the changing and difficult analgesic needs of this population.

5.1 Introduction

Palliative surgery and procedures are interventions that may improve pain, symptoms and quality of life with minimal impact on the patients' survival in carefully selected patients. Patients may need surgery for many reasons such as debulking operations (in collusion with chemotherapy and radiotherapy), surgical resection of locally advanced or metastatic cancer, management of malignant obstruction, pathological fracture management

S. Chapman, RGN, MSc, BSc • P. Farquhar-Smith, MB BChir, MA, FRCA, PhD, FFPMRCA, FFICM (✉)
Department of Anaesthetics and Pain,
The Royal Marsden NHS Foundation Trust,
Fulham Road, London SW3 6JJ, UK
e-mail: suzanne.chapman@rmh.nhs.uk;
paul.farquhar-smith@rmh.nhs.uk

M. Wichmann, G. Maddern (eds.), *Palliative Surgery*,
DOI 10.1007/978-3-642-53709-7_5, © Springer-Verlag Berlin Heidelberg 2014

and management of bleeding. However, procedures performed with palliative intent may often leave local or metastatic residual disease. Occasionally surgery may be contemplated specifically for analgesic indications.

Examples of palliative surgical procedures include:

- Colostomy to relieve tumour obstruction in the colon or rectum or for management of rectovaginal fistula
- Ileostomy for distal small bowel obstruction
- Ileal conduit for vesicovaginal fistula
- Gastric bypass for gastroduodenal outflow obstruction in advanced gastric and pancreatic cancer
- Hepatectomy (liver resection) of metastatic lesions causing pain from capsule distension and jaundice
- Pulmonary wedge resection to resect metastatic tumours or perform pleurodesis for repeated pleural effusions
- Nephrostomy tubes to relieve tumour-induced ureteric obstruction causing hydronephrosis
- Orthopaedic procedures for management of pathological fractures

Perioperative pain in palliative surgery shares the same management principles as for surgery in the general population. However, there are some special considerations that need to be considered in the palliative surgery scenario. Since palliative surgery by definition will tend to occur towards the end of the patients' cancer journey, it is imperative that the pain management promotes rapid and comfortable recovery to facilitate focus on subsequent end-of-life care.

5.2 Assessment

Holistic assessment of the patients' pain starts in the preoperative period and is key to successful pain management. All sites of the patients' pain should be assessed and this should continue postoperatively. Patients may have pain in several sites as well as metastatic disease, and management of these pains also needs to be considered with acute surgical pain. Given that pain is a major symptom of advanced cancer [1], acute pain in the palliative population is likely to be complicated by pre-existing chronic pain. Furthermore, many will be on significant opioid therapy. Palliative patients are often undertreated when they are prescribed analgesia for episodes of acute pain [2].

It is vital that the assessment includes an accurate history of current analgesia especially opioid requirements. This should include the opioid formulations the patient is taking (e.g. modified release and immediate release oral opioids, transdermal patches, transmucosal or buccal opioids). Preoperative opioid use should be assessed and recorded to estimate approximate doses of medication needed for pain control after surgery [3].

It is also being increasingly recognised that a few patients taking opioids for cancer pain may display behaviours akin to recreational drug use which may be problematic in assessment. Estimation of opioid requirements is often difficult due to the variable quality of drug and unwillingness to divulge true opioid consumption. In patients undergoing palliative surgery, a small number may also have a history of previous problematic opioid use and management may be similar to those patients taking recreational opioids. Both of these groups of patients may be relatively tolerant to opioids and the opioid dose required for acute pain management may seem very high [2, 3].

Occasionally, even patients having palliative surgery may also be on methadone or buprenorphine maintenance programmes and be under the care of drug dependency units. It is important that the patients' dose is confirmed with their prescribing centre so that this can be maintained and factored into the pain management plan [2].

Whatever the cause or extent of problematic opioid use, it is not considered appropriate to attempt rehabilitation in the postoperative period. The focus for all patients remains providing sufficient analgesia and, in those with high opioid requirements, preventing acute withdrawal symptoms.

The surgical procedure itself may allow anticipation of whether pain will be substantially reduced as a result of the procedure, but the effect of surgery on pain can be extremely variable. Patients may initially have an increase in pain due to surgery, but their overall pain may then be reduced resulting in reduced analgesic requirements. For example, patients with a pathological fracture may experience significant levels of pain preoperatively which may be substantially reduced once they have undergone fixation surgery.

For patients on substantial doses of opioids before the surgery, the focus is to manage a balance of analgesia for acute pain relief. There is a tension between the needs of acute pain management while minimising potential for withdrawal and conversely, reducing chance of opioid overdose. Opioid requirements should be assessed and reassessed frequently to allow optimal titration.

After a meticulous assessment, a perioperative analgesic plan with multidisciplinary input should be developed. Analgesic management should also include the use of non-opioid drugs and other analgesic techniques such as neuraxial and regional anaesthetic techniques all aiming to potentially reduce acute opioid requirements (vide infra). However, it must be remembered there are few experimental data from studies of the management of these patients [4].

5.3 Acute Pain Management

Analgesic medications are classed into three main groups: non-opioids, opioids and adjuvant analgesics. In addition to these three groups, local anaesthetic drugs can be administered by either peripheral or neuraxial routes. Drugs with different underlying mechanisms are used in combination to provide a synergistic effect, and this strategy is termed multimodal analgesia [5]. This approach allows lower doses of each of the drugs in the pain management plan, reducing the potential for adverse effects [6]. In patients known to be on opioids prior to surgery, a combination of drugs with different mechanisms can provide pain relief with a potential "opioid-sparing" effect where the opioid dose may be lowered or maintained without decreasing pain relief.

5.3.1 Non-opioid Analgesia

Non-opioid drugs such as paracetamol (acetaminophen) and nonsteroidal anti-inflammatory drugs (NSAIDs) are often used for the management of mild to moderate acute pain [5]. Non-opioids alone are rarely sufficient to relieve severe pain that is associated with surgery, but they are an important part of multimodal analgesia. They may also offer an opioid "dose-sparing" effect [6].

Paracetamol is an effective analgesic with few side effects with a good safety profile when taken at recommended doses. It has been shown to reduce postoperative opioid requirements by 20–30 % when given regularly [6–8]. Although the mechanism of analgesic efficacy of paracetamol remains unclear, it may involve direct and indirect inhibition of central cyclo-oxygenases (COX). The activation of the endocannabinoid system and spinal serotonergic pathways also appears to be integral to the analgesic actions of paracetamol [9–11]. Paracetamol may also enhance descending inhibitory controls [12].

Paracetamol is available in oral, intravenous and rectal preparations. The intravenous preparation provides faster, potentially more effective analgesia than the equivalent oral dose [13]. Rectal absorption of the drug is poor and subtherapeutic blood concentrations are common. The route chosen will depend on several factors such as whether the patient can take oral analgesia, what preparations are available at a local level and what type of surgery the patient has had (e.g. patients having rectal/bowel surgery or may contraindicate rectal administration).

NSAID refers to both non-selective, nonsteroidal anti-inflammatory drugs (that inhibit COX-1 and COX-2 isoenzymes) and COX-2 selective inhibitors [14]. NSAIDs inhibit COX, reduce the production of proinflammatory prostaglandins and leukotrienes, are effective analgesics and are an integral part of multimodal analgesia. In combination with paracetamol they can decrease opioid requirements [6].

Many of the adverse effects of NSAIDs are due to the physiological role of prostaglandins being inhibited including gastric mucosal protection, renal tubular function and intrarenal vasodilation, bronchodilatation and production of endothelial prostacyclin (which causes vasodilation and prevents platelet adhesion) [15]. These processes are predominantly regulated by COX-1. Tissue damage induces COX-2 production leading to synthesis of prostaglandins that result in pain and inflammation, and the COX-2 selective NSAIDs are thought to work specifically on this mechanism [16]. However, the use of COX-2 selective NSAIDs has been compromised by the potential increase in cardiac thrombotic complications [16].

NSAIDs are available in oral, parenteral and rectal preparations and are equally effective with a similar speed of onset but with no difference in side effect incidence between routes. The combination of paracetamol and NSAIDs has been found to be more effective than paracetamol alone, but compared to NSAIDs alone was less clinically significant [8, 17].

5.3.2 Opioid Analgesia

5.3.2.1 Mechanisms of Opioid Action

Opioids act via G protein coupled opioid receptors. Several types of receptor have been characterised, but the μ opioid receptor is the most important in opioid-induced analgesia. Opioid receptors are located in synapses in areas of the brain, in the spinal cord and in the periphery intimately associated with pain processing [18]. Opioid receptors are found in many areas of the brain including the periaqueductal grey and locus coeruleus which are involved in the higher processing of pain perception, emotional response and localisation. Elements of the so-called pain matrix are here and the area's importance in pain has been shown directly by functional imaging [19].

In the spinal cord opioid receptors are localised in the superficial dorsal horn, which modulates transmitter release and pain impulses, resulting in a spinally mediated analgesia. Release of the major excitatory transmitter glutamate at the spinal synapse of the primary afferent nociceptor is reduced by pre- and postsynaptic opioid mechanisms. Other transmitters are also modulated by opioid action such as substance P and calcitonin gene-related peptide [20].

Many different opioids are available for use in clinical practice such as opioids for moderate to severe pain including morphine, fentanyl and oxycodone. The opioids for mild to moderate pain (codeine, tramadol) may be used for less major palliative surgery. Choice of opioid will depend on local availability, local guideline or policy and patient tolerance to particular opioids (drug allergy or sensitivity to opioid side effects). The most common side effects are potential respiratory depression, sedation, nausea and vomiting and pruritus [21]. If a patient is on an effective dose of opioid preoperatively with a good efficacy/side effect balance, it is judicious to use the same opioid perioperatively.

Opioids can be delivered by many routes for acute pain management. The most common routes of opioid administration are intravenous, epidural or intrathecal, subcutaneous, intramuscular or oral. They can also be administered via a transdermal patch, sublingual or buccal mucosa and intranasal or rectal routes although these are more commonly used for chronic pain states. Intravenous patient-controlled analgesia (PCA) is the most frequently used method to deliver intravenous opioids postoperatively.

5.3.2.2 Patient-Controlled Analgesia (PCA)

Intravenous opioids delivered using a patient-controlled analgesia (PCA) infusion device provide the most flexible form of opioid analgesia in the postoperative period [22]. Patients have been shown to prefer PCA compared to other routes of postoperative opioid administration [23]. PCA delivers a preset bolus dose on demand with a specified lockout period between each successful dose, and a background infusion can also be administered. These variables can be adjusted according to the patients' opioid requirements.

For patients on opioid therapy prior to surgery, PCA allows higher-than-normal bolus doses to be delivered and a background infusion rate equivalent to the patient's baseline opioid requirement.

Intravenous opioid PCA provides better analgesia than conventional intramuscular and subcutaneous opioid regimens, although the magnitude of the difference in analgesia is small [24]. Although PCA administration was associated with greater opioid use, there are no differences in duration of hospital stay or opioid-related adverse effects other than pruritus, which is increased, and patient satisfaction is higher [24].

As previously discussed, for patients on preoperative opioids, there is a need to maintain a baseline level of opioid to ensure that an acute withdrawal syndrome is avoided and to ensure that pain that may be present, independent of surgery, is well managed. There are several approaches that can be taken to maintain the baseline opioid levels. As discussed previously, a background infusion can be added to a PCA and the bolus dose titrated to effect. In some cases, where the patient has a fentanyl patch, this could be left on (as long as all practitioners are aware) to maintain background requirements and PCA bolus added. Theoretically perioperative alterations in skin blood flow may result in erratic absorption from the fentanyl patch and some advocate removal of all transcutaneous medication. It should be remembered that absorption may continue after fentanyl patch removal [25]. In more minor palliative surgery, oral medications may be able to be re-established soon after surgery.

5.3.3 Adjuvant Analgesia

Adjuvant drugs such as clonidine and ketamine can also be used as part of a multimodal analgesia approach and may have a potential beneficial opioid-sparing effect.

Clonidine is an α_2-adrenoceptor agonist which produces analgesia via the descending pain pathways that modulate the transmission of pain signals in the spinal cord [26]. It can be given intravenously as a bolus dose for postoperative analgesia and is effective in reducing opioid requirements [26]. Clonidine can also be administered by other routes (neuraxial and peripheral nerve block) [27]. For patients with chronic pain having surgery, clonidine can provide effective analgesia when used in combination with other drugs although its routine use may be limited by side effects of sedation and hypotension.

Ketamine is an NMDA (*N*-methyl-D-aspartate) receptor antagonist. Pain stimuli (e.g. after surgery) can induce a so-called central sensitisation at the spinal level by (amongst other mechanisms) activation of the NMDA receptor [28]. This results in an increase in neuronal hyperexcitability and can induce further changes in the spinal cord, contributing to central sensitisation and increased perception of pain [28]. NMDA receptor function also involves pain learning and memory. Ketamine blocks the NMDA receptor, inhibits central sensitisation and potentially treats pain refractory to opioids [29].

Ketamine can be useful in the treatment of other opioid-insensitive pain, such as certain types of neuropathic pain, and cancer pain [29]. Ketamine has been used in the management of acute pain in opioid tolerance and escalating opioid requirements. In patients using opioids on a long-term basis, the administration of ketamine has been reported to lead to improved pain relief and reduced opioid requirements [30, 31]. However, the evidence base for postoperative pain has been less well established [32].

Other agents such as the gabapentinoids and steroids are beginning to accrue evidence for their efficacy in postoperative pain and may further contribute to the opioid-sparing effect of multimodal analgesia [33, 34].

5.3.4 Neuraxial (Epidural and Intrathecal) and Regional Analgesia

Neuraxial and regional analgesia can be used to provide postoperative pain relief in palliative surgery. Indeed, the opioid-sparing action potentially can minimise the issues related to management of patients on existing opioid medication.

Opioids can be given via the epidural or intrathecal (spinal) route where they bind directly with opioid receptors in the dorsal horn of the spinal cord. The main side effects are similar to parenteral administration: respiratory depression, sedation, nausea and vomiting and pruritus. Direct action on spinal opioid receptors achieves equivalent receptor occupation at a lower dose resulting in less systemic absorption and fewer systemic side effects.

Neuraxial and regional analgesia block pain impulses by administration of local anaesthetic in proximity to nerves and by virtue of blockade of the sodium channel. This approach can target either peripheral or central (neuraxial approach) nerves. Due to the differential effect on neurones of different sizes, pain impulses can be inhibited potentially retaining function in sensation and minimising the effect on muscle weakness. Neuraxial blockade can be especially effective for relief of pain provoked by movement, facilitating early postoperative mobilisation of patients, even after major surgery [35]. Infiltration of the wound with local anaesthetics may also be of merit as part of a multimodal approach [36].

Local anaesthetics and opioids are often used in combination when given epidurally as they have a synergistic pharmacological effect, allowing lower doses of each drug to be given and minimising the risk of side effects. The efficacy of epidural analgesia has been robustly demonstrated. Regardless of analgesic agent used, location of catheter, type of surgery and type or time of pain assessment, epidural analgesia provides better pain relief than parenteral opioid administration [37–39].

One meta-analysis of systemic opioids via PCA versus epidural analgesia concluded that epidural analgesia provides better pain relief at rest and with movement after all types of surgery. The epidural group had a lower incidence of nausea/vomiting and sedation, but a higher incidence of pruritus, urinary retention and motor block [37].

Other types of regional analgesia can be used for acute postoperative pain. Local anaesthetic can be administered as a single injection or as a continuous infusion in a continuous peripheral nerve block (CPNB) [40]. CPNB can also be delivered as an ambulatory service where patients are discharged home with the infusion. Examples of regional analgesia include brachial plexus blocks for upper limb surgery, and femoral blocks, lumbar plexus blocks and sciatic nerve blocks for lower limbs. Regional anaesthesia may also reduce perioperative complications in patients undergoing palliative surgery whose disease state may increase their risk [41, 42]. Reduction of sequelae will potentially allow more rapid recovery and not compromise patients' end-of-life care.

5.3.5 Non-pharmacological Approaches

Although severe acute pain clearly requires pharmacological interventions, there is a need to recognise the importance of non-pharmacological approaches that may contribute to minimising the patients' acute pain experience which may be especially pertinent in palliative surgery. Anxiety may also be an important factor in the transition from acute to chronic postoperative pain that may occur after palliative surgery [43].

5.3.5.1 Psychological Interventions

Pain is an individual experience with multifactorial influences such as previous pain experience, personal beliefs, culture, mood and ability to cope. Palliative patients undergoing surgery are likely to have previous experience of procedures and anticancer therapies, some of which may have caused pain. It is important to explore these with the patient and also concerns or expectations they may have about the current surgical procedure.

Psychological interventions include information provision, stress/tension reduction and cognitive-behavioural interventions.

Information provision consists of two strategies which target the specific sensations that will be experienced (such as "sharp", "burning" or "stinging") and a summary of the specific procedure that the patient will experience. Both are based on the assumption that providing this information will prevent the development of negative expectations that may increase anxiety and lead to increased pain sensations [44]. Information provision has been found to be effective in some studies for reducing postoperative pain reports and/or pain medication use [45, 46].

Stress/tension reduction can be provided by a range of relaxation-related techniques such as breathing relaxation, progressive muscle relaxation, imagery and hypnosis. These all involve teaching the patient how to reduce their feelings of stress, tension, anxiety and distress, so ideally the patient will need time to learn and practice them. The evidence for the effectiveness of these interventions is variable from weak to moderately strong [47].

Cognitive-behavioural interventions involve a range of behaviour change principles. These include positive reinforcement of desired behaviours, identification and modification of unhelpful thoughts (catastrophising such as "I can't stand it" or "This is unbearable") and goal setting in order to achieve a change in targeted behaviours. In acute pain this is likely to be encouraging patients to use these and other psychological strategies to meet postoperative rehabilitation goals. Training in coping methods or behavioural instruction prior to surgery has been shown to reduce pain, negative affect and analgesic use [47].

5.3.5.2 Transcutaneous Electrical Nerve Stimulation

Transcutaneous electrical nerve stimulation (TENS) delivers an electrical current across the surface of the skin via self-adhering conducting pads (electrodes) activating peripheral nerve fibres and releasing spinal inhibitory neurotransmitters resulting in pain relief [48]. Different intensity settings and stimulation patterns are effective for some acute pain settings [47] and there appears to be a potential role for TENS as an adjunct to analgesic therapy in the perioperative setting to provide pain relief for some but not all patients [48].

5.4 Summary

Pain management in palliative care surgery should utilise similar approaches to those used in the general surgical population. Consideration needs to be given to whether the patient is on opioids for pain prior to surgery and if the patient has other sites of disease that will not be improved as an outcome of surgery. However, utilising a multimodal analgesic approach and adjusting the analgesic doses to suit the patient's individual pain can provide pain relief. Consideration should be given to the role that non-pharmacological approaches may contribute to pain management.

The key points of pain management in palliative surgery are:

- Identifying patients preoperatively
- Preoperative assessment and recording of baseline opioid requirements
- Understanding the intended outcome of the surgery – will it improve all of the patient's pain?
- Development of individual patient perioperative analgesic plan
- Maintenance of baseline opioid requirements to ensure pain control and prevent withdrawal symptoms
- Use of non-opioid drugs and other techniques

References

1. van den Beuken-van Everdingen MH, de Rijke JM, Kessels AG, Schouten HC, van Kleef M, Patijn J. High prevalence of pain in patients with cancer in a large population-based study in The Netherlands. Pain. 2007;132(3):312–20.
2. Williams JE. Acute pain management in cancer patients taking regular opioid medication. In: Farquhar-Smith P, Wigmore T, editors. Anaesthesia, intensive care and pain management for the cancer patient. 1st ed. Oxford: Oxford University Press; 2011. p. 181–6.
3. De PM, Cahana A. Medical management of acute pain in patients with chronic pain. Expert Rev Neurother. 2012;12(11):1325–38.
4. Quinlan J, Carter K. Acute pain management in patients with persistent pain. Curr Opin Support Palliat Care. 2012;6(2):188–93.
5. Costantini R, Affaitati G, Fabrizio A, Giamberardino MA. Controlling pain in the post-operative setting. Int J Clin Pharmacol Ther. 2011;49(2):116–27.
6. McDaid C, Maund E, Rice S, Wright K, Jenkins B, Woolacott N. Paracetamol and selective and non-selective non-steroidal anti-inflammatory drugs (NSAIDs) for the reduction of morphine-related side effects after major surgery: a systematic review. Health Technol Assess. 2010;14(17):1–153. iii–iv.

7. Remy C, Marret E, Bonnet F. Effects of acetaminophen on morphine side-effects and consumption after major surgery: meta-analysis of randomized controlled trials. Br J Anaesth. 2005;94(4):505–13.
8. Romsing J, Moiniche S, Dahl JB. Rectal and parenteral paracetamol, and paracetamol in combination with NSAIDs, for postoperative analgesia. Br J Anaesth. 2002;88(2):215–26.
9. Bertolini A, Ferrari A, Ottani A, Guerzoni S, Tacchi R, Leone S. Paracetamol: new vistas of an old drug. CNS Drug Rev. 2006;12(3–4):250–75.
10. Pickering G, Loriot MA, Libert F, Eschalier A, Beaune P, Dubray C. Analgesic effect of acetaminophen in humans: first evidence of a central serotonergic mechanism. Clin Pharmacol Ther. 2006;79(4):371–8.
11. Mallet C, Daulhac L, Bonnefont J, Ledent C, Etienne M, Chapuy E, et al. Endocannabinoid and serotonergic systems are needed for acetaminophen-induced analgesia. Pain. 2008;139(1):190–200.
12. Pickering G, Esteve V, Loriot MA, Eschalier A, Dubray C. Acetaminophen reinforces descending inhibitory pain pathways. Clin Pharmacol Ther. 2008;84(1):47–51.
13. Moller PL, Sindet-Pedersen S, Petersen CT, Juhl GI, Dillenschneider A, Skoglund LA. Onset of acetaminophen analgesia: comparison of oral and intravenous routes after third molar surgery. Br J Anaesth. 2005;94(5):642–8.
14. Botting RM. Inhibitors of cyclooxygenases: mechanisms, selectivity and uses. J Physiol Pharmacol. 2006;57 Suppl 5:113–24.
15. Diaz G, Flood P. Strategies for effective postoperative pain management. Minerva Anestesiol. 2006;72(3):145–50.
16. Khan M, Fraser A. Cox-2 inhibitors and the risk of cardiovascular thrombotic events. Ir Med J. 2012;105(4):119–21.
17. Hyllested M, Jones S, Pedersen JL, Kehlet H. Comparative effect of paracetamol, NSAIDs or their combination in postoperative pain management: a qualitative review. Br J Anaesth. 2002;88(2):199–214.
18. Farquhar-Smith P. Anatomy, physiology and pharmacology of pain. Anaesth Intensive Care Med. 2008;9:3–7.
19. Tracey I. Neuroimaging of pain mechanisms. Curr Opin Support Palliat Care. 2007;1(2):109–16.
20. Scott K. How analgesics work. In: Cox F, editor. Perioperative pain management. Hoboken: Wiley Blackwell; 2009.
21. Benyamin R, Trescot AM, Datta S, Buenaventura R, Adlaka R, Sehgal N, et al. Opioid complications and side effects. Pain Physician. 2008;11(2 Suppl):S105–20.
22. Palmer PP, Miller RD. Current and developing methods of patient-controlled analgesia. Anesthesiol Clin. 2010;28(4):587–99.
23. Ballantyne JC, Carr DB, Chalmers TC, Dear KB, Angelillo IF, Mosteller F. Postoperative patient-controlled analgesia: meta-analyses of initial randomized control trials. J Clin Anesth. 1993;5(3):182–93.
24. Hudcova J, McNicol E, Quah C, Lau J, Carr DB. Patient controlled opioid analgesia versus conventional opioid analgesia for postoperative pain. Cochrane Database Syst Rev. 2006;4, CD003348.
25. Nelson L, Schwaner R. Transdermal fentanyl: pharmacology and toxicology. J Med Toxicol. 2009;5(4):230–41.
26. Neil MJ. Clonidine: clinical pharmacology and therapeutic use in pain management. Curr Clin Pharmacol. 2011;6(4):280–7.
27. Elia N, Culebras X, Mazza C, Schiffer E, Tramer MR. Clonidine as an adjuvant to intrathecal local anesthetics for surgery: systematic review of randomized trials. Reg Anesth Pain Med. 2008;33(2):159–67.
28. Woolf CJ. Central sensitization: implications for the diagnosis and treatment of pain. Pain. 2011;152(3 Suppl):S2–15.
29. Niesters M, Dahan A. Pharmacokinetic and pharmacodynamic considerations for NMDA receptor antagonists in the treatment of chronic neuropathic pain. Expert Opin Drug Metab Toxicol. 2012;8(11):1409–17.
30. Eilers H, Philip LA, Bickler PE, McKay WR, Schumacher MA. The reversal of fentanyl-induced tolerance by administration of "small-dose" ketamine. Anesth Analg. 2001;93(1):213–4.
31. Mitra S. Opioid-induced hyperalgesia: pathophysiology and clinical implications. J Opioid Manag. 2008;4(3):123–30.
32. Bell RF, Dahl JB, Moore RA, Kalso E. Perioperative ketamine for acute postoperative pain. Cochrane Database Syst Rev. 2006;1, CD004603.
33. Zhang J, Ho KY, Wang Y. Efficacy of pregabalin in acute postoperative pain: a meta-analysis. Br J Anaesth. 2011;106(4):454–62.
34. Dahl JB, Mathiesen O, Kehlet H. An expert opinion on postoperative pain management, with special reference to new developments. Expert Opin Pharmacother. 2010;11(15):2459–70.
35. Freise H, Van Aken HK. Risks and benefits of thoracic epidural anaesthesia. Br J Anaesth. 2011;107(6):859–68.
36. Gupta A. Wound infiltration with local anaesthetics in ambulatory surgery. Curr Opin Anaesthesiol. 2010;23(6):708–13.
37. Wu CL, Cohen SR, Richman JM, Rowlingson AJ, Courpas GE, Cheung K, et al. Efficacy of postoperative patient-controlled and continuous infusion epidural analgesia versus intravenous patient-controlled analgesia with opioids: a meta-analysis. Anesthesiology. 2005;103(5):1079–88.
38. Guay J. The benefits of adding epidural analgesia to general anesthesia: a metaanalysis. J Anesth. 2006;20(4):335–40.
39. Marret E, Remy C, Bonnet F. Meta-analysis of epidural analgesia versus parenteral opioid analgesia after colorectal surgery. Br J Surg. 2007;94(6):665–73.
40. Chelly JE, Ghisi D, Fanelli A. Continuous peripheral nerve blocks in acute pain management. Br J Anaesth. 2010;105 Suppl 1:i86–96.

41. Power I, McCormack JG, Myles PS. Regional anaesthesia and pain management. Anaesthesia. 2010;65 Suppl 1:38–47.
42. Wu CL, Raja SN. Treatment of acute postoperative pain. Lancet. 2011;377(9784):2215–25.
43. Theunissen M, Peters ML, Bruce J, Gramke HF, Marcus MA. Preoperative anxiety and catastrophizing: a systematic review and meta-analysis of the association with chronic postsurgical pain. Clin J Pain. 2012;28(9):819–41.
44. Ludwick-Rosenthal R, Neufeld RW. Stress management during noxious medical procedures: an evaluative review of outcome studies. Psychol Bull. 1988;104(3):326–42.
45. Wilson-Barnett J. Interventions to alleviate patients' stress: a review. J Psychosom Res. 1984;28(1):63–72.
46. Doering S, Behensky H, Rumpold G, Schatz DS, Rossler S, Hofstotter B, et al. Videotape preparation of patients before hip replacement surgery improves mobility after three months. Z Psychosom Med Psychother. 2001;47(2):140–52.
47. Macintyre PE, Schug SA, Scott DA, Visser EJ, Walker SM. Acute pain management: scientific evidence. 3rd ed. Melbourne: ANZCA/FRM; 2010.
48. Johnson ML, Bagley J. Transcutaneous electrical nerve stimulation in perioperative settings. In: Cox F, editor. Perioperative pain management. Hoboken: Wiley-Blackwell; 2009.

Further Readings

Cox F. Perioperative pain management. Hoboken: Wiley-Blackwell; 2009.
Davies PS, D'Arcy Y. Cancer pain management. New York: Springer; 2013.
Farquhar-Smith P, Wigmore T. Anaesthesia, intensive care, and pain management for the cancer patient. Oxford: Oxford University Press; 2011.
Pasero C, McCaffery M. Pain assessment and pharmacologic management. St. Louis: Elsevier Mosby; 2011.

Nutrition

6

Giacomo Bovio

Contents

Malnutrition and nutritional difficulties are very common in patients with advanced cancer receiving palliative care. These patients often have cancer cachexia, a multifactorial syndrome in which there is loss of skeletal muscle mass, negative protein and energy balance, alterations involving carbohydrate, lipid and protein metabolism, and neuroinflammation. The early assessment of malnutrition is particularly important in patients undergoing palliative surgery. Nutritional status can be assessed by an objective method or by validated nutritional screening tools. These tools are easy to administer even by nonexpert personnel or by the patient themselves and should be used in every surgery department. Malnutrition worsens and increases postoperative complications, surgical risk factors, and mortality. Nutritional support must be prescribed as soon as possible to malnourished patients and patients at risk of malnutrition. The main goals of perioperative nutritional support are to minimize negative protein balance by avoiding starvation; to maintain muscle, immune, and cognitive functions; and to enhance postoperative recovery. Enteral feeding is the first choice route of nutrient administration although parenteral nutrition must be recommended in cases of intestinal failure. Immunonutrition improves surgical outcomes by reducing both infectious and noninfectious complications, as well as the time spent in hospital. Nutritional support therapy is rarely indicated in terminally ill cancer patients.

G. Bovio, MD
Metabolic-Nutritional Unit and Palliative Care Unit, Fondazione Salvatore Maugeri,
Via Severino Boezio 28, Pavia 27100, Italy
e-mail: giacomo.bovio@fsm.it

M. Wichmann, G. Maddern (eds.), *Palliative Surgery*,
DOI 10.1007/978-3-642-53709-7_6, © Springer-Verlag Berlin Heidelberg 2014

Abbreviations

ASPEN	American Society for Parenteral and Enteral Nutrition
BMI	Body mass index
BMR	Basal metabolic rate
CCS	Cancer cachexia syndrome
ESPEN	European Society for Clinical Nutrition and Metabolism
MNA	Mini Nutritional Assessment
MUST	Malnutrition Universal Screening Tool
n-3 PUFAs	Omega-3 polyunsaturated fatty acids
NRI	Nutrition Risk Index
NRS-2002	Nutritional Risk Screening 2002
PG-SGA	Patient-Generated Subjective Global Assessment
SCRINIO	Screening the nutritional status in oncology
SGA	Subjective Global Assessment

6.1 Introduction

Malnutrition is "an acute, subacute or chronic state of nutrition, in which varying degrees of overnutrition or undernutrition with or without inflammatory activity have led to a change in body composition and diminished function" [1].

In palliative care patients' malnutrition is synonymous with undernutrition. Obesity can also be found in these patients, although it is uncommon and obese patients often have undernutrition. Malnutrition and nutritional difficulties are very common in patients with advanced cancer receiving palliative care [2, 3], with their prevalence in such patients depending on the site of origin of the cancer [4]. It has been reported that malnutrition may often contribute to death in cancer patients [5].

The assessment of nutritional status is very important in subjects at risk of malnutrition, such as patients receiving palliative care. Adequate nutritional support could play a fundamental role in improving the nutritional status and quality of life of such patients, especially in those undergoing surgery [6].

As well known, these patients often have cancer cachexia syndrome (CCS). CCS is a multifactorial syndrome in which there is loss of skeletal muscle mass that cannot be fully reversed by conventional nutritional support and leads to progressive functional impairment [7–9]. This syndrome also includes a negative protein and energy balance; alterations involving carbohydrate, lipid, and protein metabolism; and increased acute-phase proteins and neuroinflammation [10–12].

There are many criteria to define CCS. One easy criterion was proposed by the SCRINIO working group [13], while more recently an international consensus, reported by Fearon et al. [14], concluded that the diagnostic criterion for cachexia is weight loss greater than 5 % or weight loss greater than 2 % in individuals already showing depletion of body mass index (BMI <20 kg/m^2) or skeletal muscle mass. CCS can develop progressively through various stages (pre-cachexia to cachexia to refractory cachexia). Its classification and clinical management should be based on an assessment of anorexia or reduced food intake, catabolic drive, muscle mass and strength, and functional and psychosocial impairment.

6.2 Malnutrition: Causes and Consequences

Malnutrition can be due to reduced food intake (anorexia, nausea, dysphagia, etc.), loss of nutrients (diarrhea, malabsorption, vomiting, etc.), increased nourishment needs (surgical operations, sepsis, etc.), and metabolic alterations caused by cancer (hypermetabolism). This condition has serious consequences for all organs and systems [15].

The most significant changes occur in the cardiovascular system (decreased cardiac muscle mass and cardiac output, decreased blood pressure, conduction disorders, and arrhythmias), respiratory system (decreased vital capacity because of alterations to respiratory muscles, increased infectious complications), gastrointestinal system (reduced digestion and absorption of foods; reduced gastric, biliary, and pancreatic secretions), and urinary system (reduced glomerular filtration rate and renal plasma flow), but the muscles (muscle wasting), hematopoietic system (anemia), and immune system (increased risk of infections) may also be affected. In surgical patients, malnutrition has been demonstrated to be one of the major determinants of the development of postoperative complications, affects postoperative recovery and wound healing, prolongs the duration of hospitalization, and increases mortality [16].

6.3 Nutritional Assessment

Nutritional screening is very important in clinical practice, especially in cancer patients and hence in cancer patients undergoing surgery. All cancer patients should be submitted to nutritional assessment on admission to hospital and at least once a week thereafter. The correction of malnutrition has positive effects such as an increase in life expectancy, a reduction in the duration of hospitalization, a quicker recovery of healing after surgery, a quicker recovery from ulcers, and an improved quality of life.

A correct nutritional assessment can identify malnourished patients and those at risk of malnutrition in order to provide them with adequate nutritional support. Nutritional assessment can be done by an objective method or using nutritional screening tools.

6.3.1 Objective Method

The objective method for assessing nutritional status requires specialized personnel. Many different parameters are used in this assessment, including weight, height, sex, subcutaneous fat thickness, laboratory analyses, etc. The clinical nutritional assessment usually covers medical history, dietary records, physical examination, anthropometric measurements, body composition determination, and laboratory analyses [15]:

1. The patient's medical history can give information on the primary tumor and metastases, other pathologies, and medical treatments. An appetite assessment is of particular relevance in palliative care patients as anorexia is one of their most important problems [17]. Dietary records evaluate food consumption and dietary habits. The main tools used are 24-h food recall, a recording of food and beverage intake over the preceding 24 h; diet diaries, compiled by either the patient or the caregiver, over a week or over three nonconsecutive days; food frequency questionnaires that assess food intake over a day, a week, or a longer period; and the dietary history, which investigates food intake over the long term.
2. The physical examination evaluates indicators of malnutrition such as skin and cutaneous adnexae, muscle and fat mass, etc.
3. Anthropometric measurements are a very important part of the nutritional assessment. One of the most important parameters is body weight. This is the simplest anthropometric index giving rapid information about a patient's nutritional status. Weighing chairs or hoisting systems are used if the patient is unable to stand. It is important to determine the extent of weight variation, since an unintentional weight loss of >10 % over the preceding 6 months is a sign of malnutrition and cachexia and implies reduced survival. Body height is another important parameter in nutritional assessment. Dividing body weight in kilograms by the square of the body height in meters gives the body mass index (BMI – kg/m^2). The BMI is an important anthropometric index and immediately provides information about a patient's nutritional status. Table 6.1 shows the classification of nutritional status according to the BMI. Height can be estimated by knee height [18], ulna length [19], or demispan [20] in patients who are unable to stand. Table 6.2 reports the formulas used to calculate height in patients who cannot stand. Arm, waist, and hip circumferences are also usually measured although the last two parameters are generally more

Table 6.1 Weight classification according to BMI

BMI (kg/m^2)	Weight classification
<18.4	Underweight
18.5–24.9	Normal weight
25.0–29.9	Overweight
≥30.0	Obese

BMI body mass index

Table 6.2 Height assessment in bedridden patients

Estimating height (cm) from knee height [18]	
Females	84.88 – (0.24 × age) + (1.83 × knee height)
Males	64.19 – (0.04 × age) + (2.02 × knee height)
Estimating height (cm) from demispan [20]	
Females	(1.35 × demispan) + 60.1
Males	(1.40 × demispan) + 57.8

relevant in the assessment of obese patients than in palliative care patients.

4. Body composition can be altered as a result of physiological factors (age, sex, and physical activity) or pathological ones. It is important to determine the body composition during the nutritional assessment because malnutrition and cancer cachexia alter this composition. A reduced fat-free mass and alterations in intracellular and extracellular volumes are often seen in palliative care patients. Many techniques can be used to determine body composition. The most widely used are plicometry, bioelectrical impedance analysis, and dual-energy X-ray absorptiometry. Imaging techniques (ultrasound, computed tomography scans, and magnetic resonance imaging scans) and total body potassium measurement are expensive and generally not utilized in clinical practice. Body fat mass and hence body fat-free mass can be easily measured by plicometry. This method is inexpensive and very quick. Moreover, the triceps skinfold thickness and arm circumference can be used in formulas to give the arm muscle circumference and arm muscle area. Body impedance analysis measures the opposition of body tissues to the flow of a small alternating current and is used to determine total body water, fat-free mass, and fat mass. Dual-energy X-ray absorptiometry (DEXA) determines the body's absorption of photons when irradiated by X-rays at two different energy levels. This technique is normally used to evaluate bone mineral density. It is a widely employed method and one of the most reliable techniques for assessing body composition [21].
5. Laboratory analyses are also needed when evaluating nutritional status. Routine blood tests, urinalysis, nutrient levels, metabolic balances, immunological tests, and functional tests are used. Plasma protein levels are a part of the nutritional assessment. The levels of plasma proteins are generally lower than normal in malnutrition states since there is decreased protein synthesis in this condition. Serum albumin, transferrin, prealbumin, and retinol-binding protein are the proteins most frequently determined in a nutritional assessment. These proteins have different half-lives: albumin about 15–20 days, transferrin 8–10 days, prealbumin about 2 days, and retinol-binding protein about 10 h. Poor surgical outcomes are associated with hypoalbuminemia. Immunological tests are used in nutritional assessment since malnutrition causes immune system alterations. A lymphocyte count <1,500/mm^3 is an indicator of malnutrition. Complement fraction 3 and skin test reactivity are also determined. Finally, measurements of the blood levels of vitamins, minerals, and trace elements are included in the nutritional assessment.

It is important to appreciate that the results of anthropometric and laboratory analyses should be interpreted carefully since many alterations can be due to the neoplastic disease itself rather than to malnutrition. Body weight, BMI, and weight loss can all be affected by the dehydration or edema often found in cancer patients receiving palliative care. Levels of plasma proteins could be lower than normal as a consequence of urine and bowel leakage and interactions with acute-phase proteins. Immunological parameters, e.g., lymphocyte count, could be altered by hepatic or renal impairment or drug therapies such as steroids or immunosuppressants.

No parameter alone, except perhaps loss of body weight, can make the diagnosis of malnutrition. The diagnosis is made on the basis of many parameters and the nutritionist's experience is pivotal in this regard.

6.3.2 Nutritional Screening Tools

All patients undergoing surgery should be screened preoperatively to evaluate their nutritional status and nutritional risk, as recommended by international guidelines (American Society for Parenteral and Enteral Nutrition (ASPEN), European Society for Clinical Nutrition and Metabolism (ESPEN)). The screening is important to identify malnourished patients or those at nutritional risk. When such patients are identified, they should be addressed to nutrition specialists or to perioperative nutritional support. Nutritional status should be assessed weekly in all patients not only in the preoperative period but also after the surgical procedure. With proper nutritional support, this can help to avoid worsening of the nutritional status.

Nutritional screening tools utilize objective and subjective data to determine the patient's nutritional state. These tools are easy to use by nurses, by nonexpert personnel, and even by patients themselves and should be used in every surgery department, but especially in cancer surgery departments.

For patients receiving anticancer treatment, the ASPEN guidelines [22] recommend the Subjective Global Assessment (SGA), the Patient-Generated Subjective Global Assessment (PG-SGA) [23], and the Nutrition Risk Index (NRI) [24], while the ESPEN guidelines [25] recommend the Malnutrition Universal Screening Tool (MUST) [26], the Nutritional Risk Screening 2002 (NRS-2002) [27], and the Mini Nutritional Assessment (MNA) [28].

The SGA is a questionnaire incorporating information about medical history (weight change, dietary intake, gastrointestinal symptoms and functional impairment changes in food intake) and physical examination (muscle wasting, subcutaneous fat loss, and edema) and classifies patients into being well nourished (A), mildly to moderately undernourished (B), and severely undernourished (C). Among patients receiving palliative care, a strong correlation was found between the SGA score and nutritional status determined by the objective method [29].

The PG-SGA is an adaptation of the SGA and was developed specifically for patients with cancer. The medical history can be provided by the patient using a format of checking four boxes (weight, food intake, symptoms, activity, and functions). The physical examination (fat stores, muscle, and fluid status) is performed by a physician, nurse, or dietitian. Patients are classified as well nourished, moderately malnourished, and severely malnourished.

The NRI is based on a mathematical equation: NRI = [1,519 × albumin (g/L)] + [41.7 × (present weight − usual weight)]. An NRI >100 implies no malnutrition, between 97.5 and 100 mild malnutrition, between 83.5 and 97.5 moderate malnutrition, and <83.5 severe malnutrition.

The NRS-2002 involves an initial screening (BMI, weight loss, dietary intake, and severe illness) and a final screening considering nutritional status (weight loss, body mass index, and food intake; 1–3 points) and severity of disease (1–3 points) and patient's age (1 point if >70 years). Patients undergoing major abdominal surgery are assigned 2 points. Patients are classified as not at risk (≤3 points) or nutritionally at risk (≥3 points) and a nutritional care plan should be initiated.

The MUST considers BMI, unintentional weight loss, and the presence of an acute illness and classifies the risk of malnutrition as low (0 points), medium (1 point), or high (≥2 points).

The MNA is validated to evaluate the nutritional status of the elderly. It consists of 18 items: anthropometric data (weight, height, and weight loss), general data (medications, lifestyle, mobility), dietary data (food and fluid intake, number of meals), and autonomy of eating. Patients are classified as well nourished (≥24 points), at risk of malnutrition (17–23.5 points), or malnourished (<17 points). A Mini Nutritional Assessment short form (MNA-SF) was recently validated [30].

Every nutrition assessment should be followed by a plan of nutritional intervention or reassessment in patients at risk of malnutrition [31]. Nutritional screening tools are summarized in Table 6.3.

Table 6.3 Screening tools

Tool	Items (*N*)	Anthropometry	Diet	Others
MUST	3	BMI, weight loss		Presence of acute illness
NRS-2002	4+2	BMI, weight loss	Food intake	Severity of disease
NRI	3	Present weight, usual weight		Albumin
MNA	6+12	BMI, weight loss, mid-arm and calf circumference	Food intake (3 items), fluid intake, mode of feeding	Mobility, psychological stress, drugs, pressure sores, independence, self-consideration of health and nutritional status
SGA	7	Weight loss	Food intake	Gastrointestinal symptoms, functional impairment, physical examination (muscle and fat loss, edema)
PG-SGA	4+3	Weight history, height	Food intake	Symptoms, activities and function, disease, metabolic demand, physical examination

MUST Malnutrition Universal Screening Tool, *NRS-2002* Nutritional Risk Screening 2002, *NRI* Nutrition Risk Index, *MNA* Mini Nutritional Assessment, *SGA Subjective Global Assessment PG-SGA* Patient-Generated Subjective Global Assessment

6.4 Perioperative Nutrition

Surgical procedures cause the production of stress hormones and inflammatory substances [32]. The neuroendocrine response to stress is proportional to the extent of the surgical injury and is characterized by inflammation, reduced immune responses, and oxidative stress [33]. The metabolic response to surgical trauma is mainly characterized by an increase in basal metabolic rate (BMR), a negative nitrogen balance, increased gluconeogenesis, and increased synthesis of acute-phase proteins [34]. These changes lead to a depletion of body compartments which can impair healing and increase the risk of postoperative complications. This risk is higher in malnourished patients.

Pancreatic surgery, advanced age, weight loss, low serum albumin, and nutritional support are factors correlated with postoperative complications [35].

6.4.1 Perioperative Nutritional Support

Fast track surgery and less invasive techniques have changed the approach to the surgical patient, especially in the preoperative period. This kind of surgery allows rapid recovery of bowel function and a quick return to natural feeding within 1–3 days after surgery. The duration of preoperative fasting should be 2 h for liquids and 6 h for solids (grade A recommendation), and oral nutritional supplements should be prescribed (approximately 200 mL, energy dense, 2–3 times daily) from the day of surgery until normal food intake is achieved (grade A recommendation) [36].

However, artificial nutrition, whether enteral or parenteral, can also play an important role in improving clinical outcomes in fast track surgery. Since artificial feeding is not without risks, it should be reserved only for those patients who are malnourished or at risk of malnutrition, i.e., patients who cannot be adequately fed by mouth for 7–14 days in the postoperative period [22, 37]. Artificial nutrition is not required in well-nourished patients or in patients who do not have surgical complications and are expected to eat orally in the postoperative period.

6.4.2 Route of Administration of Nutritional Support

The first choice of route for administering nutrients in surgical patients is enteral feeding. This kind of nutrition is easiest; is less expensive than parenteral nutrition; is associated with fewer complications, particularly infectious ones; and, moreover, stimulates anastomotic healing [38]. Early enteral nutrition improves gut function and wound healing in surgical patients [39, 40]. Possible side effects of enteral nutrition are diarrhea and vomiting, which can usually be controlled with a reduction of the infusion rate and are almost always well tolerated.

Parenteral nutrition should be prescribed in cases of intestinal failure (intestinal occlusion, intestinal ischemia, etc.) or when enteral nutrition is impossible to ensure.

6.4.3 Preoperative Nutritional Support

Malnutrition worsens and increases postoperative complications, surgical risk, and mortality. The ESPEN guidelines [41, 42] recommend preoperative nutritional support for at least 7–10 days in malnourished patients and in patients at high risk of malnutrition.

A high nutritional risk is defined by the presence of one or more of the following parameters: (1) weight loss >10–15 % within the preceding 6 months, (2) a BMI <18.5 kg/m^2, (3) albumin <30 g/L, and (4) severe undernutrition determined by the SGA. If dietary supplements are insufficient to meet the patient's nutrient requirements, artificial nutrition is needed.

The main goals of perioperative nutritional support are to minimize negative protein balance by avoiding starvation and maintaining muscle, immune, and cognitive function and to enhance postoperative recovery [42].

6.4.4 Postoperative Nutritional Support

Oral feeding and oral nutritional supplements can generally be started within 1–3 days after surgery, limiting the use of artificial nutrition. Nutritional supplements enable greater energy and protein intakes in a small volume. Artificial nutrition is needed in the presence of postoperative complications such as bowel obstruction, intestinal failure, impaired gastrointestinal function, and dysphagia. This nutritional therapy is recommended in the postoperative period for patients who had severe preoperative malnutrition, metabolic stress or a septic state, an inadequate food intake (<60 % of requirements) for more than 10 days, or when there has been no oral feeding for more than 7 days (Grade C recommendation) [41].

Parenteral nutrition should be reserved for patients who cannot be fed adequately either orally or enterally. Enteral nutrition is the first choice of artificial nutrition and should be started as soon as possible. The gastric route of enteral feeding (by a nasogastric tube) is easier to achieve than post-pyloric tube feeding (by naso-jejunal or jejunostomy inserted during surgery). This latter form of enteral feeding should be started when there is a high risk of aspiration and delayed gastric emptying or when there is an intestinal anastomosis in the upper gastrointestinal tract, and it is preferable to administer the nutrients downstream of the anastomosis.

The administration of nutrients should be initiated at a low flow rate (10–20 mL/h) and increased progressively according to the patient's tolerance [41]. It can take a few days to reach the target amounts of calories and protein. If the calories that can be tolerated enterally are not sufficient, partial or peripheral parenteral nutrition should be integrated.

6.4.5 Nutritional Requirements in the Perioperative Period

Energy requirements should be 25 kcal/kg/ideal body weight but in patients with severe stress requirements may approach 30 kcal/kg/ideal body weight [42]. Energy requirements are better determined by indirect calorimetry, but it is often difficult to perform this examination in patients receiving palliative care, so BMR is almost always determined using the Harris-Benedict formula [43]. This formula is reported in Table 6.4. The BMR can be normal, decreased, or increased in cancer patients depending on the type of cancer and body composition [44].

An increase in BMR has been reported in surgical trauma [34]. The average protein requirement in the perioperative period is

Table 6.4 Harris-Benedict formula for calculating the basal metabolic rate in adults

Males	66.4730 + (13.7516 × weight in kg) + (5.0033 × height in cm) – (6.7550 × age in years)
Females	655.0955 + (9.5634 × weight in kg) + (1.8496 × height in cm) – (4.6756 × age in years)

estimated to be 1.5 g/kg/day/ideal body weight or approximately 20 % of total energy requirements (grade B recommendation), and the protein to fat to glucose calorie ratio should be approximately 20:30:50 % (grade C recommendation) [42].

To avoid the refeeding syndrome, a potentially fatal syndrome caused by intracellular loss of electrolytes, in particular phosphate, artificial nutrition should be started at a reduced calorie rate (25–50 % of estimated requirements) [45] and calorie intake should be increased gradually [46], monitoring the plasma electrolytes daily. Overfeeding should be avoided, especially in patients with impaired cardiac function or respiratory failure since overfeeding can increase both oxygen consumption and the production of carbon dioxide, with potentially severe consequences in these patients. An emerging issue is the management of nutritional support in obese patients.

6.5 Immunonutrition

As well known, major surgery is followed by a period of immunosuppression that increases the risk of morbidity and mortality due to infections. Improving immune function during this period may reduce complications due to infections. Modulating the activity of the immune system or modifying inflammatory or immune responses by specific nutrients is termed immunonutrition. This form of nutrition could improve the clinical course of surgical patients and significantly reduce postoperative morbidity [35].

Immunonutrition formulas are recommended by the 2009 ASPEN guidelines on nutritional support during anticancer treatment in adults undergoing major cancer operations [22]. This type of perioperative nutritional support in malnourished patients can decrease infectious complications and anastomotic leaks and shorten the time spent in hospital [47–50].

The main immunonutrients studied for use in the perioperative period are glutamine,omega-3 fatty acids, arginine, and nucleotides (RNA).

6.5.1 Glutamine

Glutamine is the most abundant amino acid in the body. It is an oxidative fuel for small and large bowel cells, helping to maintain the integrity of the intestinal barrier which regulates transport and host defense mechanisms at the mucosal interface with the outside world. It is a primary component of the antioxidant glutathione and is a gluconeogenic precursor. Currently glutamine is included among "conditionally essential" amino acids, becoming essential in conditions of metabolic stress such as sepsis or severe trauma. In these conditions glutamine requirements are increased [51]. Glutamine is present in many enteral formulas and in oral nutrition supplements but is not present in parenteral solutions because free glutamine is not stable in solution.

Parenteral glutamine dipeptide products (e.g., l-alanyl-l-glutamine and glycyl-l-glutamine) are available; these products are highly soluble in water [51]. The ASPEN position paper on parenteral nutrition asserts that glutamine administration is associated with a decrease in infectious complications, a shortening of time spent in hospital, and possibly a decrease in mortality in critically ill postoperative patients and in patients undergoing major abdominal surgery, although the effectiveness of glutamine has not been clearly demonstrated and requires further confirmation [52]. The recommended dose of parenteral supplementation with glutamine dipeptide is 20–40 g/24 h [54] or >0.2 g/kg/day of free glutamine [53]. At present the parenteral administration of glutamine dipeptide is only recommended for critically ill, surgical patients.

Studies on enteral supplementation of glutamine in surgical patients have provided conflicting results.

6.5.2 Omega-3 Fatty Acids

Omega-3 are polyunsaturated fatty acids (n-3 PUFAs) and are considered essential fatty acids. They play a crucial role in brain function, reduce inflammation, have immunomodulatory activities, and may lower the risk of heart disease. There is little evidence and too few studies to draw any conclusions on the effect of PUFA supplementation, administered either parenterally or enterally, in surgical patients. The ESPEN 2009 guidelines on parenteral nutrition [42] suggest (grade C recommendation) the use of lipid emulsions supplemented with fish oil for critically ill surgical patients, and a recent meta-analysis [54] concluded that the administration of a lipid emulsion containing n-3 PUFAs to patients undergoing elective major operations improves outcomes, decreases infectious complications, and reduces the time spent in hospital.

6.5.3 Arginine

Arginine serves as a substrate for the production of nitric oxide, can improve nitrogen balance, promotes wound healing, improves indices of T-cell immune function, and increases the levels of growth hormone and insulin-like growth factor-1. There are very few studies on arginine alone; almost all the studies on perioperative immunonutrition administered arginine in combination with other immunonutrients.

6.5.4 Supplements Enriched with Various Immunonutrients

Many clinical trials of immunonutrition in surgical patients have been performed using various nutrient combinations. Most studies in the perioperative period in cancer patients have been conducted with formulas containing arginine, n-3 PUFAs, and RNA and have shown improvements in the surgical outcome. Immunonutrition has this beneficial effect on surgical outcome by reducing infectious complications [55]. A recent meta-analysis [56] of 19 randomized controlled trials, involving a total of 2,331 patients with gastrointestinal cancer, concluded that perioperative immunonutrition is safe and effective at reducing postoperative infections, noninfectious complications, and time spent in hospital.

The ESPEN guidelines [41] recommended (grade A recommendation) the use of immunonutrients (arginine, n-3 PUFAs, and nucleotides) perioperatively for those patients undergoing major neck cancer surgery and major abdominal cancer surgery.

Preoperative administration of immunonutrients allows patients to face the stress response to surgery and the postoperative period with adequate tissue and plasma immunonutrient levels. Some studies have shown that administration of immunonutrients is more effective in the preoperative period than in the postoperative period [56–58].

The effectiveness of perioperative immunonutrition seems to be greater in malnourished subjects at high surgical risk. The ESPEN guidelines [59] recommend (grade A recommendation) immunonutrition for patients undergoing elective upper gastrointestinal tract surgery.

6.6 Nutrition in Terminally Ill Cancer Patients

There are limited data on the use of nutritional support in palliative care patients.

The ASPEN guidelines [22] claim that the palliative use of nutrition support therapy in terminally ill cancer patients is rarely indicated (grade B recommendation) although this issue remains controversial and is emotionally charged. The American Academy of Hospice and Palliative Medicine position statement on nutrition and hydration near the end of life (2006) is in agreement with this thought.

It is, however, necessary to consider the patient's and family's wishes, potential risks and benefits, and the patient's estimated survival and quality of life, which may worsen with artificial nutrition (e.g., because of sepsis associated with parenteral nutrition and diarrhea with tube feeding). Terminally ill cancer patients often lose the capacity to eat and drink and lose interest in food and fluids and some widely assumed benefits of artificial nutrition may be achieved by less invasive measures. Palliative care patients to submit to artificial nutrition should be carefully selected. Generally patients with a Karnofsky performance status <50 and a life expectancy of <40 days should receive only intravenous fluid therapy, although this, too, is controversial [60].

References

1. Mueller C, Compher C, Ellen DM, American Society for Parenteral and Enteral Nutrition (A.S.P.E.N.) Board of Directors. A.S.P.E.N. clinical guidelines: nutrition screening, assessment, and intervention in adults. JPEN J Parenter Enteral Nutr. 2011;35(1):16–24.
2. Sarhill N, Mahmoud F, Walsh D, Nelson KA, Komurcu S, Davis M, et al. Evaluation of nutritional status in advanced metastatic cancer. Support Care Cancer. 2003;11(10):652–9.
3. Bovio G, Bettaglio R, Bonetti G, Miotti D, Verni P. Evaluation of nutritional status and dietary intake in patients with advanced cancer on palliative care. Minerva Gastroenterol Dietol. 2008;54(3):243–50.
4. Bovio G, Fonte ML, Baiardi P. Prevalence of upper gastrointestinal symptoms and their influence on nutritional state and performance status in patients with different primary tumors receiving palliative care. Am J Hosp Palliat Care. 2013. doi:10.1177/1049909112474713.
5. Inagaki J, Rodriguez V, Bodey GP. Proceedings: causes of death in cancer patients. Cancer. 1974;33(2):568–73.
6. Lis CG, Gupta D, Lammersfeld CA, Markman M, Vashi PG. Role of nutritional status in predicting quality of life outcomes in cancer – a systematic review of the epidemiological literature. Nutr J. 2012;11:27.
7. Muscaritoli M, Bossola M, Aversa Z, Bellantone R, Rossi Fanelli F. Prevention and treatment of cancer cachexia: new insights into an old problem. Eur J Cancer. 2006;42(1):31–41.
8. Nelson KA. The cancer anorexia-cachexia syndrome. Semin Oncol. 2000;27(1):64–8.
9. Davis MP, Dickerson D. Cachexia and anorexia: cancer's covert killer. Support Care Cancer. 2000;8(3): 180–7.
10. Laviano A, Seelaender M, Rianda S, Silverio R, Rossi Fanelli F. Neuroinflammation: a contributing factor to the pathogenesis of cancer cachexia. Crit Rev Oncog. 2012;17(3):247–51.
11. Fearon KC, Glass DJ, Guttridge DC. Cancer cachexia: mediators, signaling, and metabolic pathways. Cell Metab. 2012;16(2):153–66.
12. Tisdale MJ. Metabolic abnormalities in cachexia and anorexia. Nutrition. 2000;16(10):1013–4.
13. Bozzetti F, Mariani L. Defining and classifying cancer cachexia: a proposal by the SCRINIO Working Group. JPEN J Parenter Enteral Nutr. 2009;33(4):361–7.
14. Fearon K, Strasser F, Anker SD, Bosaeus I, Bruera E, Fainsinger RL, et al. Definition and classification of cancer cachexia: an international consensus. Lancet Oncol. 2011;12(5):489–95.
15. Bovio G, Sappia T. Nutritional status and relationship to upper gastrointestinal symptoms in patients with advanced cancer receiving palliative care. In: Preedy VR, editor. Diet and nutrition in palliative care. Boca Raton: CRC Press; 2011. p. 269–81.
16. Norman K, Pichard C, Lochs H, Pirlich M. Prognostic impact of disease-related malnutrition. Clin Nutr. 2008;27(1):5–15.
17. Bovio G, Montagna G, Bariani C, Baiardi P. Upper gastrointestinal symptoms in patients with advanced cancer: relationship to nutritional and performance status. Support Care Cancer. 2009;17(10):1317–24.
18. Chumlea WC, Guo S. Equations for predicting stature in white and black elderly individuals. J Gerontol. 1992;47(6):M197–203.
19. Available at: http://www.bapen.org.uk/screening-for-malnutrition/must/must-toolkit/the-must-itself.
20. Bassey EJ. Demi-span as a measure of skeletal size. Ann Hum Biol. 1986;13(5):499–502.
21. Lee S, Gallagher D. Assessment methods in human body composition. Curr Opin Clin Nutr Metab Care. 2008;11(5):566–72.
22. August DA, Huhmann MB, American Society for Parenteral and Enteral Nutrition (A.S.P.E.N.) Board of Directors. A.S.P.E.N. clinical guidelines: nutrition support therapy during adult anticancer treatment and in hematopoietic cell transplantation. JPEN J Parenter Enteral Nutr. 2009;33(5):472–500.
23. Ottery FD. Rethinking nutritional support of the cancer patient: the new field of nutritional oncology. Semin Oncol. 1994;21(6):770–8.
24. The Veterans Affairs Total Parenteral Nutrition Cooperative Study Group. Perioperative total parenteral nutrition in surgical patients. N Engl J Med. 1991;325(8):525–32.
25. Kondrup J, Allison SP, Elia M, Vellas B, Plauth M. Educational and Clinical Practice Committee, European Society of Parenteral and Enteral Nutrition (ESPEN). ESPEN guidelines for nutrition screening 2002. Clin Nutr. 2003;22(4):415–21.
26. Stratton RJ, Hackston A, Longmore D, Dixon R, Price S, Stroud M, et al. Malnutrition in hospital outpatients and inpatients: prevalence, concurrent validity and ease of use of the "malnutrition universal screening tool" ("MUST") for adults. Br J Nutr. 2004;92(5):799–808.
27. Kondrup J, Rasmussen HH, Hamberg O, Stanga Z. Nutritional risk screening (NRS 2002): a new method based on an analysis of controlled clinical trials. Clin Nutr. 2003;22(3):321–36.
28. Vellas B, Guigoz Y, Garry PJ, Nourhashemi F, Bennahum D, Lauque S, Albarede JL. The Mini

Nutritional Assessment (MNA) and its use in grading the nutritional state of elderly patients. Nutrition. 1999;15(2):116–22.
29. Thoresen L, Fjeldstad I, Krogstad K, Kaasa S, Falkmer UG. Nutritional status of patients with advanced cancer: the value of using the subjective global assessment of nutritional status as a screening tool. Palliat Med. 2002;16(1):33–42.
30. Kaiser MJ, Bauer JM, Ramsch C, Uter W, Guigoz Y, Cederholm T et al; MNA-International Group. Validation of the Mini Nutritional Assessment short-form (MNA-SF): a practical tool for identification of nutritional status. J Nutr Health Aging 2009;13(9):782–8.
31. Huhmann MB, August DA. Perioperative nutrition support in cancer patients. Nutr Clin Pract. 2012;27(5): 586–92.
32. Desborough JP, Hall GM. Endocrine response to surgery. In: Kaufman L, editor. Anaesthesia review, vol. 10. Edinburgh: Churchill Livingstone; 1991. p. 131–48.
33. Desborough JP. The stress response to trauma and surgery. Br J Anaesth. 2000;85(1):109–17.
34. Bozzetti F. Peri-operative nutritional management. Proc Nutr Soc. 2011;70(3):305–10.
35. Bozzetti F, Gianotti L, Braga M, Di Carlo V, Mariani L. Postoperative complications in gastrointestinal cancer patients: the joint role of the nutritional status and the nutritional support. Clin Nutr. 2007; 26(6):698–709.
36. Lassen K, Soop M, Nygren J, Cox PB, Hendry PO, Spies C, et al. Enhanced Recovery After Surgery (Eras) Group Consensus review of optimal perioperative care in colorectal surgery: Enhanced Recovery After Surgery (ERAS) Group recommendations. Arch Surg. 2009;144(10):961–9.
37. American Society for Parenteral and Enteral Nutrition (A.S.P.E.N.) Board of Directors. Guidelines for the use of parenteral and enteral nutrition in adult and pediatric patients. JPEN J Parenter Enteral Nutr. 2002;26(1 Suppl):1SA–38.
38. Gabor S, Renner H, Matzi V, Ratzenhofer B, Lindenmann J, Sankin O, et al. Early enteral feeding compared with parenteral nutrition after oesophageal or oesophagogastric resection and reconstruction. Br J Nutr. 2005;93(4):509–13.
39. Braga M, Gianotti L, Gentilini O, Liotta S, Di Carlo V. Feeding the gut early after digestive surgery: results of a nine-year experience. Clin Nutr. 2002;21(1): 59–65.
40. Ward N. Nutrition support to patients undergoing gastrointestinal surgery. Nutr J. 2003;2:18.
41. Weimann A, Braga M, Harsanyi L, Laviano A, Ljungqvist O, Soeters P; DGEM (German Society for Nutritional Medicine), Jauch KW, Kemen M, Hiesmayr JM, Horbach T, Kuse ER, Vestweber KH; ESPEN (European Society for Parenteral and Enteral Nutrition). ESPEN guidelines on enteral nutrition: surgery including organ transplantation. Clin Nutr 2006;25(2):224–44.
42. Braga M, Ljungqvist O, Soeters P, Fearon K, Weimann A, Bozzetti F, ESPEN. ESPEN guidelines on parenteral nutrition: surgery. Clin Nutr. 2009;28(4): 378–86.
43. Harris JA, Benedict FG. A biometric study of human basal metabolism. Proc Natl Acad Sci U S A. 1918; 4(12):370–3.
44. Ottery FD. Cancer cachexia: prevention, early diagnosis, and management. Cancer Pract. 1994;2(2):123–31.
45. Hearing SD. Refeeding syndrome: is underdiagnosed and undertreated, but treatable. BMJ. 2004;328(7445): 908–9.
46. Palesty JA, Dudrick SJ. Cachexia, malnutrition, the refeeding syndrome, and lessons from Goldilocks. Surg Clin North Am. 2011;91(3):653–73.
47. Marik PE, Zaloga GP. Immunonutrition in high-risk surgical patients: a systematic review and analysis of the literature. JPEN J Parenter Enteral Nutr. 2010; 34(4):378–86.
48. Waitzberg DL, Saito H, Plank LD, et al. Postsurgical infections are reduced with specialized nutrition support. World J Surg. 2006;30(8):1592–604.
49. Drover JW, Dhaliwal R, Weitzel L, Wischmeyer PE, Ochoa JB, Heyland DK. Perioperative use of arginine-supplemented diets: a systematic review of the evidence. J Am Coll Surg. 2011;212(3):385–99.
50. Cerantola Y, Hubner M, Grass F, Demartines N, Schafer M. Immunonutrition in gastrointestinal surgery. Br J Surg. 2011;98(1):37–48.
51. Wernerman J. Clinical use of glutamine supplementation. J Nutr. 2008;138(10):2040S–4.
52. Vanek VW, Matarese LE, Robinson M, Sacks GS, Young LS, Kochevar M. A.S.P.E.N. position paper: parenteral nutrition glutamine supplementation. Nutr Clin Pract. 2011;26(4):479–94.
53. Singer P, Berger MM, Van den Berghe G, Biolo G, Calder P, Forbes A, et al. ESPEN guidelines on parenteral nutrition: intensive care. Clin Nutr. 2009;28(4): 387–400.
54. Wei C, Hua J, Bin C, Klassen K. Impact of lipid emulsion containing fish oil on outcomes of surgical patients: systematic review of randomized controlled trials from Europe and Asia. Nutrition. 2010;26(5): 474–81.
55. Gianotti L, Braga M. Revising concepts of artificial nutrition in contemporary surgery: from energy and nitrogen to immuno-metabolic support. Nutr Hosp. 2011;26(1):56–67.
56. Zhang Y, Gu Y, Guo T, Li Y, Cai H. Perioperative immunonutrition for gastrointestinal cancer: a systematic review of randomized controlled trials. Surg Oncol. 2012;21(2):e87–95.
57. Braga M, Gianotti L, Nespoli L, Radaelli G, Di Carlo V. Nutritional approach in malnourished surgical patients: a prospective randomized study. Arch Surg. 2002;137(2):174–80.
58. Gianotti L, Braga M, Nespoli L, Radaelli G, Beneduce A, Di Carlo V. A randomized controlled trial on preoperative oral supplementation with a

specialized diet in patients with gastrointestinal cancer. Gastroenterology. 2002;122(7):1763–70.

59. Kreymann KG, Berger MM, Deutz NE, Hiesmayr M, Jolliet P, Kazandjiev G, et al; DGEM (German Society for Nutritional Medicine), Ebner C, Hartl W, Heymann C, Spies C; ESPEN (European Society for Parenteral and Enteral Nutrition). ESPEN guidelines on enteral nutrition: intensive care. Clin Nutr 2006;25(2):210–23.

60. American Academy of Hospice and Palliative Medicine. Position statements. Statement on artificial nutrition and hydration near the end of life approved by the board of directors. December 8, 2006. http://www.aahpm.org/positions/default/nutrition.html. Accessed on 22 Jan 2013.

Medical Oncology

7

Peter S. Savas and Timothy J. Price

Contents

The focus of this chapter is to discuss the impact of modern systemic therapy on the outcomes of patients with advanced malignancy. Gastrointestinal cancer is an ideal example where outcomes have improved and opportunities for surgery of palliative benefit have therefore multiplied. For advanced colorectal cancer in particular, where without effective systemic therapy the median survival was 6 months, there is now the potential for cure when surgery and chemotherapy are incorporated into the treatment plan. Here we will give a concise review of systemic agents along with their potential toxicities and highlight interventions that have now become evermore relevant for the surgeon to consider given the longer survival times of patients with advanced cancer.

P.S. Savas, MBBS, BMedSci (✉)
Department of Medical Oncology,
The Queen Elizabeth Hospital,
Woodville South 5011, SA, Australia
e-mail: psavas@gmail.com

T.J. Price, MBBS, FRACP (✉)
Department of Medical Oncology,
The Queen Elizabeth Hospital and University of Adelaide, Woodville Road,
Adelaide 5011, SA, Australia
e-mail: timothy.price@health.sa.gov.au

M. Wichmann, G. Maddern (eds.), *Palliative Surgery*,
DOI 10.1007/978-3-642-53709-7_7,

Abbreviations

CT	Computed tomography
EGFR	Epidermal growth factor receptor
FDG-PET	Fluorodeoxyglucose positron emission tomography
FOLFIRINOX	5-fluorouracil irinotecan, oxaliplatin
HER2	Human epidermal growth factor receptor 2
VEGF	Vascular endothelial growth factor

7.1 Introduction

The overall survival of patients with advanced malignancies from the time of diagnosis has been improving in the modern era of multimodality treatment. As an example, the median overall survival of patients with metastatic colorectal carcinoma enrolled in contemporary clinical trials is now at least 24 months, with a 5-year survival of 12 % [1, 2]. This improvement in most cancer types, but particularly gastrointestinal cancers, relates to the optimisation of cytotoxic chemotherapy, the advent of biological agents and increasing recognition of the role for surgery in patients with advanced, incurable disease. Improvements in survival with systemic therapy have also been paralleled by improvements in quality of life [3–5]. Chemotherapy regimens have become sufficiently tolerable to permit continuous maintenance administration particularly in lung [6] and colorectal carcinoma [7], strategies which further improve survival and quality of life. These improving outcomes for many patients with cancer provide multiple opportunities throughout the treatment course where surgical management may be necessary or desirable for palliative benefit. This is particularly relevant to gastrointestinal cancers, which will be used here as an example to illustrate various medical oncology considerations pertinent to palliative surgery. We will also discuss the relevance of "prognosis" prediction and provide a broad overview of some of the frequently used chemotherapy and newer biological or targeted agents.

7.2 Defining Prognosis and Its Relevance to Surgical Considerations

It is worth considering at this point the role of prognosis in deciding the management of patients with advanced cancer. The gross 5-year survival from the time of diagnosis for advanced solid tumours remains generally below 25 %, particularly for gastrointestinal cancers [2]. A single value such as this, however, does not capture the wide variation in the natural history of advanced malignancy. Multiple lines of evidence indicate that even within cancer histological subtypes, there are many subgroups distinguishable only at a genomic level that have different prognoses and responses to treatment [3–5, 8, 9]. The data used to estimate prognosis are derived from large cohorts of patients and represent merely an average value across these subgroups. The problem with broad and oversimplified estimates of survival is exemplified by the concept of conditional survival. Conditional survival is the expected survival of a patient after they have already survived for a period of time from diagnosis. It has been demonstrated in all common solid tumours across multiple studies [10–12] that the longer a patient survives from the time of diagnosis, the more likely they are to survive the next 5 years. Although counterintuitive, this is a reflection of the fact that some patients have tumours with indolent biology, and these patients make up the majority of long-term survivors with incurable disease. It is often impossible to identify those with indolent tumour biology from the outset. It is therefore presumptive to assume that a patient who has lived with an advanced malignancy for a period of time is unlikely to survive much longer, particularly if they have clinical evidence of disease stability. The conditional survival in the next 5 years after patients with various gastrointestinal

Table 7.1 Conditional survival in common gastrointestinal cancers

Estimated survival over the next 5 years (%)				
Cancer	From diagnosis	1 year already survived	3 years already survived	5 years already survived
Stomach	5	21	81	93
Colorectal	12	24	56	83
Pancreas	2	20	62	83

Adapted with permission from Yu et al. [11]

cancers have already survived 1, 3 and 5 years can be seen in Table 7.1.

Response to treatment is also an important determinant of survival [13]. Any cohort of patients will exhibit a variable response to chemotherapy, and this translates into differing outcomes of significant magnitude. In a study investigating the prognostic impact of an early response to chemotherapy in advanced colorectal cancer, there was a twofold increase in median survival for patients with an early response on computed tomography (CT) imaging compared to those with stable disease [14]. Beyond CT, imaging of tumour metabolism with fluorodeoxyglucose positron emission tomography (FDG-PET) permits the identification of a response to treatment early in the treatment course, although resource constraints have limited widespread adoption of this modality [15]. Studies using FDG-PET have determined that an early metabolic response to treatment is correlated with improved survival in multiple tumour types, including colorectal and pancreatic cancer [16, 17]. Chemo-responsiveness is hence an important and useful predictor of prognosis with great relevance to surgical decision making.

These complexities highlight that when weighing the risks and benefits of surgical intervention in a patient with advanced cancer, the nuances of prognostication are best handled by the multidisciplinary team. Multidisciplinary teams have been shown to be more accurate at predicting survival than individual clinicians [18], and oversimplified predictions of "prognosis" alone may not be helpful.

Table 7.2 Chemotherapy and targeted agents and their common toxicities

Agent	Common toxicities
5-fluorouracil, oxaliplatin, irinotecan, carboplatin, cisplatin, gemcitabine, doxorubicin, docetaxel, paclitaxel, cyclophosphamide, capecitabine, temozolomide	Anaemia, neutropenia, thrombocytopenia Fatigue Nausea, vomiting, diarrhoea Oral mucositis Neuropathy, nephropathy, ototoxicity
Bevacizumab	Bleeding Delayed wound healing Hypertension Cardiovascular/cerebrovascular acute events
Sunitinib, sorafenib, pazopanib	Bleeding Delayed wound healing Cardiovascular/cerebrovascular acute events Cutaneous toxicity Liver function abnormalities Diarrhoea Oral mucositis Fatigue Thrombocytopenia Hypertension
Cetuximab, erlotinib, gefitinib	Skin rash, hypomagnesaemia Diarrhoea Pneumonitis, liver function abnormalities

7.3 The Oncology Patient Undergoing Surgery

7.3.1 An Overview of Chemotherapy and Targeted Agents

It is important to consider the current systemic therapeutic regimen when contemplating elective surgery for an oncology patient. Common cancer therapies and their toxicities are presented in Table 7.2. Chemotherapy has traditionally consisted of cytotoxic agents with broad efficacy across tumour types. The mechanism of action in general relates to inducing DNA damage or inhibiting progression through the cell cycle such that malignant cells die by apoptosis or necrosis [19]. Most chemotherapy agents are given intravenously as single doses separated by 1–4 weeks, to permit recovery from side effects and haematological abnormalities. Combinations of two or more agents are commonly used to improve response rates and circumvent drug resistance. Of note, 5-fluorouracil is often given in continuous infusions lasting days or weeks requiring central venous access. Surgically inserted venous access devices are potentially one of the most common "palliative" surgical interventions. Oral chemotherapeutic agents, such as capecitabine and temozolomide, are given in continuous or interrupted schedules lasting 5 days or more. Capecitabine is an oral 5-fluorouracil derivative which in theory reduces the need for venous access although only if taken as a single agent, which in today's practice is less common.

The haematological and mucosal toxicities of cytotoxic chemotherapy are likely to be of most concern to the surgeon. Neutropenia and thrombocytopenia may affect the timing of surgery but usually resolve within a 1–2-week time frame. Mucosal toxicities such as chemotherapy-related diarrhoea and cutaneous toxicities are commonly mild but in some cases can be severe and create unfavourable conditions for surgery. It is likely that surgeons today have had experience with the reversible toxicity of standard chemotherapy.

Newer so-called biological or targeted agents have differing toxicity profiles that may also differ in severity and time to recovery compared to what would be considered typical for conventional anticancer therapies. These agents target particular molecular abnormalities present in the tumour that provide a growth advantage. The target for some tumours can be identified pretreatment with mutation testing of pathology specimens, such as the *absence* of mutations in the KRAS oncogene in colorectal cancer, indicating sensitivity to cetuximab [20]. Immunohistochemical procedures may also identify a target such as human epidermal growth factor receptor 2 (HER2) overexpression in breast cancer, indicating sensitivity to trastuzumab [21]. In other cases the presence of the target is assumed. This is often the case for currently available oral targeted agents which are all inhibitors of the tyrosine kinase domain. This functional domain of various cellular receptors and proteins is mutated or overexpressed in multiple tumour types causing unhindered proliferative signalling and malignant transformation [22]. Agents that inhibit these tyrosine kinase domains have demonstrated efficacy in multiple advanced malignancies (Table 7.3).

Table 7.3 Description of targeted agents

Agent	Target	Tumour
Monoclonal antibodies – intravenous agents		
Trastuzumab	Amplification of the human epidermal growth factor receptor 2 (HER2)	Breast carcinoma Gastric carcinoma
Bevacizumab	Vascular endothelial growth factor (VEGF)	Colorectal carcinoma
Cetuximab Panitumumab	Epidermal growth factor receptor (EGFR)	Colorectal carcinoma with nonmutant KRAS gene Head and neck squamous cell carcinoma
Tyrosine kinase inhibitors – oral agents		
Sunitinib Pazopanib Sorafenib	Multiple tyrosine kinases associated with the vascular endothelial growth factor receptor, platelet-derived growth factor receptor and others	Renal cell carcinoma Gastrointestinal stromal tumour Renal cell carcinoma Hepatocellular carcinoma Renal cell carcinoma
Erlotinib, gefitinib	Mutant overactive epidermal growth factor receptor (EGFR)	Lung adenocarcinoma
Imatinib	Mutant C-KIT	Gastrointestinal stromal tumour

Anti-angiogenic therapies that target vascular endothelial growth factor (VEGF) are particularly relevant to the surgeon. They include the anti-VEGF monoclonal antibody bevacizumab and the anti-VEGF tyrosine kinase inhibitors sunitinib, sorafenib and pazopanib. Anti-VEGF agents have been associated with excess bleeding risk, and they may impair wound healing [23–26]. Where possible, surgery should be delayed until a suitable treatment-free period to prevent complications. Data suggest that a 6–8-week interval from the last dose of bevacizumab is sufficient to prevent surgical complications for major abdominal procedures requiring laparotomy [27] and bevacizumab treatment may be commenced 4 weeks after surgery [28]. For minor procedures such as surgical insertion of vascular access devices, a 14-day interval from the last bevacizumab treatment is sufficient [29]. Potent anti-VEGF activity of bevacizumab is still detectable in blood and tissue at 6 weeks from the last treatment, but this is not associated with wound healing complications [30]. There is less evidence regarding the timing of surgery and the use of anti-VEGF tyrosine kinase inhibitors, but the short half-life of these drugs in contrast to bevacizumab suggests that shorter intervals are acceptable. Studies of neoadjuvant administration of these agents in renal cell carcinoma provide evidence that an interval of anywhere between 1 and 16 days from the last dose to major surgery is safe and feasible and that treatment can be restarted 2–6 weeks after surgery if the wound is well healed [31–33].

There is a paucity of data regarding the peri-operative safety of agents that target the epidermal growth factor receptor (EGFR) in colon and lung cancer (such as cetuximab, panitumumab, erlotinib) or C-KIT in gastrointestinal stromal tumours (imatinib), but they appear to have less impact on healing and bone marrow function, and thus significant delays in surgery are not considered necessary. Potential cytopenias should, however, be evaluated with a full blood examination and differential count immediately prior to surgery, as imatinib in particular can cause neutropenia [34]. Cetuximab appeared safe when used prior to resection of hepatic metastases from colorectal cancer in a study where surgery was performed a mean of 32 days after chemotherapy (range 12–56 days), with no increase in surgical complications and no evidence of excess hepatotoxicity [35].

7.4 Management of the Patient with Advanced Colorectal Cancer

7.4.1 Modern Chemotherapy Regimens in Advanced Colorectal Cancer and Impact on Outcome

Improved outcomes have resulted from the incorporation of multi-agent chemotherapy regimens into the treatment of metastatic colorectal cancer, combining oxaliplatin or irinotecan with 5-fluorouracil or capecitabine [36]. These regimens yield response rates of approximately 40–50 % in patients not previously treated and 10 % in those already treated with chemotherapy, with a median overall survival of around 20 months [1]. The addition of the targeted agents bevacizumab (anti-VEGF) and, for KRAS wild-type tumours, cetuximab or panitumumab (anti-EGFR) has brought about further incremental improvements in response rates and progression-free and overall survival [37]. In general the order of the regimens used is considered less important than exposing a patient to all agents [38], although the potential for hepatic surgery or the presence of an in situ primary lesion does play a role in drug choice and hence timing. Since patients undergoing resection of hepatic metastases have been consistently shown to have improved survival [39], the response rate of a chosen regimen becomes relevant as it may be possible to convert a borderline resectable lesion to one where resection is possible. Adding an anti-EGFR agent in this setting can be considered given the higher response rates reported [40]. Additionally, as a consequence of improved therapies and longer survival, there is greater opportunity for surgical intervention in managing the complications of an in situ primary tumour or metastatic disease.

7.4.2 The Role of Primary Tumour Resection in Patients with Metastatic Colorectal Cancer: A Multidisciplinary Perspective

Most patients presenting with metastatic disease in colon cancer do not require urgent surgery. For those patients with malignant bowel obstruction, tumour perforation or bleeding, the value of urgent surgical intervention is not in doubt. Alternatively for symptomatic but well patients, chemotherapy has a 40–50 % chance of shrinking the primary tumour [1], which may improve symptoms of itself. Colonic stenting has also emerged as a feasible alternative that may avoid extensive surgery and improve obstructive symptoms [41, 42]. Stenting has the advantage that observational studies suggest chemotherapy may be administered promptly after stenting without apparent excess risk [43, 44].

There is considerable debate about the risks and benefits of elective resection of the primary tumour in asymptomatic patients with clearly incurable disease. The rationale for this approach is threefold. Firstly, it may prevent development of acute complications during the lifetime of the patient, which as noted previously is now significantly longer. In patients with metastatic colorectal cancer where the primary tumour remains in situ and there are no symptoms, only 11–14 % experience morbidity related to the primary tumour that may require surgical or nonsurgical intervention such as stenting or radiotherapy [45–48]. Secondly, primary tumour resection may prevent treatment complications such as haemorrhage or perforation that arise due to the use of the anti-VEGF agent bevacizumab. In a meta-analysis not incorporating individual patient data, bevacizumab was associated with an increased risk of gastrointestinal perforation in patients with metastatic colorectal carcinoma [49]. However, data pertaining specifically to primary tumour complication rates in patients with asymptomatic primary tumours receiving bevacizumab do not show increased rates of perforation or haemorrhage [47]. Thirdly, primary resection may improve the efficacy of systemic treatment and prolong survival. There are, however, conflicting data on the survival benefit of primary tumour resection and no prospective randomised trials [50], although recent retrospective studies have suggested a survival benefit [51, 52]. These data are tempered by the significant post-operative complication rates for primary tumour resection in patients with stage IV disease, with a 12 % major complication rate reported in one large retrospective study [45]. Retrospective studies have identified various factors that are associated with better survival after primary tumour resection including younger age, few comorbidities, liver-only metastases and lower serum carcinoembryonic antigen level [51–54]. Evidence from trials of neoadjuvant chemotherapy indicates that the primary tumour may be less sensitive to chemotherapy than metastatic lesions [55], but whether this difference is relevant to modern chemotherapy regimens with response rates of 40 % or more is unclear. In summary, it is likely that carefully selected patients may benefit from primary tumour resection followed by systemic therapy, but this patient population remains undefined.

7.4.3 Multidisciplinary Management of Colorectal Cancer Metastases

As mentioned earlier with regard to surgical resection of hepatic metastases, metastectomy has a role in the management of advanced colorectal cancer and permits some patients with few sites of metastatic disease to achieve prolonged disease-free survival without chemotherapy. The most robust evidence exists for patients with metastases limited to the liver. In these patients who undergo resection of metastatic lesions, 5-year overall survival may average 40 %, with a median survival of 65 months [39, 56–58]. For patients considered borderline resectable or unresectable, there is a further subgroup that may be converted to resectable with systemic therapy [40, 59]. Improved outcomes are evident for patients converted to resectable and undergoing surgery, with a median survival of 40 months in one study, double the expected median survival for metastatic colorectal cancer [59]. This approach has not been validated in large randomised controlled trials, however. Less robust data also exist for the benefits of resection of limited pulmonary metastases [60, 61], although this consists mainly of retrospective analyses subject to bias and in theory randomised trials are needed [62].

7.5 Management of the Patient with Advanced Upper Gastrointestinal Cancer

7.5.1 Modern Chemotherapy Regimens in Advanced Gastric Cancer

Multi-agent chemotherapy is associated with improved outcomes in gastric cancer [63]. The most active regimens are considered to consist of capecitabine, a platinum compound such as cisplatin or oxaliplatin, and epirubicin, with response rates of around 40–48 % [64]. Trastuzumab in combination with capecitabine/5-fluorouracil and cisplatin has also shown efficacy in tumours that overexpress HER2 although this equates to only 20–25 % of patients [65]. More recently evidence from randomised phase III trials of chemotherapy with irinotecan or docetaxel versus best supportive care alone has shown the survival benefits of further treatment after the failure of first-line therapy [66, 67]. As with colorectal cancer, survival has now improved, and in particular for HER2-positive patients, median survival is reported as greater than 14–16 months [65], and thus the potential for late-stage events requiring surgery increases.

7.5.2 Modern Chemotherapy Regimens in Advanced Pancreatic Cancer

Pancreatic cancer is considered among the most lethal upper gastrointestinal malignancies. With treatment, median survival for locally advanced inoperable disease approaches 12 months in contemporary clinical trials [68] and 6–8 months for metastatic disease [69]. Chemoradiotherapy is the standard of care for patients with good performance status and inoperable disease, usually following several months of chemotherapy alone to determine if the tumour is responsive to chemotherapy. Compared to chemotherapy alone, chemoradiotherapy prolongs survival but may not improve quality of life [68]. Radiological response rates to chemoradiotherapy are less than 10 % [68]. For metastatic disease, single-agent gemcitabine is commonly used but suffers from poor response rates and an uncertain impact on quality of life [70, 71]. Recently a multi-agent regimen consisting of 5-fluorouracil, oxaliplatin and irinotecan (FOLFIRINOX) has produced the most promising results to date in metastatic pancreatic cancer, with a median survival of 11 months and response rate of 30 % [72]. FOLFIRINOX also prevented degradation in quality of life compared with gemcitabine [73]. Significant toxicity was associated with FOLFIRINOX, and it is considered suitable only for fit patients without troublesome biliary obstruction. That said, favouring surgical palliation of biliary obstruction to avoid the risk of infected biliary stents may become a more frequent discussion point to facilitate greater use of this regimen. Furthermore, the higher response rates seen with FOLFIRINOX warrant investigation in the preoperative setting with the hope that some patients may be down staged and become resectable.

7.6 Multidisciplinary Management of the Complications of Gastrointestinal Malignancy

7.6.1 Malignant Gastric Outlet Obstruction

Gastric outlet obstruction may develop later in the natural history of gastric cancer and pancreatic cancer or at presentation. It is typically associated with a decline in the patient's functional status and nutritional state. In these unwell patients, the response rates expected with the available chemotherapy regimens for gastric, and in particular pancreatic, cancer are often inadequate to effectively palliate outlet obstruction. Although gastrectomy remains a successful intervention for gastric outlet obstruction related to gastric cancer, endoscopic stenting may be a preferable option for patients with more limited life expectancy or where surgery is not possible [74]. There are, however, no data on quality of life outcomes post-endoscopic stenting [75], and some authors have suggested the technology of duodenal stenting lags behind that of biliary stents, and thus laparoscopic or open gastric bypass remains an important consideration [76]. Radiation has been associated with good palliation in gastric cancer causing obstruction with symptom control rates of 80 % in a small series and has the advantage of also controlling bleeding [77]. Management of gastric outlet obstruction may then permit the administration of systemic chemotherapy.

7.6.2 Malignant Biliary Obstruction

The presence of uncontrolled biliary obstruction due to upper gastrointestinal malignancy or other disease metastatic to the liver renders systemic therapy problematic, affecting the excretion and toxicity profile of several agents active in gastrointestinal cancers such as epirubicin, gemcitabine, irinotecan and sorafenib [78]. Uncontrolled biliary obstruction also predisposes patients to cholangitis which is undesirable during potentially immunosuppressive chemotherapy and often excludes patients from inclusion in clinical trials. The alleviation of biliary obstruction is therefore preferable prior to instituting systemic therapy if possible. Stenting endoscopically or percutaneously is an effective and less invasive option than surgical bypass, having been shown to have fewer short-term complications, although a higher re-occlusion rate [79]. For patients with bulky metastatic disease, a borderline performance status or poorly controlled symptoms, stenting procedures allow prompt institution of systemic therapy without the need for recovery from surgery. In one small retrospective study in patients with metastatic colorectal or gastric cancer, chemotherapy administration was feasible in approximately half of patients who underwent successful percutaneous biliary drainage [80]. Factors associated with a poor outcome after the percutaneous procedure in this study included extensive liver metastases, poor performance status, prior chemotherapy and ascites [80]. Patients with a poor prognosis and limited life expectancy are also candidates for stenting for palliative benefit. Alternatively, in patients with low-volume disease and good functional status who are candidates for intensive chemotherapy such as FOLFIRINOX, the better long-term outcomes and theoretically lower risk of sepsis may favour surgical bypass, although stenting remains the preferred procedure for the majority of patients [79]. The multidisciplinary setting is the ideal environment to weigh these factors prior to intervention.

7.6.3 Malignant Bowel Obstruction

Malignant bowel obstruction typically develops in advanced disease due to peritoneal dissemination of malignancy. It is of course not limited to upper gastrointestinal malignancy. It may occur when a patient still has viable options for systemic therapy or in patients with a very limited life expectancy and no treatment options, and this context is crucial to deciding on an appropriate management strategy. Patients with active bowel obstruction unable to eat are rarely able to receive any systemic therapy, and thus careful consideration should be given to whether overcoming the obstruction may lead to future palliative systemic therapy. Although malignant bowel obstruction may improve with conservative measures and bowel rest, the possibility of surgery is often raised and carries with it the caveats of high recurrence rates and high perioperative morbidity and mortality, even in selected patients [81]. The use of parenteral nutrition prior to surgery is only likely to be beneficial in an extremely small subset of patients with advanced malignancy, particularly if they are refractory to known systemic treatments [82]. Multidisciplinary consultation including palliative care is vital to avoid futile intervention and similarly to avoid withholding treatment from a patient who may still benefit.

7.6.4 Malignant Pleural Effusion

Pleural effusions are a common consequence of metastases to the pleural space from colon and upper gastrointestinal cancers. They also occur not infrequently in lung, breast and gynaecological cancers. Accumulation of the effusion is associated with distressing symptoms of dyspnoea and is invariably recurrent without further intervention. Systemic therapy is able to delay recurrence of a malignant pleural effusion, but rapidly accumulating symptomatic effusions are an indication to consider local intervention. Pleurodesis with talc administered through a chest tube or at the time of thoracoscopy is an effective procedure in preventing recurrence of effusions [83]. Indwelling pleural catheters may also achieve this purpose, however, and seem equivalent in efficacy [84]. They have the advantage of less recurrent procedures and a shorter hospital stay than talc pleurodesis but are associated with more adverse events after insertion [84]. Indwelling catheter placement may be a preferable option for patients with poor functional status and very limited life expectancy. For patients with adequate functional reserve and performance status, surgical pleurodesis potentially offers a more definitive intervention allowing subsequent systemic therapy to be delivered [83].

Conclusion

With improved systemic therapies the survival for patients with advanced incurable cancer has improved significantly over the last decade, as has been illustrated here. With prolonged survival comes a change in the needs of these patients and a greater likelihood that surgical intervention may be required, both in the initial phase of disease and in the later stages of the patient's journey. Furthermore there is a need to understand the potential interaction of surgery and current or planned systemic therapy. Multidisciplinary consultation is increasingly considered vital for the initial management plan for a patient, but we would argue that multidisciplinary care remains relevant throughout the patient's life. Balancing potential responses to systemic therapy with the risks of palliative interventions such as surgical bypass of gastric outlet obstruction requires careful and timely discussion to ensure the best outcome for the patient. As systemic therapy continues to improve, it is clear that there should be an ongoing multidisciplinary approach for patients with advanced cancer, which brings together the surgeon and other oncology and palliative care professionals.

References

1. Tournigand C, André T, Achille E, Lledo G, Flesh M, Mery-Mignard D, et al. FOLFIRI followed by FOLFOX6 or the reverse sequence in advanced colorectal cancer: a randomized GERCOR study. J Clin Oncol. 2004;22(2):229–37.
2. Siegel R, Naishadham D, Jemal A. Cancer statistics, 2013. CA Cancer J Clin. 2013;63(1):11–30.
3. Glimelius B, Hoffman K, Graf W, Påhlman L, Sjödén PO. Quality of life during chemotherapy in patients with symptomatic advanced colorectal cancer. The Nordic Gastrointestinal Tumor Adjuvant Therapy Group. Cancer. 1994;73(3):556–62.
4. Bennett L, Zhao Z, Barber B, Zhou X, Peeters M, Zhang J, et al. Health-related quality of life in patients with metastatic colorectal cancer treated with panitumumab in first- or second-line treatment. Br J Cancer. 2011;105(10):1495–502.
5. Kabbinavar FF, Wallace JF, Holmgren E, Yi J, Cella D, Yost KJ, et al. Health-related quality of life impact of bevacizumab when combined with irinotecan, 5-fluorouracil, and leucovorin or 5-fluorouracil and leucovorin for metastatic colorectal cancer. Oncologist. 2008;13(9):1021–9.
6. Belani CP, Brodowicz T, Ciuleanu TE, Krzakowski M, Yang SH, Franke F, et al. Quality of life in patients with advanced non-small-cell lung cancer given maintenance treatment with Pemetrexed versus placebo (H3E-MC-JMEN): results from a randomised, double-blind, phase 3 study. Lancet Oncol. 2012;13(3):292–9.
7. Chibaudel B, Maindrault-Goebel F, Lledo G, Mineur L, André T, Bennamoun M, et al. Can chemotherapy be discontinued in unresectable metastatic colorectal cancer? The GERCOR OPTIMOX2 study. J Clin Oncol. 2009;27(34):5727–33.

8. The Cancer Genome Atlas Network. Comprehensive molecular characterization of human colon and rectal cancer. Nature. 2012;487(7407):330–7.
9. The Cancer Genome Atlas Network. Comprehensive molecular portraits of human breast tumours. Nature. 2012;490(7418):61–70.
10. Merrill RM, Hunter BD. Conditional survival among cancer patients in the United States. Oncologist. 2010;15(8):873–82.
11. Yu XQ, Baade PD, O'Connell DL. Conditional survival of cancer patients: an Australian perspective. BMC Cancer. 2012;12(1):460.
12. Wang SJ, Emery R, Fuller CD, Kim J-S, Sittig DF, Thomas CR. Conditional survival in gastric cancer: a SEER database analysis. Gastric Cancer. 2007;10(3): 153–8.
13. Buyse M, Thirion P, Carlson RW, Burzykowski T, Molenberghs G, Piedbois P. Relation between tumour response to first-line chemotherapy and survival in advanced colorectal cancer: a meta-analysis. Meta-Analysis Group in Cancer. Lancet. 2000;356(9227): 373–8.
14. Suzuki C, Blomqvist L, Sundin A, Jacobsson H, Byström P, Berglund Å, et al. The initial change in tumor size predicts response and survival in patients with metastatic colorectal cancer treated with combination chemotherapy. Ann Oncol. 2012;23(4):948–54.
15. Wahl RL, Jacene H, Kasamon Y, Lodge MA. From RECIST to PERCIST: evolving considerations for PET response criteria in solid tumors. J Nucl Med. 2009;50 Suppl 1:122S–50.
16. Von Hoff DD, Ramanathan RK, Borad MJ, Laheru DA, Smith LS, Wood TE, et al. Gemcitabine plus nab-paclitaxel is an active regimen in patients with advanced pancreatic cancer: a phase I/II trial. J Clin Oncol. 2011;29(34):4548–54.
17. Hendlisz A, Golfinopoulos V, Garcia C, Covas A, Emonts P, Ameye L, et al. Serial FDG-PET/CT for early outcome prediction in patients with metastatic colorectal cancer undergoing chemotherapy. Ann Oncol. 2012;23(7):1687–93.
18. Gwilliam B, Keeley V, Todd C, Roberts C, Gittins M, Kelly L, et al. Prognosticating in patients with advanced cancer – observational study comparing the accuracy of clinicians' and patients' estimates of survival. Ann Oncol. 2013;24(2):482–8.
19. Chabner BA. Clinical strategies for cancer treatment: the role of drugs. In: Chabner BA, Longo DL, editors. Cancer chemotherapy and biotherapy: principles and practice. Philadelphia: Lippincott Williams & Wilkins; 2010. p. 3–14.
20. Karapetis CS, Khambata-Ford S, Jonker DJ, O'Callaghan CJ, Tu D, Tebbutt NC, et al. K-ras mutations and benefit from cetuximab in advanced colorectal cancer. N Engl J Med. 2008;359(17):1757–65.
21. Seidman AD, Fornier MN, Esteva FJ, Tan L, Kaptain S, Bach A, et al. Weekly trastuzumab and paclitaxel therapy for metastatic breast cancer with analysis of efficacy by HER2 immunophenotype and gene amplification. J Clin Oncol. 2001;19(10):2587–95.
22. Baselga J. Targeting tyrosine kinases in cancer: the second wave. Science. 2006;312(5777):1175–8.
23. Bhojani N, Jeldres C, Patard J-J, Perrotte P, Suardi N, Hutterer G, et al. Toxicities associated with the administration of sorafenib, sunitinib, and temsirolimus and their management in patients with metastatic renal cell carcinoma. Eur Urol. 2008;53(5):917–30.
24. Sternberg CN, Davis ID, Mardiak J, Szczylik C, Lee E, Wagstaff J, et al. Pazopanib in locally advanced or metastatic renal cell carcinoma: results of a randomized phase III trial. J Clin Oncol. 2010;28(6):1061–8.
25. Je Y, Schutz FAB, Choueiri TK. Risk of bleeding with vascular endothelial growth factor receptor tyrosine-kinase inhibitors sunitinib and sorafenib: a systematic review and meta-analysis of clinical trials. Lancet Oncol. 2009;10(10):967–74.
26. Hapani S, Sher A, Chu D, Wu S. Increased risk of serious hemorrhage with bevacizumab in cancer patients: a meta-analysis. Oncology. 2010;79(1–2):27–38.
27. Kesmodel SB, Ellis LM, Lin E, Chang GJ, Abdalla EK, Kopetz S, et al. Preoperative bevacizumab does not significantly increase postoperative complication rates in patients undergoing hepatic surgery for colorectal cancer liver metastases. J Clin Oncol. 2008;26(32):5254–60.
28. Scappaticci FA, Fehrenbacher L, Cartwright T, Hainsworth JD, Heim W, Berlin J, et al. Surgical wound healing complications in metastatic colorectal cancer patients treated with bevacizumab. J Surg Oncol. 2005;91(3):173–80.
29. Erinjeri JP, Fong AJ, Kemeny NE, Brown KT, Getrajdman GI, Solomon SB. Timing of administration of bevacizumab chemotherapy affects wound healing after chest wall port placement. Cancer. 2011;117(6):1296–301.
30. Starlinger P, Alidzanovic L, Schauer D, Maier T, Sommerfeldt S, Herberger B, et al. Activity of bevacizumab at the time of surgery after 6 weeks of preoperative cessation. J Clin Oncol. 2012;30 Suppl 4:abstract 455.
31. Boleti E, Sarwar N, Jones RR, Chowdhury S, Crabb SJ, Shamash J, et al. The safety and efficacy of pazopanib prior to planned nephrectomy in metastatic clear cell renal cancer. J Clin Oncol. 2012;30 Suppl 5:abstract 427.
32. Powles T, Kayani I, Blank C, Chowdhury S, Horenblas S, Peters J, et al. The safety and efficacy of sunitinib before planned nephrectomy in metastatic clear cell renal cancer. Ann Oncol. 2011;22(5):1041–7.
33. Cowey CL, Amin C, Pruthi RS, Wallen EM, Nielsen ME, Grigson G, et al. Neoadjuvant clinical trial with sorafenib for patients with stage II or higher renal cell carcinoma. J Clin Oncol. 2010;28(9):1502–7.
34. Demetri GD, Von Mehren M, Blanke CD, Van den Abbeele AD, Eisenberg B, Roberts PJ, et al. Efficacy and safety of imatinib mesylate in advanced gastrointestinal stromal tumors. N Engl J Med. 2002;347(7): 472–80.
35. Pessaux P, Marzano E, Casnedi S, Bachellier P, Jaeck D, Chenard M-P. Histological and immediate

postoperative outcome after preoperative cetuximab: case-matched control study. World J Surg. 2010; 34(11):2765–72.
36. Meyerhardt JA, Mayer RJ. Systemic therapy for colorectal cancer. N Engl J Med. 2005;352(5):476–87.
37. Cunningham D, Atkin W, Lenz H-J, Lynch HT, Minsky B, Nordlinger B, et al. Colorectal cancer. Lancet. 2010;375(9719):1030–47.
38. Grothey A, Sargent D, Goldberg RM, Schmoll H-J. Survival of patients with advanced colorectal cancer improves with the availability of fluorouracil-leucovorin, irinotecan, and oxaliplatin in the course of treatment. J Clin Oncol. 2004;22(7):1209–14.
39. Kopetz S, Chang GJ, Overman MJ, Eng C, Sargent DJ, Larson DW, et al. Improved survival in metastatic colorectal cancer is associated with adoption of hepatic resection and improved chemotherapy. J Clin Oncol. 2009;27(22):3677–83.
40. Folprecht G, Gruenberger T, Bechstein WO, Raab H-R, Lordick F, Hartmann JT, et al. Tumour response and secondary resectability of colorectal liver metastases following neoadjuvant chemotherapy with cetuximab: the CELIM randomised phase 2 trial. Lancet Oncol. 2010;11(1):38–47.
41. Fiori E, Lamazza A, Schillaci A, Femia S, Demasi E, Decesare A, et al. Palliative management for patients with subacute obstruction and stage IV unresectable rectosigmoid cancer: colostomy versus endoscopic stenting: final results of a prospective randomized trial. Am J Surg. 2012;204(3):321–6.
42. Meisner S, González-Huix F, Vandervoort JG, Repici A, Xinopoulos D, Grund KE, et al. Self-expanding metal stenting for palliation of patients with malignant colonic obstruction: effectiveness and efficacy on 255 patients with 12-Month's follow-up. Gastroenterol Res Pract. 2012;2012:296347.
43. Karoui M, Charachon A, Delbaldo C, Loriau J, Laurent A, Sobhani I, et al. Stents for palliation of obstructive metastatic colon cancer: impact on management and chemotherapy administration. Arch Surg. 2007;142(7):619–23.
44. Bielawska B, Hookey LC, Jalink D. Large-diameter self-expanding metal stents appear to be safe and effective for malignant colonic obstruction with and without concurrent use of chemotherapy. Surg Endosc. 2010;24(11):2814–21.
45. Scheer MGW, Sloots CEJ, Van der Wilt GJ, Ruers TJM. Management of patients with asymptomatic colorectal cancer and synchronous irresectable metastases. Ann Oncol. 2008;19(11):1829–35.
46. McCahill LE, Yothers G, Sharif S, Petrelli NJ, Lai LL, Bechar N, et al. Primary mFOLFOX6 plus bevacizumab without resection of the primary tumor for patients presenting with surgically unresectable metastatic colon cancer and an intact asymptomatic colon cancer: definitive analysis of NSABP trial C-10. J Clin Oncol. 2012;30(26):3223–8.
47. Poultsides GA, Servais EL, Saltz LB, Patil S, Kemeny NE, Guillem JG, et al. Outcome of primary tumor in patients with synchronous stage IV colorectal cancer receiving combination chemotherapy without surgery as initial treatment. J Clin Oncol. 2009;27(20):3379–84.
48. Tebbutt NC, Norman AR, Cunningham D, Hill ME, Tait D, Oates J, et al. Intestinal complications after chemotherapy for patients with unresected primary colorectal cancer and synchronous metastases. Gut. 2003;52(4):568–73.
49. Hapani S, Chu D, Wu S. Risk of gastrointestinal perforation in patients with cancer treated with bevacizumab: a meta-analysis. Lancet Oncol. 2009; 10(6):559–68.
50. Damjanov N, Weiss J, Haller DG. Resection of the primary colorectal cancer is not necessary in nonobstructed patients with metastatic disease. Oncologist. 2009;14(10):963–9.
51. Karoui M, Roudot-Thoraval F, Mesli F, Mitry E, Aparicio T, Des Guetz G, et al. Primary colectomy in patients with stage IV colon cancer and unresectable distant metastases improves overall survival: results of a multicentric study. Dis Colon Rectum. 2011; 54(8):930–8.
52. Faron M, Bourredjem A, Pignon J-P, Bouche O, Douillard J-Y, Adenis A, et al. Impact on survival of primary tumor resection in patients with colorectal cancer and unresectable metastasis: pooled analysis of individual patients' data from four randomized trials. J Clin Oncol. 2012;30 Suppl 15:abstract 3507.
53. Costi R, Mazzeo A, Di Mauro D, Veronesi L, Sansebastiano G, Violi V, et al. Palliative resection of colorectal cancer: does it prolong survival? Ann Surg Oncol. 2007;14(9):2567–76.
54. Gonsalves WI, Wolpert J, Tashi T, Ganti AK, Subbiah S, Ternent C, et al. Assessment of prognostic factors after primary tumor resection in metastatic colon cancer patients: a Veteran's Affairs Central Cancer Registry (VACCR) analysis, 1995–2008. J Surg Oncol. 2012;106(4):486–90.
55. Gervaz P, Rubbia-Brandt L, Andres A, Majno P, Roth A, Morel P, et al. Neoadjuvant chemotherapy in patients with stage IV colorectal cancer: a comparison of histological response in liver metastases, primary tumors, and regional lymph nodes. Ann Surg Oncol. 2010;17(10):2714–9.
56. Fernandez FG, Drebin JA, Linehan DC, Dehdashti F, Siegel BA, Strasberg SM. Five-year survival after resection of hepatic metastases from colorectal cancer in patients screened by positron emission tomography with F-18 fluorodeoxyglucose (FDG-PET). Ann Surg. 2004;240(3):438–50.
57. Scheele J, Stang R, Altendorf-Hofmann A, Paul M. Resection of colorectal liver metastases. World J Surg. 1995;19(1):59–71.
58. Steele BG, Bleday R, Mayer RJ, Lindblad A, Petrelli N, Weaver D. A prospective evaluation of hepatic resection for colorectal carcinoma metastases to the liver: Gastrointestinal Tumor Study Group Protocol 6584. J Clin Oncol. 1991;9(7):1105–12.
59. Delaunoit T, Alberts SR, Sargent DJ, Green E, Goldberg RM, Krook J, et al. Chemotherapy permits

resection of metastatic colorectal cancer: experience from Intergroup N9741. Ann Oncol. 2005;16(3): 425–9.
60. Gonzalez M, Robert JH, Halkic N, Mentha G, Roth A, Perneger T, et al. Survival after lung metastasectomy in colorectal cancer patients with previously resected liver metastases. World J Surg. 2012;36(2):386–91.
61. Iida T, Nomori H, Shiba M, Nakajima J, Okumura S, Horio H, et al. Prognostic factors after pulmonary metastasectomy for colorectal cancer and rationale for determining surgical indications: a retrospective analysis. Ann Surg. 2013;257(6):1059–64.
62. Fiorentino F, Hunt I, Teoh K, Treasure T, Utley M. Pulmonary metastasectomy in colorectal cancer: a systematic review and quantitative synthesis. J R Soc Med. 2010;103(2):60–6.
63. Wagner AD, Unverzagt S, Grothe W, Kleber G, Grothey A, Haerting J et al. Chemotherapy for advanced gastric cancer. Cochrane Database Syst Rev 2010;(3):CD004064.
64. Cunningham D, Starling N, Rao S, Iveson T, Nicolson M, Coxon F, et al. Capecitabine and oxaliplatin for advanced esophagogastric cancer. N Engl J Med. 2008;358(1):36–46.
65. Bang Y-J, Van Cutsem E, Feyereislova A, Chung HC, Shen L, Sawaki A, et al. Trastuzumab in combination with chemotherapy versus chemotherapy alone for treatment of HER2-positive advanced gastric or gastro-oesophageal junction cancer (ToGA): a phase 3, open-label, randomised controlled trial. Lancet. 2010;376(9742):687–97.
66. Thuss-Patience PC, Kretzschmar A, Bichev D, Deist T, Hinke A, Breithaupt K, et al. Survival advantage for irinotecan versus best supportive care as second-line chemotherapy in gastric cancer – a randomised phase III study of the Arbeitsgemeinschaft Internistische Onkologie (AIO). Eur J Cancer. 2011;47(15):2306–14.
67. Kang JH, Lee II S, Lim DH, Park K-W, Oh SY, Kwon H-C, et al. Salvage chemotherapy for pretreated gastric cancer: a randomized phase III trial comparing chemotherapy plus best supportive care with best supportive care alone. J Clin Oncol. 2012;30(13):1513–8.
68. Loehrer PJ, Feng Y, Cardenes H, Wagner L, Brell JM, Cella D, et al. Gemcitabine alone versus gemcitabine plus radiotherapy in patients with locally advanced pancreatic cancer: an Eastern Cooperative Oncology Group trial. J Clin Oncol. 2011;29(31):4105–12.
69. Moore MJ, Goldstein D, Hamm J, Figer A, Hecht JR, Gallinger S, et al. Erlotinib plus gemcitabine compared with gemcitabine alone in patients with advanced pancreatic cancer: a phase III trial of the National Cancer Institute of Canada Clinical Trials Group. J Clin Oncol. 2007;25(15):1960–6.
70. Burris HA, Moore MJ, Andersen J, Green MR, Rothenberg ML, Modiano MR, et al. Improvements in survival and clinical benefit with gemcitabine as first-line therapy for patients with advanced pancreas cancer: a randomized trial. J Clin Oncol. 1997;15(6): 2403–13.
71. Romanus D, Kindler HL, Archer L, Basch E, Niedzwiecki D, Weeks J, et al. Does health-related quality of life improve for advanced pancreatic cancer patients who respond to gemcitabine? Analysis of a randomized phase III trial of the cancer and leukemia group B (CALGB 80303). J Pain Symptom Manage. 2012;43(2):205–17.
72. Vaccaro V, Sperduti I, Milella M. FOLFIRINOX versus gemcitabine for metastatic pancreatic cancer. N Engl J Med. 2011;365(8):768–9.
73. Gourgou-Bourgade S, Bascoul-Mollevi C, Desseigne F, Ychou M, Bouché O, Guimbaud R, et al. Impact of FOLFIRINOX compared with gemcitabine on quality of life in patients with metastatic pancreatic cancer: results from the PRODIGE 4/ACCORD 11 randomized trial. J Clin Oncol. 2013;31(1):23–9.
74. Jeurnink SM, Van Eijck CHJ, Steyerberg EW, Kuipers EJ, Siersema PD. Stent versus gastrojejunostomy for the palliation of gastric outlet obstruction: a systematic review. BMC Gastroenterol. 2007;7:18–27.
75. Larssen L, Medhus AW, Hauge T. Treatment of malignant gastric outlet obstruction with stents: an evaluation of the reported variables for clinical outcome. BMC Gastroenterol. 2009;9:45–50.
76. Conrad C, Lillemoe KD. Surgical palliation of pancreatic cancer. Cancer J. 2012;18(6):577–83.
77. Tey J, Back MF, Shakespeare TP, Mukherjee RK, Lu JJ, Lee KM, et al. The role of palliative radiation therapy in symptomatic locally advanced gastric cancer. Int J Radiat Oncol Biol Phys. 2007;67(2):385–8.
78. Field KM, Michael M. Part II. Liver function in oncology: towards safer chemotherapy use. Lancet Oncol. 2008;9(12):1181–90.
79. Moss AC, Morris E, Mac Mathuna P. Palliative biliary stents for obstructing pancreatic carcinoma. Cochrane Database Syst Rev 2006;(2):CD004200.
80. Kasuga A, Ishii H, Ozaka M, Matsusaka S, Chin K, Mizunuma N, et al. Clinical outcome of biliary drainage for obstructive jaundice caused by colorectal and gastric cancers. Jpn J Clin Oncol. 2012;42(12): 1161–7.
81. Feuer DJ, Broadley KE, Shepherd JH, Barton DP. Surgery for the resolution of symptoms in malignant bowel obstruction in advanced gynaecological and gastrointestinal cancer. Cochrane Database Syst Rev. 2000;4, CD002764.
82. Hoda D, Jatoi A, Burnes J, Loprinzi C, Kelly D. Should patients with advanced, incurable cancers ever be sent home with total parenteral nutrition? A single institution's 20-year experience. Cancer. 2005;103(4): 863–8.
83. Shaw P, Agarwal R. Pleurodesis for malignant pleural effusions. Cochrane Database Syst Rev. 2004;1, CD002916.
84. Davies HE, Mishra EK, Kahan BC, Wrightson JM, Stanton AE, Guhan A, et al. Effect of an indwelling pleural catheter vs chest tube and talc pleurodesis for relieving dyspnea in patients with malignant pleural effusion: the TIME2 randomized controlled trial. JAMA. 2012;307(22):2383–9.

8 Radiation Oncology

Scott A. Carruthers

Contents

S.A. Carruthers, FRANZCR
Department of Radiation Oncology, Royal Adelaide Hospital, Adelaide 5000, SA, Australia
e-mail: scott.carruthers@health.sa.gov.au

Radiotherapy (RT) is an integral part of the palliative management of malignancy. Delivery of palliative RT is a simpler process than with curative RT, as the treatment is less complex in planning and delivery, with the treatment course generally much shorter and of lower radiation dose, and associated with less toxicity as a result. Palliative RT is applicable to a wide range of pathologies and to both primary and secondary sites. Commonly treated primary sites include the bronchus, oesophagus, rectum, bladder, and cervix. Secondary sites most often treated are skeletal, brain, and epidural (spinal cord compression). Palliative RT can be delivered in conjunction with surgical management or as an alternative management approach.

8.1 Introduction

Radiation oncology plays an integral role in cancer management as one of the three recognised disciplines together with surgical oncology and medical oncology. Radiation oncology is responsible for delivery of the treatment modality of radiotherapy (RT), principally used for neoplastic conditions, but much less frequently, benign conditions are also managed with RT. RT is an effective management for cancer in both the curative and palliative settings. The optimal utilisation rate of radiotherapy, prescribed at least once over the cancer journey for all patients diagnosed with cancer, has been calculated at 52 % [1].

M. Wichmann, G. Maddern (eds.), *Palliative Surgery*,
DOI 10.1007/978-3-642-53709-7_8, © Springer-Verlag Berlin Heidelberg 2014

Similar to surgery, RT is a local therapy with treatment effects limited to the organ/site treated, and toxicities are dependent upon a number of factors such as total radiation dose, dose per daily treatment, volume of normal tissue irradiated, and concurrent systemic therapy, in addition to patient factors of age, performance status, and comorbidity.

RT as a palliative modality can be used both as an addition to palliative surgery, such as following the resection of a cerebral metastasis, and as an alternative to surgery, such as resection for malignant epidural spinal cord compression.

This chapter provides a general introduction to the principles of radiotherapy, and palliative radiotherapy in particular, including discussion of various primary and secondary organ subsites where radiotherapy has a specific palliative role.

8.2 General Principles of Radiotherapy

8.2.1 Physics and Radiobiology

Therapeutic radiation is ionising, describing its capability of interacting with biological molecules to cause breaks in chemical bonds, either directly or via production of free radicals. DNA in the nucleus of the cancer cell is considered the most important biological target, with mitotic cell death due to radiation more common than apoptotic death [2].

The energy of therapeutic radiation is in a far higher range than diagnostic radiation, which uses low energy kilovoltage radiation. The majority of RT is delivered via photons produced electronically by linear accelerators of energy range 4–18 MV (megavoltage energy). Production of gamma rays by cobalt units is no longer a feature of contemporary radiation oncology departments. Electrons of similar energy range are also produced and are suitable for treating more superficially placed disease sites. The advantage of megavoltage photons is the ability to treat locations deep in the body, with relative sparing of the overlying skin due to the phenomenon of "build up" with higher energies. Less often radiotherapy is delivered with lower energy superficial (30–100 kV), or the poorly named deep X-rays (200–300 kV), or via brachytherapy using radioisotopes of kilovoltage range energies, such as iridium-192 of average 370 kV.

Radiation dose is measured in the unit Gray (Gy), which is a very small amount of energy (1 Gy = 1 J/kg). The historical unit of the Rad is smaller than the Gray (1 Gy = 100 Rads). The unit Gray is thus a measure of concentration, rather than a measure of total quantity of dose administered. By way of example, the mean lethal total body dose for humans (LD50) is 4 Gy, [2], but 4 Gy delivered to a small volume, such as one litre of lung, is a dose than can be safely delivered once daily for 5 consecutive days.

Typically RT is administered as a course of treatment in daily doses, known as fractions, as they represent fractions of the whole (total) dose prescribed. Single doses delivered as sole treatment are often used for palliation in circumstances, where the prognosis is particularly poor, and are commonly referred to as "single fractions", although this sounds a misnomer.

Fractionation of radiotherapy has a very important radiobiological basis. Generally, for a single dose, malignant cell populations differ from normal tissue populations in regard to their degree of cellular damage at low dose levels. This is due to differing balances of lethal and sublethal damage at the cellular level. The relative lethal effect on malignant cell populations is greater at these low dose levels. To exploit these differences, an interval of at least 6 h between low doses allows recovery of sublethal damage, such that the effect of low dose levels is repeated to the advantage of the normal tissue population. Fractionation thus allows relative sparing of effects on normal tissues relative to malignant cells. Although some of this advantage of fractionation is lost with palliative schedules using larger daily doses, the total dose remains low and hence minimises the potential for normal tissue toxicity.

Other advantages of fractionation are to allow redistribution of the malignant cell population to more radiosensitive phases of the cell cycle and reoxygenation of less oxygenated regions, which improves the radiosensitivity of malignant cells. A treatment course cannot be extended indefinitely with very small doses, however, as repopulation of malignant clonogens would exceed cell death achieved due to treatment.

8.2.2 Radiotherapy Planning and Delivery

Most radiotherapy is delivered as external beam radiotherapy (EBRT), while internal radiotherapy (brachytherapy) is a more subspecialised treatment, often involving greater preparation. The process of planning and delivering a course of radiotherapy may involve a number of steps. Palliative RT is generally more simplified, and so does not involve all of the complex preparation steps outlined next, and thus is less time-consuming and resource dependent and allows for RT to be delivered sooner.

The initial preparation involves simulating the proposed treatment position/setup to ensure a comfortable and accurately reproducible position for treatment. This may be achieved with particular devices such as head or body casts and shoulder or hip cradles and confirmed using wall-mounted laser lines and discreet skin ink tattoo points. Generally, computerised tomography (CT) images are obtained to allow determination of both treatment volume(s) and tissue electron densities for computerised dosimetry. A planning target volume (PTV) is determined based on all available clinical, radiological, and pathological information on the macroscopic and microscopic tumour location, including use of magnetic resonance imaging (MRI) and positron emission tomography (PET) fusion where beneficial. The particular technique then chosen will aim to deliver a uniform dose to the PTV, with the least possible dose beyond this volume. Organs at risk (OARs) are identified to determine toxicity risks based on dose and volume irradiated. Contemporary treatment planning uses computerised dosimetry with a wide number of commercial planning systems, capable of generating complex plans in very short periods of time, allowing an increased number of alternative plans for consideration. Planning can be simply two dimensional (2D) (Fig. 8.1) or three dimensional (3D) where multiple axial levels are calculated.

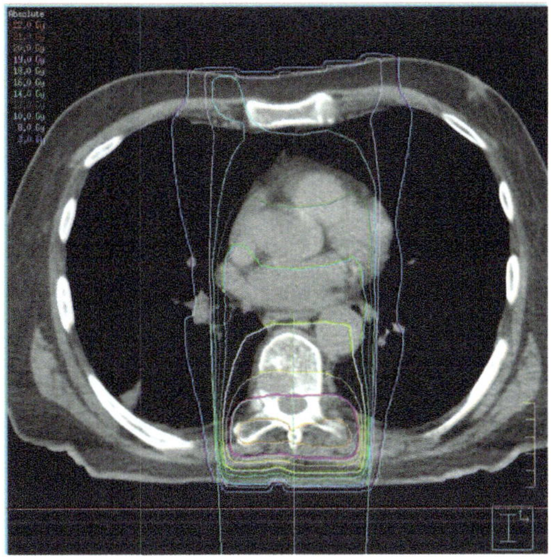

Fig. 8.1 Two-dimensional treatment dosimetry plan for treatment of a vertebral body metastasis

Higher-level planning includes intensity modulated radiotherapy (IMRT), where the fluence of the photon beam may be manipulated by static or dynamic multi-leaf collimation, to produce a dose distribution more conformal, or shaped, to the tumour position. IMRT is not a process that is applicable to lower doses of RT used for palliative intent.

In order to achieve the planning outcomes on the treatment couch, multiple quality assurance (QA) processes are needed, both at daily and less regular intervals, on the treatment equipment and for the individual patient. The individual patient setup is confirmed, including regular radiographic images. A modern multiple energy linear accelerator is capable of delivering a wide range of photon and electron energies (Fig. 8.2).

8.2.3 General Clinical Considerations

8.2.3.1 Palliative Radiotherapy Versus Curative Radiotherapy

A broad distinction is generally made between curative radiotherapy, where the goal of therapy

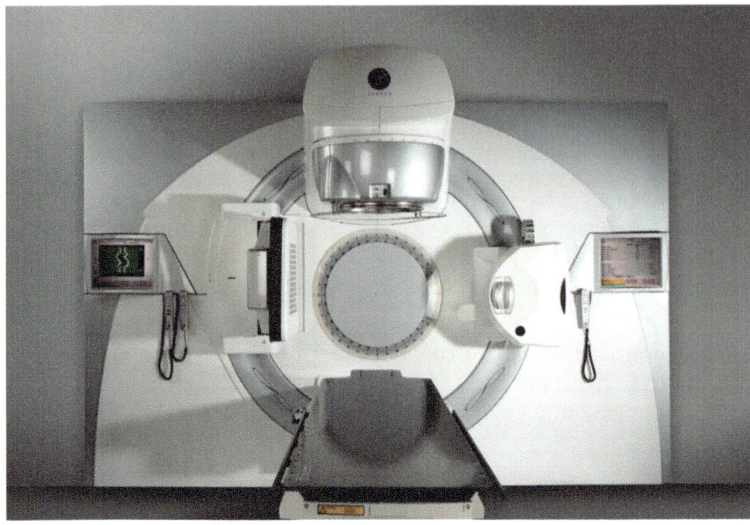

Fig. 8.2 An example of a modern linear accelerator (Elekta, Sweden)

is eradication of all malignant clonogens to effect cure, and palliative radiotherapy, where the general principle is symptom control, with the lowest effective dose. Symptom control can be achieved at lower radiation doses without the requirement of complete sterilisation of the malignant population. By way of example, pain control of symptomatic bony metastases has been achieved in a high proportion of studies with low doses such as a single dose of 8 Gy, compared to effective curative doses of 60 Gy or more for the same pathological cell population.

Palliative radiotherapy enjoys a number of considerable logistical advantages relative to curative radiotherapy:

- Lower total doses with fewer daily treatments per total dose
  - For example, a typical dose scheduled for brain metastases is 20 Gy in 5 daily fractions at 4 Gy/day delivered over 5 consecutive days
- Shorter schedules, leading to easier treatment schedules for less fit patients
- Simpler techniques for delivery of radiotherapy allowing a shorter period for treatment planning and thus earlier delivery of treatment
- Reduced toxicities (short and long term) due to lower total doses

8.2.3.2 Symptom Management

There are a number of common symptoms due to advanced cancer where palliative radiotherapy has an established role. These symptoms can exist at a variety of sites and be due to either primary or secondary disease. The most commonly encountered symptoms are those of pain, bleeding, obstruction, and compression.

Commonly encountered symptoms where radiotherapy is an effective treatment option include:

- Pain from skeletal metastases
- Bleeding from a variety of epithelial carcinomas such as within the bronchus, cervix, bladder, or rectum
- Obstruction of a lumen such as the bronchus or oesophagus
- Compression of normal tissues such as the brain parenchyma, spinal cord, and superior vena cava

8.2.3.3 Primary Versus Secondary Sites

Although the doses of radiotherapy to deliver effective palliation do not differ with respect to the site being either primary or secondary, it is important to consider this aspect when determining the radiation schedule. Patients with incurable but only local disease may benefit from a higher yet palliative dose to deliver more durable symptom control. Generally, the prognosis is better in the absence of significant metastatic burden, and recurrence of symptoms over time is more likely with lower radiation doses. For a terminal patient with symptomatic secondary disease, the lowest effective dose to achieve symptomatic relief is chosen.

8.2.3.4 Pathology Type

Inherent radiosensitivity between different pathological diagnoses influences the radiotherapy dose prescription. Non-Hodgkin's lymphoma (NHL) and Hodgkin's disease are particularly radiosensitive malignancies, and very effective palliation can be achieved with low doses. A retrospective study of 54 patients with indolent NHL found a dose of 4 Gy in two doses of 2 Gy each achieved an overall response rate of 81 %, with a 2-year rate for freedom from local progression of 50 %. Complete response rates of 57 and 27 % were achieved in masses <5 cm and >10 cm respectively. Symptom improvement was recorded in 92 % of sites [3]. The significance of such radiosensitivity is achievement of sustained palliation with minimal toxicity impact, such that large abdominal masses, for example, can be managed effectively. The radiobiological basis to explain such radiosensitivity of follicular NHL has been reported as apoptosis of NHL cells and an elicited immune response [4].

Other pathological diagnoses, although without such inherent radiosensitivity, can be effectively palliated with acceptably low doses of radiation, including carcinoma, melanoma, and sarcoma.

Melanoma has historically been viewed as a radioresistant malignancy based in part on early in vivo cell survival data for cultured cells. This resulted in the recommendation of large individual fraction sizes for melanoma, with the clinical basis for this recommendation based on studies with small patient numbers, heterogeneous doses, and tumour sizes and with short follow-up [5]. The impact of large fraction sizes is potentionally greater toxicity to normal tissues. In support of the radioresponsiveness of melanoma to conventional RT, a review of 26 patients with 39 bone metastases found a palliative response rate of 85 %, with fraction sizes of up to 3 Gy effective in 15 of 19 bony lesions [6].

A randomised study of 137 patients [7] comparing a few large doses (32 Gy in 4 fractions of 8 Gy) with a higher number of smaller doses (50 Gy in 20 fractions of 2.5 Gy) demonstrated meaningful responses for melanoma. For a variety of sites, the majority being soft tissue/skin, equivalent response rates of 60 % versus 58 % and equivalent complete response rates of 24 and 23 % were found. Thus, large fraction sizes above 4 Gy are not necessary to achieve palliative end points for melanoma. What is not immediately obvious is that the trial 32 Gy schedule is calculated as a much greater dose to normal tissues (due to the radiobiological impact of large doses), and as such the 50 Gy schedule achieved palliation with significantly less risk to normal tissue. It is also worth noting the response rate that was achieved, which is highly superior to historical systemic cytotoxic therapies.

8.3 Primary Site Palliation

8.3.1 Lung/Respiratory

A systematic review of palliative thoracic RT for lung cancer [8] examined 13 studies with 3,473 patients included. Complete response rates for palliation of haemoptysis ranged from 68 to 73 %, complete response rates for chest pain ranged from 51 to 57 %, and improvement in cough ranged from 48 to 53 %. Total symptom score and survival were both significantly improved in the higher RT dose group. The lack of quality of life assessment in this review is a limitation, but it can be concluded that patients with better performance status have a modest benefit with a longer course of RT [9].

Brachytherapy is an option for palliation of endobronchial tumours where airway obstruction exists. The dosimetric advantage of brachytherapy relates to the avoidance of delivering radiation through normal lung tissue to access the disease site. Thus retreatment of the lung may be better tolerated with reduced lung and adjacent tissue toxicity. A study of 406 patients [10] treated with intraluminal brachytherapy of the bronchus included 324 patients having initial treatment with this approach. Response rates for haemoptysis (82 %) and stridor (92 %) at 6 weeks were maintained at similar levels at 4 months posttreatment. Similarly a smaller study of 76 patients [11] found excellent response rates for intraluminal brachytherapy. Haemoptysis responded in 95 % of cases, with bronchoscopic assessment at 1–3 months finding a total response rate of 87 %. In a series of 175 patients [12] where the vast majority had received previous external RT, 66 % showed symptomatic improvement, with bronchoscopic improvement in obstruction, to at least 50 % of lumen reopened, reported in 78 %. Survival was significantly improved in the symptomatic responders. Brachytherapy is, however, a more resource-intensive treatment than EBRT, requiring bronchoscopic access, and is used less often due to such factors.

Superior vena cava obstruction (SVCO) occurs with a variety of malignancies, but lung cancer is the principal cause. Provided that no airway obstruction/respiratory compromise exists, therapy can be delayed to allow a histological diagnosis to be made in advance of treatment. Effective palliation can be achieved with RT, with a systematic review of lung cancer patients with SVCO [13] finding complete relief of symptoms within 2 weeks in 78 % of small-cell and 63 % of non-small-cell lung cancer. Endovascular stenting was also reviewed, achieving relief of symptoms in 95 % of more than 150 patients stented. Stenting allows rapid relief of symptoms and as such is very useful for severely symptomatic patients, particularly with non-chemotherapy-sensitive pathologies, and relapsed previously treated patients. Chemosensitive malignancies (small-cell lung cancer, NHL, germ cell tumours) are managed systemically, with the expectation of a rapid response.

Reirradiation of locally recurrent lung cancer can achieve effective palliation of symptoms with low rates of high-grade toxicity, based on a review of published studies [14], with a haemoptysis response rate of 83–100 %.

8.3.2 Gastrointestinal

Oesophageal cancer most commonly presents with dysphagia due to partial or complete obstruction. A review of 127 patients [15] treated with RT found an overall improvement in dysphagia in 70 % with maintenance of food passage to death in 54 %. Higher doses of RT achieved much more durable palliation of dysphagia. A randomised comparison of single-dose brachytherapy with metal stent placement included 209 patients with dysphagia of the oesophagus or oesophagogastric junction [16]. Although relief of dysphagia was slower with brachytherapy than stenting, long-term relief of dysphagia and quality of life scoring were better with brachytherapy, with complications more often with stenting. The presence of a malignant fistula with oesophageal cancer is not a contraindication for RT. Successful fistula closure with combined chemoradiotherapy has been recorded in 17 of 24 patients, with 16 returning to oral nutrition [17].

Locally advanced or recurrent colorectal cancer may present with pain, bleeding, and/or obstruction. In a review of 80 patients with a symptomatic pelvic mass due to metastatic colorectal cancer [18], with symptoms of pain (68 cases), bleeding (18 cases), and obstruction (9 cases), RT achieved symptom palliation in 80 % of cases. Median duration of symptom control was 5 months, with significant factors for duration of symptom control being higher RT dose and concurrent chemotherapy. Reirradiation is feasible for rectal cancer. A review of 50 patients reirradiated for rectal cancer found that a dose of 30–39 Gy was well tolerated, with 3-year local control rate of 21 % for patients not receiving further surgery [19].

8.3.3 Genitourinary/Gynaecological

Locally advanced bladder cancer may often present with haematuria. Patients may not be fit for repeated cystoscopic resection, with palliative RT a less invasive option for palliation. In a randomised study of patients unsuitable for radical management of muscle invasive bladder cancer

[20], data on 274 patients analysed at 3 months following randomisation to either 35 Gy in 10 daily treatments with 21 Gy in 3 daily doses of 7 Gy found improvement in haematuria at 3 months in 63 % with no difference detected in efficacy or toxicity between the 2 arms.

Cervix cancer may present as locally advanced disease and be unsuitable for curative treatment due to metastatic disease and/or poor performance status. Pelvic symptoms of bleeding or pain are often the presenting symptoms. A systematic review [21] analysed five series using multiple doses of 10 Gy, separated over one or more weeks, for response of symptoms of bleeding and pain, with partial (>50 %) or complete improvement for bleeding of 80–100 % and pain of 50–100 %. Although this review supports repeated large doses for symptom improvement, durations of improvement and toxicities were poorly recorded, and for patients with a better immediate prognosis, a more conventional dose may be preferable.

8.4 Metastatic Site Palliation

8.4.1 Brain Metastases

Brain metastases are a common problem in a variety of malignancies, and more common than primary intracranial tumours, with 25 % of patients with lung cancer developing brain metastases [22]. The central nervous system (CNS) is also a sanctuary site for cytotoxic agents, which is a factor in the development of brain metastases. Commonly patients present with symptoms due to effects of raised intracranial pressure (headache, vomiting) or neurological loss.

Optimal management depends on assessment of a number of factors, including the patient's performance status, age, and presence or otherwise of extracranial disease. Prognostic classes (classes 1, 2, and 3) have been created based on these factors [23], with validation in a further trial [24].

Neurosurgical resection and stereotactic radiosurgery (SRS) are both options for patients in the better prognostic class 1. Whole brain RT (WBRT) is generally recommended following surgery or SRS. Randomised trials have studied surgery and postoperative WBRT, compared to WBRT alone. Patchell et al. [25] found that surgery significantly improved survival (40 vs. 15 weeks), control of recurrence, and quality of life, with Noordijk et al. [26] finding significantly improved survival (10 months vs. 6 months) also with surgery. Better outcomes occurred with less active extracranial disease. Kocher et al. [27] reported on a randomised study of 359 patients who underwent surgery or SRS for one to three brain metastases and then randomised to WBRT or observation. Adjuvant RT reduced intracranial relapses, but overall survival was similar.

Patients in a poorer prognostic class are not suitable for surgery or SRS and better managed with WBRT or supportive care alone as options. Median survival with supportive care alone is generally 1–2 months, with WBRT increasing median survival to 3–6 months.

Two randomised WBRT studies comparing commonly used schedules [28] assessed neurological symptom relief, finding an overall rate of improvement in neurological function of 47 and 52 % for the two studies. Median duration of improvement for neurological function was 10–12 weeks and overall survival 15 weeks and 18 weeks for the two studies. Partial or complete relief of specific neurological symptoms occurred in 60–90 % of patients. For the different dose schedules studied, none had an advantage with respect to frequency or duration of improvement or survival.

A recent randomised study of higher doses of WBRT in more favourable patients [29] has compared 40 Gy in 20 twice-daily fractions with 20 Gy in 4 daily fractions, with 36 % of patients receiving prior resection of a solitary brain lesion. Late toxicity was uncommon, and no different between the arms. Intracranial progression and salvage surgery or RT were all significantly less frequent in the higher dose arm of the trial, without any survival difference. In conclusion it was commented that for subgroups of better prognosis patients, a higher dose schedule should be considered. A further randomised study of 90 patients [30], with similar treatment arms, also found improved control of CNS progression with a higher dose schedule, but with no survival advantage.

Typically WBRT schedules of 20 Gy in 5 daily doses or 30 Gy in 10 daily doses are prescribed. Treatment is generally well tolerated, with side effects of alopecia and possible fatigue.

Reirradiation may be beneficial for some patients who have a longer progression-free interval after initial WBRT. A review of 86 retreated patients with a median retreatment dose of 20 Gy found a neurological symptom overall response rate of 70 %, with a median survival of 4 months [31]. Less encouraging results were found in a review of 44 reirradiated patients, receiving cumulative WBRT doses of 38–75 Gy, with partial neurological improvement in only 27 %, median survival of 8 weeks, and 3 of 8 brain necropsies demonstrating brain necrosis [32]. Partial brain radiation is better tolerated than WBRT, and the risk of late toxicity is assessed against the risk of neurological loss due to disease progression.

8.4.2 Metastatic Spinal Cord Compression (MSCC)

Malignant spinal cord compression is recognised as an emergency condition due to the irreversible neurological effect of prolonged compression. It is a common complication from a variety of primary cancers, affecting 5–14 % of cancer patients at some stage in the disease course [33], with the clinical outcome dependent on factors of degree, rate and duration of neurological loss, histopathology type, and rapidity of treatment. Patients may present after a period of days or weeks of increasing spinal pain, possibly with a radicular pattern, followed by neurological deficit, featuring as leg weakness and paraesthesia, with urinary retention, or as an acute presentation with leg weakness or paraplegia.

Early diagnosis is important for prognosis [34, 35], with neurological function at the time of diagnosis predicting for the success of treatment for recovery of neurological loss [36]. Magnetic resonance imaging (MRI) is the optimal method of diagnosis (Fig. 8.3), and the possibility of multiple levels of compression requires imaging of the length of the spine. Initial treatment is with glucocorticoids, typically dexamethasone at doses of 16 mg daily, with opiate-based analgesia. A Cochrane meta-analysis of three trials of differing dose levels was unable to determine clinical benefit and optimal dosage [37], with higher doses associated with serious toxicities [38].

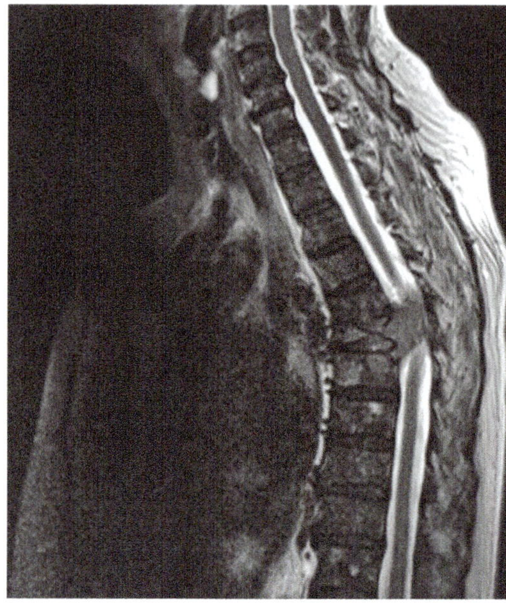

Fig. 8.3 MRI demonstrating extradural cord compression

Treatment options include surgery, radiotherapy, and supportive care alone. Surgery as a treatment option for MSCC using laminectomy with postoperative RT failed to show an advantage compared to RT alone [39]. A randomised study of aggressive surgical debulking with postoperative RT versus RT alone of 30 Gy in 10 fractions [40] found that significantly more surgical patients were able to walk after treatment (84 % vs. 57 %), surgical patients retained the ability to walk for significantly longer (median 122 days vs. 13 days), and significantly more surgical patients regained the ability to walk (62 % vs. 19 %), necessitating early trial closure at interim analysis. In contrast, a matched pair analysis [33] found similar outcomes for improvement in motor function and ambulatory rate post treatment for the surgical and RT alone groups, but with surgical complications an additional factor.

Surgery is a more demanding management approach where patients may already be of poor performance status due to advanced malignancy. The general cancer prognosis and suitability for surgery must be considered alongside other factors of MSCC site, duration of neurological loss, and histopathological type. Radiotherapy is more frequently the sole method of treatment for MSCC. EBRT also produces effective palliation of pain in a significant proportion of patients.

In a randomised trial of two dose schedules with 276 patients with MSCC [41], pain relief (complete or partial) was achieved in 57 %, 90 % of ambulatory patients maintained this level of function, and 35 % of non walking patients regained function. This trial also found a shorter schedule of 2 doses of 8 Gy as effective as an 8 day schedule for response and duration of response. A variety of EBRT dose schedules have been used, and an ongoing randomised trial (SCORAD III) is recruiting patients to either a single-dose schedule or a conventional fractionated schedule.

Retreatment of MSCC is possible with EBRT, with a small review finding maintenance of walking in six of seven patients for a median duration of 4.5 months [42]. Above doses of 50 Gy at conventional daily doses of 2 Gy, there is an increasing risk of radiation myelitis; however, in general the malignancy represents a much greater risk to neurological function than the potential risk of exceeding radiotolerance.

8.4.3 Skeletal Metastases

Bone metastases are a common development in a high proportion of cancer diagnoses, with pain and reduction in quality of life a frequent occurrence. Skeletal metastases may cause complications of pathological fracture, nerve root irritation/compression, and epidural spinal cord compression. Radiotherapy is a highly effective method of palliation for pain, resulting in an improvement in quality of life, with an analgesic benefit at relatively low doses. Comparison in randomised trials of single doses with fractionated schedules has consistently found equivalent palliation, but with improved patient convenience and reduced costs with the shorter schedule. These trials have compared a single dose of 8 Gy with a variety of schedules, including 20 Gy in 4 or 5 daily doses, 24 Gy/6, and 30 Gy/10 [43–47] (Table 8.1).

In summary, pain responses of 62–78 % were recorded, with no differences for single versus fractionated schedules. The requirement for retreatment was consistently higher for the single-dose arms, although greater physician willingness to retreat after a lower dose has been postulated as a factor to explain the variability in retreatment rates [45]. Lutz et al. [48] documented the ASTRO evidence-based guidelines where pain relief equivalency was shown between fractionated and single 8 Gy fractions, with a systematic review by Chow et al. [49] supporting this conclusion.

Retreatment with radiation for initially unresponsive or relapsed pain can achieve beneficial

Table 8.1 Randomised trials of single-dose versus fractionated RT for painful bone metastases

Author	RT schedules	Patient numbers	Overall pain response (%)	Complete pain response (%)
Steenland et al. [43]	8 Gy	585	72	37
	4 Gy × 6	586	69	33
Hartsell et al. [45]	8 Gy	455	66	15
	3 Gy × 10	443	66	18
Yarnold [46]	8 Gy	383	78	57
	4 Gy × 5[a]	378	78	58
Nielsen et al. [47]	8 Gy	122	62	15
	5 Gy × 4	119	71	15

[a]2 % of multifraction received 3 Gy × 10

results. A systematic review and meta-analysis of reirradiation of 2,694 patients across 7 studies [50] found that 527 received repeat radiation, with a demonstrated pain response in 58 %. The duration of response ranged from 15 to 22 weeks. Retreatment of pain relapse with a dose as low as 4 Gy has shown a 74 % response rate and a response rate of 46 % for patients initially not responding [51]. There is an ongoing international randomised trial currently addressing the question of the optimal fractionation schedule for reirradiation of skeletal metastases.

Neuropathic pain due to skeletal metastases is a common complication, presenting with referred pain. RT is effective in achieving analgesia, with a randomised comparison [52] of a single 8 Gy versus 20 Gy in 5 daily doses demonstrating analgesic benefit, with a nonsignificant difference between the two arms (53 % vs. 61 %).

Therapeutic radioisotopes of strontium-89 and samarium-153 have been used successfully as intravenous radiopharmaceuticals to target osteoblastic bone metastases, particularly for prostate and breast cancer. Strontium-89 is a pure beta emitter (electrons), meaning a short range of radiation effect, and is biologically treated as an imitator of calcium [53], with incorporation into the bony structure by osteoblasts. Due to uptake throughout the skeleton at sites of osteoblastic activity, widespread metastases may be treated rather than the limited site(s) of external beam RT. Myelosuppression is the principal toxicity, with thrombocytopenia and leucopenia relative contraindications to treatment.

The TransCanada Strontium-89 Study [53], where 126 patients were randomised to placebo or strontium-89 after local field EBRT, demonstrated the ability of strontium in addition to local field EBRT to significantly reduce the future intake of analgesics and development of new sites of pain. Comparison of strontium-89 with EBRT in a randomised comparison [54] found similar pain improvement sustained to 3 months of 66 % versus 63 % but also a delay in the development of new pain sites with strontium-89. Average falls in platelet and white cell counts of 30–40 % were found with strontium-89. A randomised comparison of samarium-153 with placebo for a variety of malignancies [55] demonstrated significant benefits with the active treatment. Pain relief of 62–72 % was observed in the first month, with maintenance of analgesia in 43 % at 4 months.

Surgical management is often required for a pathological fracture involving a long bone or as prophylaxis for a fracture risk. Postoperative radiotherapy is routinely delivered postoperatively.

8.4.4 Hepatic Metastases

RT can offer palliation of painful hepatic metastases, as shown in a prospective study of 103 patients with solid hepatic metastases [56]. RT was delivered with a number of dose schedules. Pain improved in 55 % of patients, with treatment well tolerated and with no cases of radiation-induced hepatitis. There are many possible therapeutic modalities on offer for hepatic metastases, with RT possibly underutilised, but further study is needed to gain a clearer understanding of the role for RT.

8.5 Summary

Palliative RT has widespread application as an effective modality for symptom management of primary and secondary disease. A typical palliative treatment involves simple preparation and is delivered as a short course, aiming for minimal demands upon the palliative patient.

References

1. Delaney G, Jacob S, Featherstone C, Barton M. The role of radiotherapy in cancer treatment: estimating optimal utilization from a review of evidence-based clinical guidelines. Cancer. 2005;104(6):1129–37.
2. Hall EJ. Radiobiology for the radiologist. Philadelphia: Lippincott Williams and Wilkins; 2000.
3. Chan EK, Fung S, Gospodarowicz M, Hodgson D, Wells W, Sun A, Pintile M, Tsang RW. Palliation by low-dose local radiation therapy for indolent non-Hodgkin lymphoma. Int J Radiat Oncol Biol Phys. 2011;81(5):e781.
4. Ganem G, Cartron G, Girinsky T, Haas RL, Cosset JM, Solal-Celigny P. Localized low-dose radiotherapy for follicular lymphoma: history, clinical results,

mechanisms of action, and future outlooks. Int J Radiat Oncol Biol Phys. 2010;78(4):975.

5. Trott K-R. The optimal radiation dose per fraction for the treatment of malignant melanomas. Int J Radiat Oncol Biol Phys. 1991;20:905–7.
6. Rate WR, Solin LJ, Turrisi AT. Palliative radiotherapy for metastatic malignant melanoma: brain metastases, bone metastases, and spinal cord compression. Int J Radiat Oncol Biol Phys. 1988;15(4):859.
7. Sause WT, Cooper JS, Rush S, Ago CT, Cosmatos D, Coughlin CT, JanJan N, Lipsett J. Fraction size in external beam radiation therapy in the treatment of melanoma. Int J Radiat Oncol Biol Phys. 1991;20(3):429–32.
8. Fairchild A, Harris K, Barnes E, Wong R, Lutz S, Bezjak A, Cheung P, Chow E. Palliative thoracic radiotherapy for lung cancer: a systematic review. J Clin Oncol. 2008;26(24):4001–11.
9. Wagner Jr H. Just enough palliation: radiation dose and outcome in patients with non-small-cell lung cancer. J Clin Oncol. 2008;26(24):3920–2.
10. Gollins SW, Burt PA, Barber PV, Stout R. High dose rate intraluminal radiotherapy for carcinoma of the bronchus: outcome of treatment of 406 patients. Radiother Oncol. 1994;33:31–40.
11. Chang Li-Fen L, Horvath J, Peyton W, Ling SS. High dose rate afterloading intraluminal brachytherapy in malignant airway obstruction of lung cancer. Int J Radiat Oncol Biol Phys. 1994;28(3):589–96.
12. Kelly JF, Delclos ME, Morice RC, Huaringa A, Allen PK, Komaki R. High dose rate endobronchial brachytherapy effectively palliates symptoms due to airway tumors: the 10-year M.D. Anderson Cancer Centre experience. Int J Radiat Oncol Biol Phys. 2000;48(3):697–702.
13. Rowell NP, Gleeson FV. Steroids, radiotherapy, chemotherapy and stents for superior vena caval obstruction in carcinoma of the bronchus: a systematic review. Clin Oncol (R Coll Radiol). 2002;14(5):338–51.
14. Jeremić B, Videtic GMM. Chest reirradiation with external beam radiotherapy for locally recurrent non-small-cell lung cancer: a review. Int J Radiat Oncol Biol Phys. 2011;80(4):969–77.
15. Caspers RJ, Welvaart K, Verkes RJ, Hermans J, Leer JW. The effect of radiotherapy on dysphagia and survival in patients with esophageal cancer. Radiother Oncol. 1988;12(1):15.
16. Homs MY, Steyerberg EW, Eijkenboom WM, Tilanus HW, Stalpers LJ, Bartelsman JF, van Lanschot JJ, Wijrdeman HK, Mulder CJ, Reinders JG, Boot H, Aleman BM, Kuipers EJ, Siersema PD. Single-dose brachytherapy versus metal stent placement for the palliation of dysphagia from oesophageal cancer: multicentre randomised trial. Lancet. 2004;364(9444):1497.
17. Muto M, Ohtsu A, Miyamoto S, Muro K, Boku N, Ishikura S, Satake M, Ogino T, Tajiri H, Yoshida S. Concurrent chemoradiotherapy for esophageal carcinoma patients with malignant fistulae. Cancer. 1999;86(8):1406.
18. Bae SH, Park W, Choi DH, Nam H, Kang WK, Park YS, Park JO, Chun HK, Lee WY, Yun SH, Kim HC. Palliative radiotherapy in patients with a symptomatic pelvic mass of metastatic colorectal cancer. Radiat Oncol. 2011;6:52.
19. Das P, Delclos ME, Skibber JM, Rodriguez-Bigas MA, Feig BW, Chang GJ, Eng C, Bedi M, Krishnan S, Crane CH. Hyperfractionated accelerated radiotherapy for rectal cancer in patients with prior pelvic irradiation. Int J Radiat Oncol Biol Phys. 2010;77(1):60–5.
20. Duchesne GM, Bolger JJ, Griffiths GO, Trevor Roberts J, Graham JD, Hoskin PJ, Fosså SD, Uscinska BM, Parmar MKB. A randomized trial of hypofractionated schedules of palliative radiotherapy in the management of bladder carcinoma: results of Medical Research Council trial BA09. Int J Radiat Oncol Biol Phys. 2000;47(2):379–88.
21. van Lonkhuijzen L, Thomas G. Palliative radiotherapy for cervical carcinoma, a systematic review. Radiother Oncol. 2011;98:287–91.
22. Ellis R, Gregor A. The treatment of brain metastases from lung cancer. Lung Cancer. 1998;20:81–4.
23. Gaspar L, Scott C, Rotman M, Asbell S, Phillips T, Wasserman T, Gillies McKenna W, Byhardt R. Recursive partitioning analysis (RPA) of prognostic factors in three Radiation Therapy Oncology Group (RTOG) brain metastases trials. Int J Radiat Oncol Biol Phys. 1997;37(4):745–51.
24. Gaspar LE, Scott C, Murray K, Curran W. Validation of the RTOG recursive partitioning analysis (RPA) classification for brain metastases. Int J Radiat Oncol Biol Phys. 2000;47(4):1001–6.
25. Patchell RA, Tibbs PA, Walsh JW, Dempsey RJ, Maruyama Y, Kryscio RJ, Markesbery WR, Macdonald JS, Young B. A randomized trial of surgery in the treatment of single metastases to the brain. N Engl J Med. 1990;322:494–500.
26. Noordijk EM, Vecht CJ, Haaxma-Reiche H, Padberg GW, Voormolen JHC, Hoekstra FH, Tans JTJ, Lambooij N, Metsaars JAL, Wattendorff AR, Brand R, Hermans J. The choice of treatment of single brain metastasis should be based on extracranial tumor activity and age. Int J Radiat Oncol Biol Phys. 1994;29(4):711–7.
27. Kocher M, Soffietti R, Abacioglu U, Villà S, Fauchon F, Baumert BG, Fariselli L, Tzuk-Shina T, Kortmann R-D, Carrie C, Hassel MB, Kouri M, Valeinis E, van den Berge D, Collette S, Collette L, Mueller R-P. Adjuvant whole-brain radiotherapy versus observation after radiosurgery or surgical resection of one to three cerebral metastases: results of the EORTC 22952–26001 study. J Clin Oncol. 2011;29(2):134–41.
28. Borgelt B, Gelber R, Kramer S, Brady LW, Chang CH, Davis LW, Perez CA, Hendrickson FR. The palliation of brain metastases: final results of the first two studies by the Radiation Therapy Oncology Group. Int J Radiat Oncol Biol Phys. 1980;6(1):1–9.
29. Graham PH, Bucci J, Browne L. Randomized comparison of whole brain radiotherapy, 20 Gy in four

daily fractions versus 40 Gy in 20 twice-daily fractions, for brain metastases. Int J Radiat Oncol Biol Phys. 2010;77(3):648–54.
30. Davey P, Hoegler D, Ennis M, Smith J. A phase III study of accelerated versus conventional hypofractionated whole brain irradiation in patients of good performance status with brain metastases not suitable for surgical excision. Radiother Oncol. 2008;88:173–6.
31. Wong WW, Schild SE, Sawyer TE, Shaw EG. Analysis of outcome in patients reirradiated for brain metastases. Int J Radiat Oncol Biol Phys. 1996;34(3):585–90.
32. Hazuka MB, Kinzie JJ. Brain metastases: results and effects of re-irradiation. Int J Radiat Oncol Biol Phys. 1988;15(2):433–7.
33. Rades D, Huttenlocher S, Dunst J, Bajrovic A, Karstens JH, Rudat V, Schild SE. Matched pair analysis comparing surgery followed by radiotherapy and radiotherapy alone for metastatic spinal cord compression. J Clin Oncol. 2010;28(22):3597–604.
34. Leviov M, Dale J, Stein M, Ben-Shahar MB, Ben-Arush M, Milstein D, Goldsher D, Kuten A. The management of metastatic spinal cord compression: a radiotherapeutic success ceiling. Int J Radiat Oncol Biol Phys. 1993;27(2):231–4.
35. Latini P, Maranzano E, Ricci S, Aristei C, Checcaglini F, Panizza BM, Perrucci E. Role of radiotherapy in metastatic spinal cord compression: preliminary results from a prospective trial. Radiother Oncol. 1989;15(3):227–33.
36. Maranzano E, Latini P. Effectiveness of radiation therapy without surgery in metastatic spinal cord compression: final results from a prospective trial. Int J Radiat Oncol Biol Phys. 1995;32(4):959–67.
37. George R, Jeba J, Ramkumar G, Chacko AG, Leng M, Tharyan P. Interventions for the treatment of metastatic extradural spinal cord compression in adults. The Cochrane Library (Internet) 20 Jan 2010. Available from http://onlinelibrary.wiley.com/doi/10.1002/14651858.CD006716.pub2/full
38. Sorensen S, Helweg-Larsen S, Mouridsen H, Hansen HH. Effects of high-dose dexamethasone in carcinomatous metastatic spinal cord compression treated with radiotherapy: a randomised trial. Eur J Cancer. 1994;30A(1):22–7.
39. Young RF, Post EM, King GA. Treatment of spinal epidural metastases. Randomized prospective comparison of laminectomy and radiotherapy. J Neurosurg. 1980;53(6):741–8.
40. Patchell RA, Tibbs PA, Regine WF, Payne R, Saris S, Kryscio RJ, Mohiuddin M, Young B. Direct decompressive surgical resection in the treatment of spinal cord compression caused by metastatic cancer: a randomised trial. Lancet. 2005;366:643–8.
41. Maranzano E, Bellavita R, Rossi R, De Angelis V, Frattegiani A, Bagnoli R, Mignogna M, Beneventi S, Lupattelli M, Ponticelli P, Biti GP, Latini P. Short-course versus split-course radiotherapy in metastatic spinal cord compression: results of a phase III, randomized, multicenter trial. J Clin Oncol. 2005;23(15):3358–65.
42. Maranzano E, Trippa F, Casale M, Anselmo P, Rossi R. Irradiation of metastatic spinal cord compression: definitive results of two randomized trials. Radiother Oncol. 2011;98:234–7.
43. Steenland E, Leer J, van Houwelingen H, Post WJ, van den Hout WB, Kievit J, de Haes H, Martijn H, Oei B, Vonk E, van der Steen-Banasik E, Wiggenraad RGJ, Hoogenhout J, Wárlám-Rodenhuis C, van Tienhoven G, Wanders R, Pomp J, van Reijn M, van Mierlo T, Rutten E. The effect of a single fraction compared to multiple fractions on painful bone metastases: a global analysis of the Dutch Bone Metastasis Study. Radiother Oncol. 1999;52:101–9.
44. van der Linden YM, Lok JJ, Steenland E, Martijn H, van Houwelingen H, Marijnen CAM, Leer JWH. Single fraction radiotherapy is efficacious: a further analysis of the Dutch Bone Metastasis Study controlling for the influence of retreatment. Int J Radiat Oncol Biol Phys. 2004;59(2):528–37.
45. Hartsell WF, Scott CB, Bruner DW, et al. Randomized trial of short versus long-course radiotherapy for palliation of painful bone metastases. J Natl Cancer Inst. 2005;97:798.
46. Yarnold JR. 8 Gy single fraction radiotherapy for the treatment of metastatic skeletal pain: randomised comparison with a multifraction schedule over 12 months of patient follow-up on behalf of the Bone Pain Trial Working Party. Radiother Oncol. 1999; 52(2):111–21.
47. Nielsen OS, Bentzen SM, Sandberg E, Gadeberg CC, Timothy AR. Randomized trial of single dose versus fractionated palliative radiotherapy of bone metastases. Radiother Oncol. 1998;47(3):233–40.
48. Lutz S, Berk L, Chang E, Chow E, Hahn C, Hoskin P, Howell D, Konski A, Kachnic L, Lo S, Sahgal A, Silverman L, von Gunten C, Mendel E, Vassil A, Bruner DW, Hartsell W. Palliative radiotherapy for bone metastases: an ASTRO evidence-based guideline. Int J Radiat Oncol Biol Phys. 2011;79(4): 965–76.
49. Chow E, Harris K, Fan G, Tsao M, Sze WM. Palliative radiotherapy trials for bone metastases: a systematic review. J Clin Oncol. 2007;25(11):1423–36.
50. Huisman M, van den Bosch MAAJ, Wijlemans JW, van Vulpen M, van der Linden YM, Verkooijen HM. Effectiveness of reirradiation for painful bone metastases: a systematic review and meta-analysis. Int J Radiat Oncol Biol Phys. 2012;84(1):8–14.
51. Jeremic B, Shibamoto Y, Igrutinovic I. Single 4 Gy re-irradiation for painful bone metastasis following single fraction radiotherapy. Radiother Oncol. 1999;52:123–7.
52. Roos DE, Turner SL, O'Brien PC, Smith JG, Spry NA, Burmeister BH, Hoskin PJ, Ball DL. Randomized trial of 8 Gy in 1 versus 20 Gy in 5 fractions of radiotherapy for neuropathic pain due to bone metastases (Trans-Tasman Radiation Oncology Group, TROG 96.05). Radiother Oncol. 2005;75:54–63.
53. Porter AT, McEwan AJB, Powe JE, Reid R, McGowan DG, Lukka H, Sathyanarayana JR, Yakemchuk VN,

Thomas GM, Erlich LE, Crook J, Gulenchyn KY, Hong KE, Wesolowski C, Yardley J. Results of a randomized Phase-III trial to evaluate the efficacy of Strontium-89 adjuvant to local field external beam irradiation in the management of endocrine resistant metastatic prostate cancer. Int J Radiat Oncol Biol Phys. 1993;25:805–13.
54. Quilty PM, Kirk D, Bolger JJ, Dearnaley DP, Lewington VJ, Mason MD, Reed NSE, Russell JM, Yardley J. A comparison of the palliative effects of strontium-89 and external beam radiotherapy in metastatic prostate cancer. Radiother Oncol. 1994;31:33–40.
55. Serafino AN, Houston SJ, Resche I, Quick DP, Grund FM, Ell PJ, Bertrand A, Ahmann FR, Orihuela E, Reid RH, Lerski RA, Collier BD, McKillop JH, Purnell GL, Pecking AP, Thomas FD, Harrison KA. Palliation of pain associated with metastatic bone cancer using Samarium-153 Lexidronam: a double-blind placebo-controlled clinical trial. J Clin Oncol. 1998;16(4):1574–81.
56. Borgelt BB, Gelber R, Brady LW, Griffin T, Hendrickson FR. The palliation of hepatic metastases: results of the Radiation Therapy Oncology Group pilot study. Int J Radiat Oncol Biol Phys. 1981;7(5):587–91.

Image-Guided Interventions 9

Oliver Ayres and Frank Voyvodic

Contents

O. Ayres, MBBS, FRANZCR (✉)
Department of Medical Imaging, Flinders Medical Centre, Bedford Park 5042, SA, Australia

Benson Radiology, 229 Melbourne Street, North Adelaide 5006, SA, Australia
e-mail: oliver.ayres@health.sa.gov.au

F. Voyvodic, MBBS(Hons), FRANZCR
Benson Radiology, 229 Melbourne Street, North Adelaide 5006, SA, Australia

Department of Medical Imaging, Flinders Medical Centre, Bedford Park 5042, SA, Australia
e-mail: voyvodicfrank@bensonradiology.com.au

Image-guided procedures are increasingly utilised in oncology patients in diagnosis and management, with both curative and palliative intent, and are often performed in interventional radiology. Interventional radiologists, given their background in diagnostic imaging, can provide useful input to the multidisciplinary team caring for oncology patients with regard to technical feasibility of diagnostic and therapeutic interventions and their likely outcomes. This chapter aims to outline available interface between interventional radiology and the rest of the multidisciplinary team in caring for palliative patients, focusing on common conditions and how imaging can be used in assessment.

M. Wichmann, G. Maddern (eds.), *Palliative Surgery*,
DOI 10.1007/978-3-642-53709-7_9, © Springer-Verlag Berlin Heidelberg 2014

9.1 Introduction

Image-guided procedures are increasingly utilised in oncology patients in diagnosis and management, with both curative and palliative intent [1–3], and are often performed in interventional radiology [4]. Diagnostic procedures and those with therapeutic palliative intent shall be discussed in a variety of conditions. Interventional radiologists, given their background in diagnostic imaging, can provide useful input to the multidisciplinary team caring for oncology patients with regard to technical feasibility of interventions and their likely outcomes [5]. This chapter aims to outline available interface between interventional radiology and the rest of the multidisciplinary team in caring for palliative patients, focusing on common conditions and how imaging can be used in assessment.

9.2 Background

As with all interventions in palliative care, image-guided procedures aim to provide symptom relief and/or improvement in quality of life without adding to patient morbidity, so the overall benefits of the intervention should outweigh the risks [1, 5, 6]. Image-guided procedures can be performed with ultrasound (US), fluoroscopy, computed tomography (CT) and less commonly magnetic resonance imaging (MRI) [7]. Each modality has its strengths and weaknesses, and some procedures utilise a combination of modalities, for example, ultrasound for initial bile duct access in percutaneous biliary drainage followed by fluoroscopic guidance for the remainder of the procedure [7].

The majority of therapeutic image-guided procedures utilise a technique of gaining needle access to a body structure or cavity, maintaining access via insertion of a wire through the needle and then insertion of a device (catheter or drain) over the wire [7, 8]. This concept was initially developed by Sven-Ivar Seldinger for angiographic vascular access and first reported in 1953 [8]. The technique has since been modified for other body sites and structures, and is now commonly known as the modified Seldinger technique [7, 9].

It is common to think of radiological interventional procedures as minimally invasive just because they do not take place in an operating theatre per se. Many of the procedures described in this text can be performed under local anaesthetic, but some of the procedures are more invasive than others and can require a general anaesthetic, with others best performed with a combination of analgesia and sedation [7]. It is important to provide adequate procedural and periprocedural analgesia, and this is a dual responsibility of the referrer or treating team, as well as the operator of the procedure (interventional radiologist). Coagulation parameters should be optimised before any invasive procedure, and a useful reference was published in the *Journal of Vascular and Interventional Radiology* [10].

9.3 Diagnosis and Staging

Patients presenting with untreatable disease but without a histological diagnosis may need biopsy to confirm histological diagnosis prior to commencement of palliative therapies (e.g. some chemotherapies). Image-guided percutaneous biopsy is increasingly used to confirm histological diagnosis (Fig. 9.1a, b) [2, 11] and can even help to stage a malignancy, if sampling a metastatic lesion [2, 12]. Nearly any organ or body site can be accessed accurately and safely via percutaneous approach under image guidance, either using direct or coaxial technique [7, 11]. Percutaneous biopsy can be performed under US [7, 13], CT [7, 13], MRI [14] or fluoroscopy [7].

Newly developed technologies exist enabling fusion of previously acquired CT images with procedural US images or MR images with procedural CT to facilitate accurate and safe biopsy procedures by optimising tumour localisation, with potential for reduced radiation dose [14, 15]. Functional information from positron emission tomography (PET) can also be fused with anatomical detail from either CT or MRI to facilitate biopsy procedures performed under CT, MRI or US guidance [14, 15].

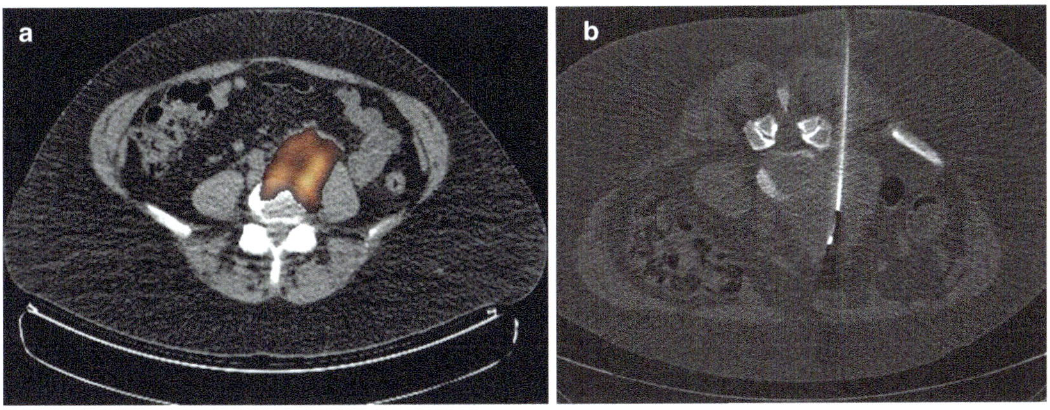

Fig. 9.1 (**a**, **b**) Percutaneous lymph node biopsy. (**a**) Axial PET/CT fusion image demonstrating active nodal disease adjacent/enveloping left common iliac artery due to lymphoma. (**b**) Axial non-contrast CT with patient prone, demonstrating biopsy needle within the left para-aortic/iliac chain nodal disease

9.4 Vascular Access

9.4.1 Central Venous Catheters (CVCs)

Indications: Short-term vascular access for medications (e.g. antibiotics), chemotherapy, total parenteral nutrition (TPN) and atraumatic/needleless venous sampling [2].

Results: Image-guided central vascular access has been shown to be more efficient and safer than venous access based on external landmarks [16].

Technique: Involves placement of a catheter with its tip at the atriocaval junction or within the right atrium, usually using a modified Seldinger technique via the internal jugular vein, with a combination of real-time US and fluoroscopic guidance [17, 18].

Complications: Intraprocedural/early complications relate to surrounding tissue injury such as pneumothorax (<1 %), arterial puncture (1–2 %), haematoma or haemorrhage (up to 2 %) and air embolism (up to 1 %). These potential complications are common to other centrally inserted central venous access devices including tunneled haemodialysis catheters and implantable ports, and are less common when using image guidance [2, 18]. Longer-term problems unaffected by technique of insertion include infection (local infection 1–7 %, catheter-related bacteraemia 1–4 %) and thrombosis (up to 28 % of cancer patients) [2, 18]. Reported pulmonary embolus rates vary between 15 and 25 % of those with CVC-related thrombosis [2, 19, 20]. Thrombosis risk is greater in those with multi-lumen catheters [2, 21].

9.4.2 Peripherally Inserted Central Catheters (PICCs)

PICCs are inserted via a peripheral upper arm vein into the central venous system and range from single to triple lumen catheters up to 7 Fr in size [18]. PICCs are designed for intermediate term use up to 2 months and can be used for venous sampling and TPN also. Recent advancements in PICC design allow for high-pressure injections such as in contrast CT studies. Risk of blood stream infection is low at around 2.1 infections per 1,000 catheter days [18].

Tunneled PICCs can also be performed if peripheral venous access is too difficult to achieve. This method involves initial venous puncture into the jugular or subclavian vein before creating a subcutaneous tunnel in the anterior chest wall. This is similar to the insertion method of tunneled haemodialysis and apheresis catheters.

9.4.3 Infusaport

Another device providing long-term central venous access, but with a reservoir (port) that sits in a subcutaneous pouch in the anterior chest, connecting to catheter tubing with tip in the atriocaval junction. The port can be accessed using a non-coring (Huber) needle through the skin [18]. Ports have now been developed that can tolerate high-pressure injections for contrast CT studies. The port insertion procedure is usually performed under light sedation with ample local anaesthetic using ultrasound guidance for initial venous puncture and fluoroscopy for catheter tip placement.

The infection rate is lower than for external catheters, but the consequences of infection are more troublesome, potentially requiring port removal and alternate siting of the device (e.g. contralateral chest or arm) or obtaining alternate access (e.g. PICC). The lowest risk of bloodstream infection amongst the aforementioned central venous access devices at 0.1 infections per 1,000 catheter days [18].

9.4.4 Tunneled Haemodialysis and Apheresis Catheters

This is a larger calibre (up to 14.5 Fr) double lumen central access catheter mainly used for dialysis access in the setting of renal failure or plasmapheresis in the setting of haematological malignancy and stem cell transplant therapy [2, 18]. Insertion is in the same way as a tunneled PICC with majority of access via the jugular vein with a subcutaneous tunnel over the anterior chest wall. The procedure is usually performed with light sedation and ample local anaesthetic. The subclavian vein can also be utilised but has higher rate of associated central venous stenosis or occlusion (up to 50 %) [18]. Translumbar access of the inferior vena cava (IVC) has also been described [18].

9.5 Nutritional Support

Nutrition is an important and ongoing issue for cancer patients, particularly towards the end of life, and especially in patients with head and neck malignancy [22]. Adequate nutrition has been shown to improve therapeutic tolerance and chemotherapy response [22]. Options include TPN that is utilised for those patients without adequately functioning gastrointestinal tracts, or enteral routes for those with functioning bowel [23]. Enteral nutrition has fewer complications than TPN [18]. Enteral feeding tubes can be inserted via an oral/nasal approach or percutaneously into the stomach or small bowel, using fluoroscopic techniques (Fig. 9.2a, b) [1, 18].

9.5.1 Oropharyngeal Tubes

Indications: Short-term enteral feeding (or gastric decompression) with tip placement in the stomach or post-pyloric small bowel (jejunum).

Complications: Long-term placement is associated with high complication rates including aspiration pneumonitis in 9.8 % in a study by Ryu et al. [24], local erosions and mechanical problems such as tube blockage [18, 22].

9.5.2 Radiologically Inserted Gastrostomy (RIG)

Indications: Long-term or permanent feeding in patients with swallowing difficulties and end stage malignancy, most commonly head and neck cancers, who are unsuitable for percutaneous endoscopic gastrostomy (PEG) insertion due to pharyngeal or oesophageal obstruction [1, 18, 22, 25].

Absolute contraindications: Unsatisfactory anatomy (e.g. overlying transverse colon), uncorrectable coagulopathy and very short life expectancy [18].

Results: With meta-analysis, technical success of RIG placement nears 100 % with low procedure-related mortality (0.3 %) and less complications than other insertion methods [1, 18, 22]. No prospective randomised control

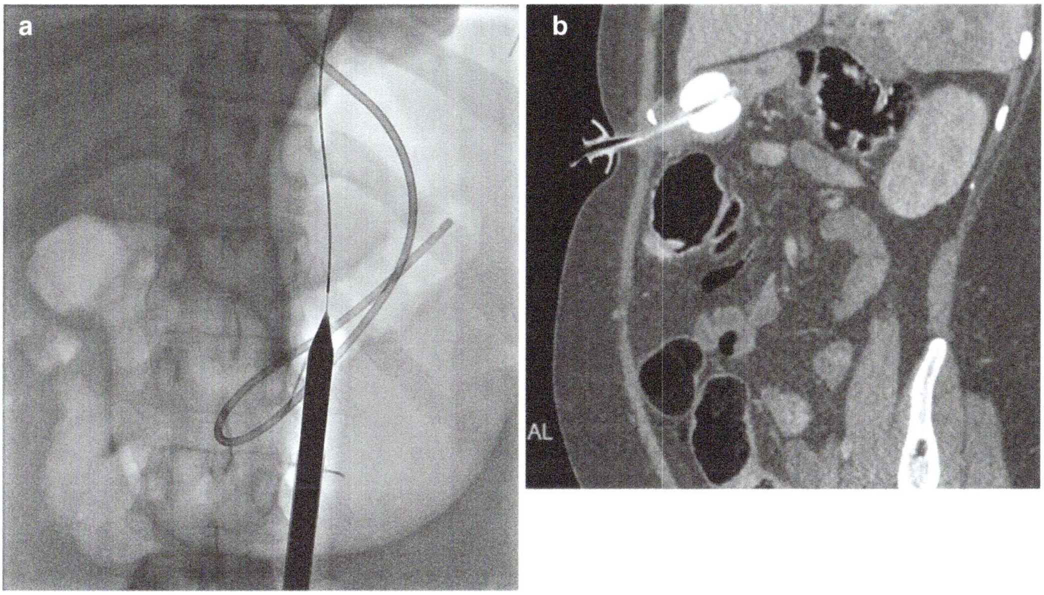

Fig. 9.2 (**a**, **b**) Gastrostomy insertion. (**a**) Demonstrates gastric distension via gas inflation through existing nasogastric tube, with guidewire and percutaneous dilator in place. (**b**) Oblique Sagittal CT shows satisfactory position of radiologically inserted percutaneous gastrostomy

trials (RCTs) compare RIG, PEG and surgical gastrostomy insertion, but multiple studies have indicated RIG is superior and is the most cost-effective approach, once endoscopic failures are considered [1, 22, 26, 27].

Complications: Complications are uncommon (5.9 %) but early on include mild discomfort with infusions and infection [2, 18]. Peritonitis can occur from leakage of gastric juices into the peritoneal cavity or incorrect tube placement [18]. If tube dislodgement occurs 2 weeks or more after insertion, then the tract is usually sufficiently matured to enable replacement without need for repuncture or procedural sedation [2, 18]. RIG techniques often incorporate gastropexy with insertion of small metallic stay/anchor sutures to maintain access to the stomach wall in the short term and prevent tube dislodgement [1, 18]. The sutures are usually cut after 1–2 weeks, allowing the anchors to pass into the bowel [1, 18].

9.5.3 Gastrojejunostomy and Jejunostomy Tubes

These tubes can be placed in those patients who have significant gastroesophageal reflux or are at risk of aspiration pneumonitis, noting that gastrostomies do not eliminate aspiration risk and may even increase the risk due to effect on gastric emptying [18, 28]. They may be placed directly into the jejunum or be converted from existing gastrostomy, which is more successful after initial fluoroscopic insertion (93 % success) compared to a primary endoscopic or surgical approach (68 % success) [1, 29]. Complication rates are similar to gastrostomy [2].

9.6 Symptom Relief

9.6.1 Pain

Pain is a common symptom amongst oncology patients and a significant cause of morbidity, particularly in advanced disease [2, 30, 31]. Cancer pain can be multifactorial, acute and chronic and related to the primary disease process or treatment effects, but the most common pain issue in advanced disease is bone and visceral pain [30–32].

In a significant amount of cancer patients (5–14 %), pain is not adequately controlled with medical treatment [30, 33, 34]. Interventional pain management techniques are an additional option in such patients. These procedures incorporate drug delivery to the spinal cord or major nerve plexuses, application of neurolytic agents to neural structures and can provide short-term or permanent pain relief [30, 35]. These procedures can be performed under ultrasound for superficial structures or under CT guidance for deeper targets.

Vertebroplasty as a treatment method for bone pain will be discussed later in this section.

Image guidance for pain interventions has not been demonstrated in the literature to be more effective or safer than without guidance. However, the lack of supportive evidence is unlikely to change practice given the inherent logic that image guidance should help.

9.6.1.1 Central Neural Blockade

Intrathecal opioids have been used in cancer patients for pain control since the late 1970s [30, 35]. Addition of adjuvant drugs such as local anaesthetics and/or steroids to the injectate provides more effective analgesia than single agent injections [34]. Opioid dosing requirements are greater in the epidural space compared with the intrathecal administration, either as single injection or via infusion catheters [34]. When used, image guidance for epidural or intrathecal injections can be with CT or fluoroscopy for thoracic or lumbar region injections, whilst fluoroscopy is more often used for cervical injections. Epidural blocks with steroid and local anaesthetic are usually performed for vertebral cancer-induced bone pain, although evidence is limited [34].

Indications: Pain not adequately covered with oral analgesics or where the side effects of treatment are too inconvenient. Head and neck cancer patients with pain can benefit from cervical epidural steroid injection in particular.

Results: Intrathecal opioids are effective in treatment of cancer pain, and a small survival benefit has also been shown [30, 34].

Complications: The most feared complication is that of infection but fortunately is of low incidence up to 4.6 % superficial infections and 1.2 % deep infections (increased with longer duration of catheter placement) [30, 34]. Other self-limiting complications include dural puncture headache (15 %), epidural haematoma (0.5–0.9 %) and cerebrospinal fluid (CSF) leak [30, 34]. Medication effects also warrant consideration including respiratory depression due to cephalad spread of opioids, weakness and sensory disturbance (from local anaesthetics at higher doses) [34]. Complications of epidural injection of steroid are usually a result of misplacement of the needle (e.g. intrathecal injection, epidural haematoma, vascular injury).

9.6.1.2 Neurolysis

Permanent pain relief with intrathecal injection of alcohol, particularly in advanced disease.

9.6.1.3 Neural Blockade

Coeliac Plexus Block

Located anterior to the coeliac trunk at the L1 vertebral body level and supplying most of the abdominal viscera, the coeliac plexus can be blocked by anterior or posterior approaches, most commonly under CT guidance, using alcohol or phenol injectates, from a posterior approach [30, 34–36].

Indications: Intractable pain caused from abdominal tumours arising from the upper and lower gastrointestinal tract, pancreas, kidney and adrenal origin may benefit from a coeliac plexus ganglion block [30, 31, 34–36].

Results: Pain reduction can be expected in the majority of patients (up to 90 % in meta-analysis) [37], especially in those with pancreatic cancer [30, 31, 34–36].

Superior Hypogastric Plexus Block

Located in the retroperitoneum on both sides of the midline at the L5/S1 disc level close to the bifurcation of common iliac vessels [34].

Indications: Pelvic pain due to gynaecological, colorectal and genitourinary cancers [34].

Results: Up to 80 % of patients get significant pain relief [30, 34]. No block-related complications reported.

Ganglion Impar Block

Retroperitoneal in location at the termination of paired vertebral sympathetic chains at the sacrococcygeal junction. CT, fluoroscopic and even ultrasound guidance can be used to facilitate needle placement anterior to the sacrococcygeal junction [38].

Indications: Rectal or perineal pain from genitourinary and colorectal cancers [38].

Results: Effective pain relief in vast majority of cancer patients without adverse effects [30, 38].

Lumbar Sympathetic Chain Block

Lumbar sympathetic chain block can be considered for inoperable peripheral vascular disease, less commonly visceral abdominal and pelvic cancer pain (urological) and rectal tenesmus [34].

Stellate Ganglion Block

Stellate ganglion block is used for temporary relief or autonomic pains in the head, neck and upper limbs, either by single or repeated injections [34]. This can be safely performed under US guidance, which is safer than fluoroscopic guidance [39]. Neurolysis is generally not performed due to risk of inadvertent arterial puncture in this location with potential for neural injury or stroke [34, 39].

Splanchnic Nerve Block

Not performed as routinely as the coeliac plexus block, the splanchnic nerve block can be considered in those whom have failed coeliac plexus block [31]. The splanchnic nerves arise from the thoracic sympathetic trunk and join the coeliac ganglion after piercing the diaphragm at T11 and T12 levels [31, 36]. The nerves can be targeted under CT guidance with anterior or posterior approach, or with fluoroscopy for posterior approach [31, 36]. Effective in up to 70 % of patients. Complications include pneumothorax, diarrhoea (self-limiting), diaphragmatic paralysis and cardiac arrhythmias [31, 36].

Complications: Coeliac plexus commonly postural hypotension and diarrhoea which are usually self-limiting and transient [30, 31, 34]. Major complications are rare and usually due to suboptimal placement of phenol injectate. This includes anterior spinal artery spasm causing anterior cord ischaemia with permanent paraplegia (0.15 %) [30, 34]. Aortic dissection, haematoma and retroperitoneal abscess formation have also been reported. There is not sufficient evidence to prove that image guidance is safer than blind techniques for injection, but it is postulated that better visualisation of needle tip and critical adjacent structures (e.g. arteries, organs) should improve accuracy of needle placement with reduced risk of complications due to misplacement [39].

9.6.1.4 Peripheral Nerve Blockade

This has a more limited role in the palliative setting and is technically possible for most neural structures using predominantly US guidance for selective injections. Common targets include the suprascapular, paravertebral, intercostal, lumbar, obturator, sciatic and femoral nerves with blockade performed using a long-acting local anaesthetic (e.g. bupivacaine) with or without corticosteroid. Steroids are particularly effective when the peripheral nerve is involved by the disease process. The risk of peripheral nerve neurolysis is neuritis [34].

9.6.2 Pleural Effusions

Malignant pleural effusion is seen in approximately 50 % of patients with widespread malignancy at some stage during their disease [40, 41]. Associated morbidity and mortality is significant, with 30 days mortality between 29 and 50 %, and mean survival of 3 months [2, 40].

The aetiology is lung cancer or breast cancer in 75 %, but also seen in lymphoma, ovarian cancer and gastric cancer [40, 41]. Dyspnoea is the most common symptom affecting quality of life, also cough and chest pain [2, 40–42].

Treatment is usually palliative, aiming for rapid symptomatic relief (reexpansion of underlying lung), whilst minimising discomfort, inconvenience and disruption of daily activities (Fig. 9.3a, b) [2, 40, 41].

US can be utilised for drainage of most pleural effusions and has been shown to save time and improve first puncture success of thoracocentesis, with reduced risk of pneumothorax [40]. CT is also effective for image guidance in more difficult cases [40].

9.6.2.1 Thoracocentesis

Indications: Exudative pleural effusion or loculated effusion. Simple method for diagnosis

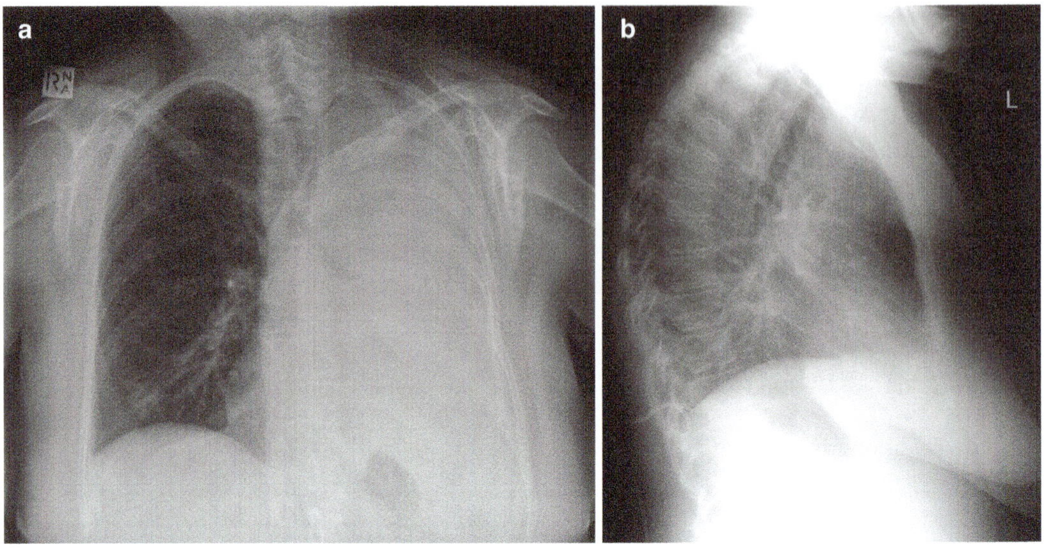

Fig. 9.3 (**a**, **b**) Pleural effusion and drainage. (**a**) Frontal CXR demonstrates large left pleural effusion with left hemithorax whiteout, in patient with left hilar non-small cell lung cancer. (**b**) Lateral CXR post-insertion of pigtail drain shows tip of drain in the posterior costophrenic recess

and immediate short-term symptom relief, but repeated thoracocentesis is not optimal for rapidly reaccumulating malignant effusions [40]. It may be of benefit in those with short survival expectancy or where fluid reaccumulation is slow [40].

Results: Success with US increased up to 88 %, with reduced pneumothorax rate [40]. Malignant pleural effusion will recur within 30 days post-thoracocentesis in nearly all patients [41].

Complications: Uncommon with low rate of pneumothorax (up to 6 %), haemothorax, reexpansion pulmonary oedema, organ laceration, intercostal artery injury and intercostal neuralgia [40]. Approximately half of patients with pneumothorax require formal drainage tube [40]. The bleeding risk is reduced by correcting coagulation parameters prior to the procedure and by ensuring needle placement above the rib margin to avoid the neurovascular bundle [10, 40, 41]. Risks of the procedure increase with repeated thoracocentesis [41].

9.6.2.2 Nontunneled and Tunneled Drainage Catheters

Pigtail drainage tube insertion is commonly performed with US guidance using a modified Seldinger technique following dilatation of the tract, although some direct stick catheters are available [1, 41]. Tunneled catheters are inserted via a similar technique, with the proximal catheter tunneled in subcutaneous tissues to enable longer-term management of effusion due to reduced infection and dislodgement rates [40, 41, 43].

Indications: Long-term management of malignant pleural effusion enabling outpatient management, best with tunneled catheter [40, 41]. Tunneled drains can still be effective after failed formal pleurodesis [40].

Results: Symptomatic relief and control of malignant effusion occurs in 90–95 % of patients with tunneled catheter technique [40]. Spontaneous pleurodesis occurs in approximately 40 %, mostly within 1 month of the tube insertion [40, 41]. Tunneled catheters are safe, cost-effective and enable outpatient management of effusion [40, 43].

Complications: Most common is fluid loculation (8 %), with incomplete drainage [41]. Less commonly empyema, cellulitis, tube dislodgement, bleeding, tumour seeding and extrapleural migration of the catheter [40, 43]. Long-term non-tunneled catheter placement may eventually lead to empyema [1]. Tunneled catheters have the advantage of reduced risk for dislodgement and low risk of complications including tunnel or pleural infections or pericatheter leakage, due to development of a fibrous cuff around proximal portion of catheter, and a one-way valve at proximal hub of the catheter [40].

9.6.2.3 Pleurodesis

Pleurodesis obliterates the pleural space to prevent pleural effusion from reaccumulation [1, 40, 41]. Approximately two thirds of patients with malignant pleural effusion fail to respond to thoracocentesis or drainage catheters, without pleurodesis [40].

Chest tube insertion with pleurodesis and thoracoscopy can require hospitalisation for up to 1 week, which is neither desirable nor cost-effective as a palliative management in patients with a short life expectancy [40]. Intrapleural instillation of sclerosant material can be used to facilitate pleurodesis, and this can be performed as an outpatient, with small drainage catheter pleurodesis as effective as traditional large bore catheter use [2, 40, 41, 44, 45]. The procedure can be undertaken after one or two consecutive drainages of fluid [40]. Sclerosing agents include talc, tetracycline, doxycycline and bleomycin, with talc being the most commonly used [1, 41, 44, 46]. The chest tube can be removed when drainage is less than 50–100 ml/day, although protocols vary by institution [1, 18, 40].

Indications: Recurrent malignant pleural effusion.

Results: Recurrence rates of effusion can be as low as 10 % using talc slurry pleurodesis [1].

Complications: In addition to complications of drain insertion, minimal discomfort and mild fever are common side effects, with talc pneumonitis and respiratory failure less commonly observed [40].

9.6.3 Ascites

Abnormal volume of fluid in the peritoneal cavity as a result of cancer is termed malignant ascites and is a common presentation of malignancy in up to 50 % [1, 47]. Common underlying neoplasms include breast, ovarian, gastric, pancreas and colon cancer, with up to 20 % of unknown primary [1, 41, 48]. Associated life expectancy is short, less than 4 months, with breast and ovarian cancer as exceptions where survival is usually more prolonged [1, 49].

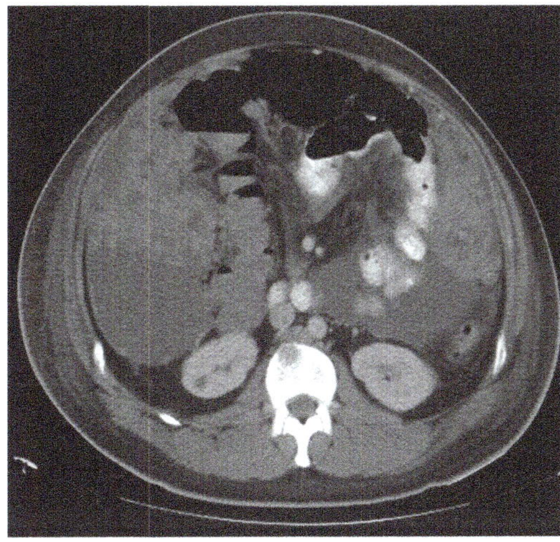

Fig. 9.4 Peritoneal carcinomatosis. Axial CT abdomen demonstrating large volume ascites, omental caking and peritoneal disease in a patient with melanoma

With the exception of those awaiting liver transplant, treatment of recurrent ascites is palliative [1]. Temporary relief of malignant ascites with either blind- or US-guided paracentesis is effective in reducing pain, shortness of breath, anorexia, nausea and improving mobility, although swift reaccumulation of fluid is likely (Fig. 9.4) [1, 41].

Repeated paracentesis can cause significant morbidity through bleeding, organ injury or infection, dehydration and malnutrition, although the overall complication rate is low (around 1 %) [1, 41].

9.6.3.1 Nontunneled and Tunneled Catheters

Single drainage of ascites with nontunneled catheters is effective but if left in place long term are prone to complications such as infection (35 %), accidental removal, leakage (20 %) and occlusion (30 %) [1, 41]. As a result, unless the patient has a short life expectancy, tunneled catheters are preferred for long-term management of malignant ascites, as they have reduced infection risk [1, 41].

Indications: Malignant ascites.

Results: US-guided tunneled catheters have similar complication rates and patient satisfaction when compared to large volume paracentesis, although the reduced need for hospital visits to undergo paracentesis is an obvious advantage of a tunneled drain [41].

Complications: Peritonitis, leakage and loculation are all uncommon [41].

9.6.4 Collections

Whilst generalised accumulation of fluid in the abdomen can be a cause for presentation or deterioration in a patient's condition, so too can complications of underlying disease (e.g. cystic liver metastases causing capsular distension and pain, liver abscess in patients with hepatopancreatobiliary malignancy) or treatment complications, such as intra-abdominal or pelvic collections in the setting of debulking surgery or targeted invasive organ therapies (e.g. liver abscess post-ablation or chemoembolisation) [7, 18, 50–53].

Whilst diagnostic aspirations can be performed under local anaesthetic with small calibre needles, symptomatic benefit usually requires percutaneous 6–8 Fr drain insertion (10 Fr or larger for more complex collections) for several days [7]. As with drainage of ascites, collection drainage can be performed percutaneously under US or CT guidance using a modified Seldinger technique. US is suitable for superficial collections or when angled access is required and allows real-time guidance, whereas CT fluoroscopy is safer for deeper collections or those containing gas and gives better anatomical detail [7, 18].

9.6.4.1 Abdominal Fluid Collections and Abscess

Common locations include hepatic, perihepatic (subphrenic and subhepatic), gallbladder bed, splenic bed, lesser sac, paracolic and the retroperitoneum [7].

Indications: Collection greater than 4 cm, symptomatic [7]. Collections <4 cm in diameter may well respond to conservative treatment, although aspiration when symptomatic can be beneficial [7].

Results: Percutaneous drainage is a safe, effective alternative to surgery with low complication rate (5 %), morbidity and likely a shorter hospital stay [7]. Multiple or multi-loculated collections are more challenging, and although there are high success rates for drainage in the noncancer setting up to 90 %, outcomes are not as impressive in infected tumour drainage, with higher rates of secondary or permanent drainage being required [7, 54, 55]. This relates to infected tumour tending to be a preterminal entity, with complete drainage unlikely unless the underlying tumour resolves, and these patients are often unfit for surgery to definitively treat the tumour [54]. Those with underlying hepatopancreatobiliary malignancy have poorer outcomes of drainage than in other malignancies [50].

Complications: Although uncommon, the major complications are haemorrhage (2 %), bowel or organ injury (~1 %) and sepsis (1–5 %) [7, 18]. In subphrenic abscess drainage, pneumothorax due to pleural transgression is possible with or without development of pleural effusion or empyema [7, 54].

9.6.4.2 Pelvic Fluid Collections

Indications: Postoperative collections or lymphoceles, diverticular abscess, cystic tumour or infected tumour are common indications for drainage in patients with malignancy [7, 18]. Whilst infected collections can be symptomatic due to sepsis, other presentations can relate to mass effect of the collection, such as intractable pain and bowel obstruction [7, 18, 56].

Contraindications: Lack of safe access route and irreversible coagulopathy.

Modality for drainage: Collections superficial to the abdominal muscles can be drained with US guidance. Deeper collections may require CT to identify collection as separate from the bowel [7]. Posterior transgluteal approach via the greater sciatic foramen can be used in deep pelvic abscesses [7, 56]. Alternatively, transrectal (if adjacent rectum) or transvaginal (if in contact with vagina) drainage may be more feasible or even transperineal [7, 18, 56].

Results: Successful in up to 90 % in the noncancer setting and best if the collection is postsurgical, with slightly poorer outcomes associated with infected tumour or fistula [7, 56].

Complications: Rare (<5 %) including haemorrhage, bacteraemia, pain (particularly in transgluteal approach), organ injury, bowel injury and drain kinking or blockage [7, 56].

9.6.5 Biliary Obstruction

9.6.5.1 Biliary Drainage and Stent

Obstructive jaundice can cause pruritus, cholangitis, sepsis, hepatic dysfunction and malnutrition and is associated with short life expectancy if untreated [1]. Endoscopic treatment of distal biliary obstruction due to pancreatic neoplasm is an effective treatment for the majority of patients [2, 57]. The role of percutaneous treatment is for effective primary or palliative management in those who fail endoscopic intervention, are unfit for endoscopy, or in those with proximal duct obstruction (due to hilar lymphadenopathy, hilar metastatic liver disease) [2, 57]. The efficacy of nonsurgical palliative treatments varies according to the location of obstruction, the technique and extent of decompression and the biliary stent prosthesis used, but biliary stents improve quality of life [1, 57].

Percutaneous drainage can be performed using a combination of US and fluoroscopic guidance [7]. Once biliary access is established, it may be possible to traverse the obstruction/stricture (using catheters and wires) to enable insertion of a stent or placement of an internal-external biliary drain as a temporising measure prior to stent insertion (Figs. 9.5a–d and 9.6a–c) [7, 57]. Percutaneous stent placement is less preferred than endoscopic metal stent placement due to theoretically more bleeding and pain complications, but this has not been confirmed in RCTs [1]. If the obstruction cannot be passed, then an external biliary drain is the only option, and this will likely be permanent, requiring regular drain exchanges to reduce infection risk and maintain patency [1, 7, 57].

Another topic of debate is that of metal versus plastic stents. Self-expanding metal stents have been shown to have better patency rates than plastic drains and plastic stents [1]. An advantage of plastic drains is that the patient is aware of blockage as soon as it happens due to bile leakage through the drainage bag or around the drain catheter [1]. Post-procedure pain associated with percutaneous drainage can usually be controlled with oral analgesia [1].

Less commonly, combined procedures with an endoscopist can be performed with side by side insertion of a duodenal or hepaticoduodenal stent. A problem with stent insertion is that they can block and need redilatation with a balloon catheter.

Indications: Biliary obstruction in patients not fit for or amenable to endoscopic decompression [1, 2, 7].

Contraindications: Massive ascites, uncorrectable coagulopathy, uncooperative patient and progressive hepatic failure [7].

Results: Metallic biliary stents have been shown to provide best palliative treatment for unresectable malignant obstructive jaundice, allowing longer patency rates than plastic endoprostheses [7]. Technical success nears 100 % (depending on operator experience) with lower clinical efficacy but still over 90 % [7]. Stent patency depends on the cause and site of stenosis, with a 6-month patency rate for metallic stents of 50 % [2]. Plastic stents are of smaller calibre and occlude sooner, but can be exchanged, unlike metallic stents, so are preferred if patient life expectancy is greater than 6 months [57]. Biliary stents have been shown to improve quality of life in patients with biliary obstruction [57].

Complications: Generally a low rate of minor and major complications, including intra-abdominal infection, sepsis and haemorrhage, with a low mortality rate less than 4 % [2, 7, 58]. Stent occlusion or misplacement can be corrected with second stent placement [7]. Complication rates are higher in oncology patients than in the general setting [57–59]. Incidence of cholangitis in oncology patients is 50 % with drainage, being twice as common with internal-external drains as with external drains, and directly correlates with duration of drain placement [2, 60]. If the patient has uncorrectable coagulopathy, or no safe hepatic access, then a percutaneous cholecystostomy is a safe alternative [7].

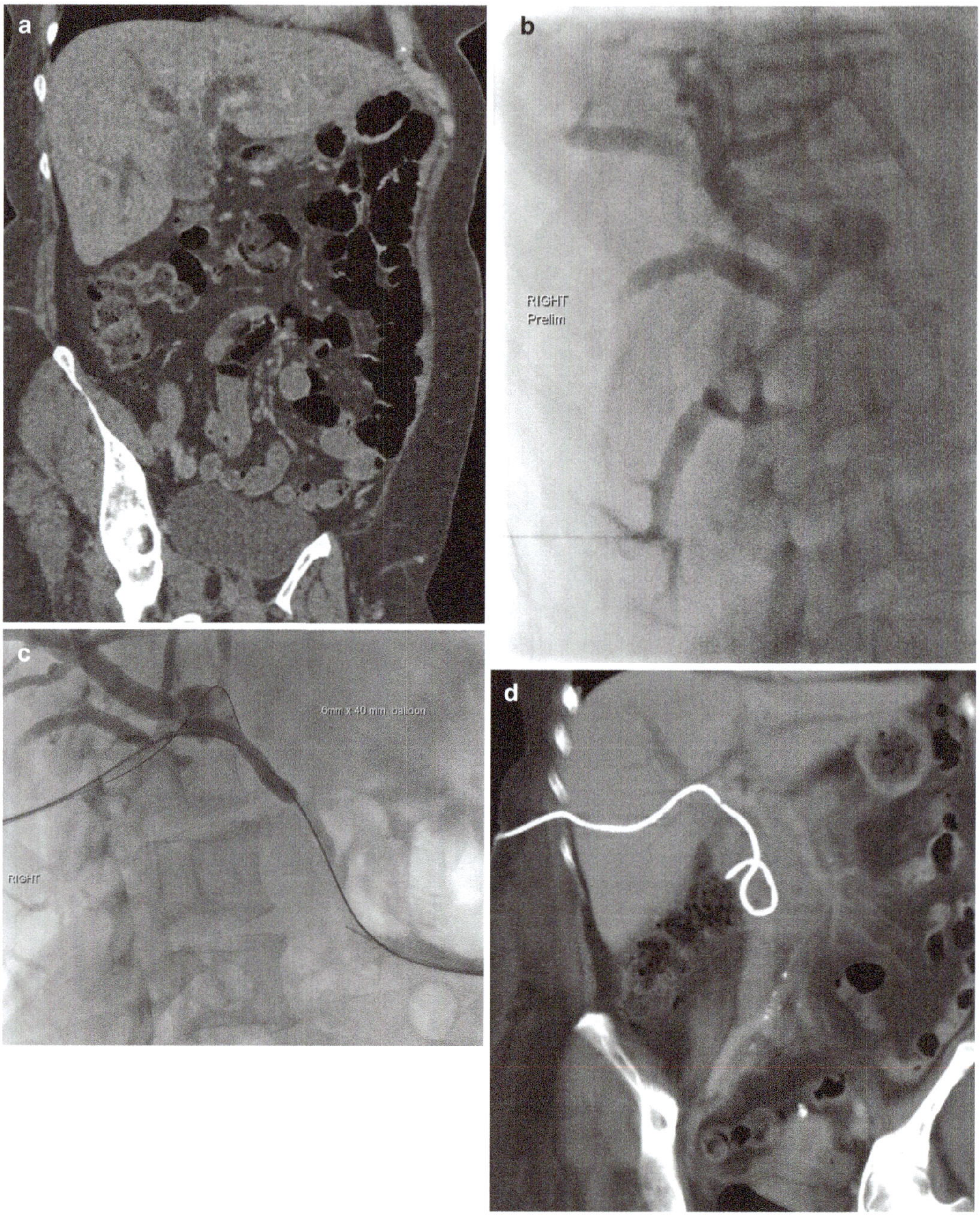

Fig. 9.5 (**a**–**d**) Biliary drain. (**a**) Coronal portal venous phase CT abdomen demonstrating marked intrahepatic biliary dilatation due to gallbladder carcinoma infiltrating ducts at the hilum. (**b**) Percutaneous cholangiogram with contrast identifying dilated intrahepatic ducts, but no drainage into the common bile duct (CBD). (**c**) Balloon dilatation of the tract in the region of the hilum and CBD having crossed the stenosis with wire placement across CBD and into the duodenum. (**d**) Demonstration of drain position on coronal portal venous phase CT abdomen with some associated reduction in degree of biliary dilatation

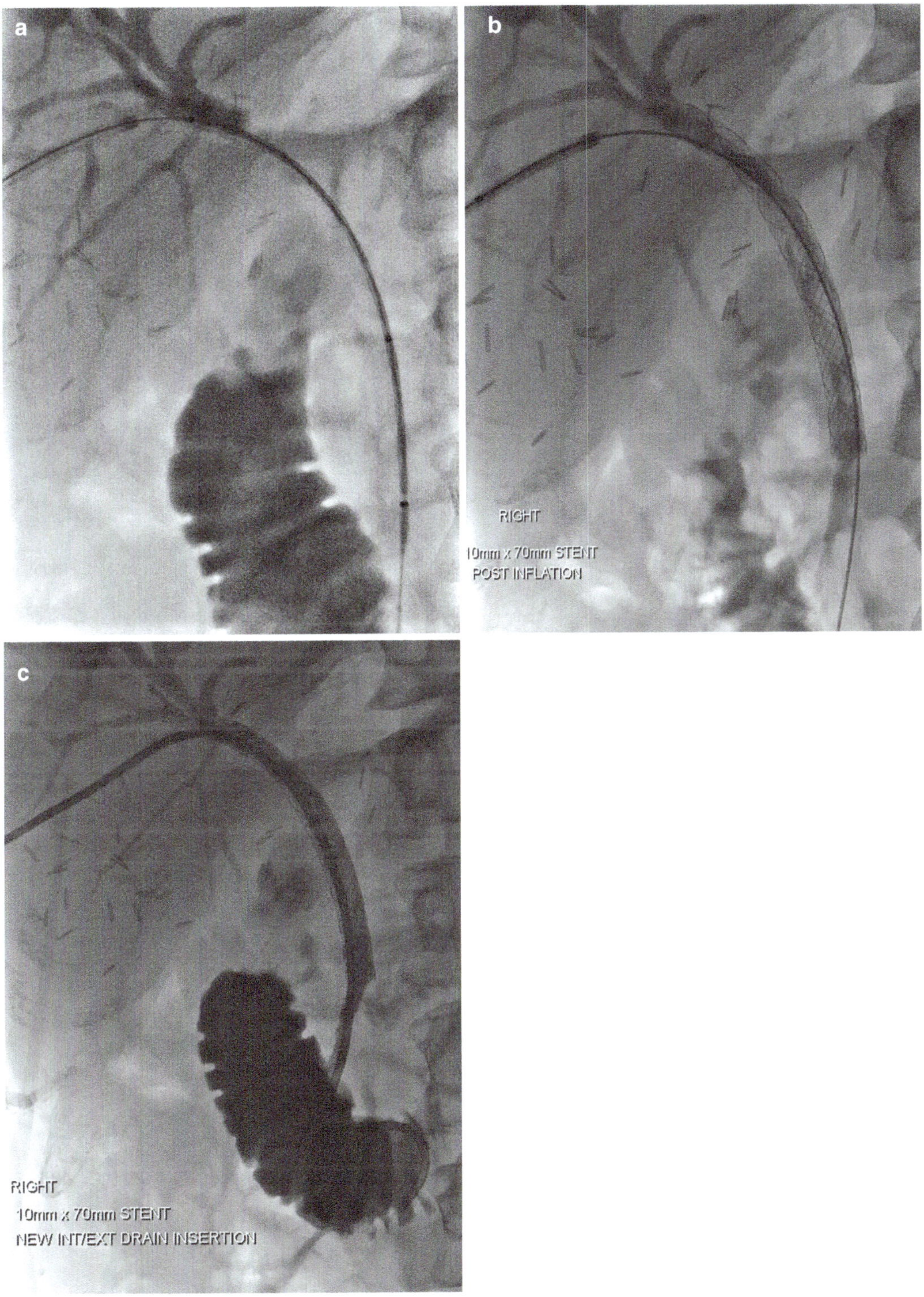

Fig. 9.6 (**a–c**) Biliary stent. (**a**) Procedural x-ray with wire and catheter across hilar and CBD stricture following percutaneous cholangiogram. (**b**) Post deployment and balloon dilatation of the stent. (**c**) Final stent position with insertion of additional internal-external biliary drain as a precaution to maintain access, in case of early stent blockage

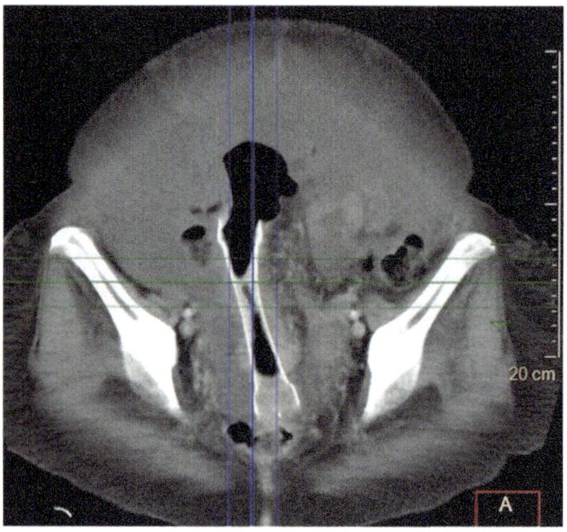

Fig. 9.7 Colonic stent. Oblique axial CT reformat demonstrating stent position

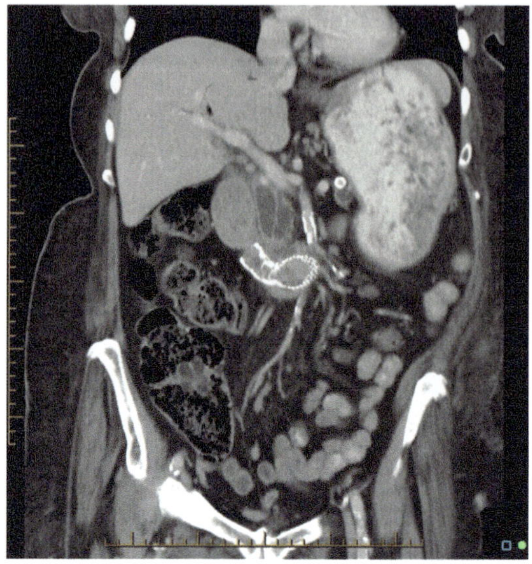

Fig. 9.8 Duodenal stent. Coronal portal venous phase CT abdomen demonstrates common bile duct and pancreatic duct dilatation in a patient with pancreatic ampullary carcinoma

9.6.6 Gastrointestinal Obstruction

9.6.6.1 Colonic Stent

Malignant colonic obstruction in a patient not suitable for surgery can be managed effectively with a self-expanding colonic stent, under fluoroscopic guidance (Fig. 9.7) [57, 61]. With this method, stents can be inserted into the rectum and distal sigmoid, but with combined colonoscopic guidance stents can be placed through the caecum and more proximal colon [57].

Indications: Malignant colonic obstruction in palliative patients or those not fit for emergency surgery but who may undergo elective surgery [57, 61].

Results: Success rate is high (80–100 %) with symptomatic relief and improved quality of life [57]. There is no difference in mortality and morbidity rates compared with surgery, but the advantage of stenting is a shorter hospital stay with less procedure time and blood loss [61].

Complications: Stent migration (most common but reduced with larger diameter stents), recurrent obstruction, transient anorectal pain, tenesmus, rectal bleeding, perforation and death [57, 61].

9.6.7 Gastroduodenal Obstruction

Gastric outlet obstruction is frequently seen in end stage advanced gastric, duodenal and biliary disease with these patients often not candidates for palliative surgical therapy [57]. Simple decompressive techniques such as nasogastric tube and gastrostomy placement can provide effective palliation [57]. A longer-term solution is gastroduodenal stenting which can be performed endoscopically or percutaneously with a self-expanding metal stent (Fig. 9.8) [57].

Indications: Malignant gastric outlet obstruction.

Results: High technical success between 92 and 100 %, with improved quality of life, but unfortunately such patients still have a short life expectancy of between 7 and 14 weeks [57].

Complications: Overall low complication rates, most commonly stent obstructions, stent migration and duodenal stenosis.

9.6.8 Oesophageal Stent and Balloon Dilatation

The aim of palliation in patients with oesophageal cancer is to maintain swallowing, access for nutrition and pain management [62]. Balloon dilatation of oesophageal tumoural strictures provides immediate relief of dysphagia in most patients, but recurrence of symptoms is often rapid due to lack of effect on the underlying tumour, with repeat dilatation usually needed [62]. The procedure is associated with a small risk of perforation, which is reduced with use of fluoroscopy and guidewires [62].

Oesophageal stenting provides symptomatic improvement in patients with malignant oesophageal obstruction [62]. Numerous stenting options are available from covered or uncovered plastic or self-expanding metal stents [62]. Covered stents have the advantage of resisting tumour ingrowth and can be used to cover fistulas and leaks, but these have a higher migration rate [62]. Uncovered stents are less likely to migrate but are subject to tumour ingrowth and obstruction [62].

Indications: Dysphagia due to unresectable oesophageal tumour or in patients who are not candidates for other therapies. Stenting is also indicated in oesophageal perforation and tracheooesophageal fistula.

Relative contraindication: Oesophageal disease abutting the thoracic aorta due to risk of aortooesophageal fistula.

Results: Success rates similar between plastic stents and self-expanding metal stents although more migration with plastic stents [62]. Stenting is effective for all indications, although recurrent obstruction is an issue in 50 % who require subsequent interventions [62].

Complications: The rate of serious complications is low, but the mortality rate is between 0.5 and 2 % [62]. Intraprocedural complications include aspiration, malposition, oesophageal perforation; post-procedural include chest pain, bleeding, tracheal compression, with delayed findings of stent migration, fistula, recurrent dysphagia, stent occlusion [62].

9.6.9 Urological Obstruction

Acute urinary obstruction can be treated with percutaneous nephrostomy (PCN) insertion, usually under ultrasound and/or fluoroscopic guidance, or less commonly CT (Fig. 9.9) [2, 7]. The procedure is usually performed under local anaesthetic and light sedation and in the urological malignancy setting is usually a temporising measure to facilitate later ureteric stent insertion, performed either as a urological surgical procedure or in radiology [7, 18]. Untreated, urinary obstruction can lead to uraemia, renal failure and death [57]. Prompt decompression of the system preserves renal function, reduces pain and reduces potential infection [2].

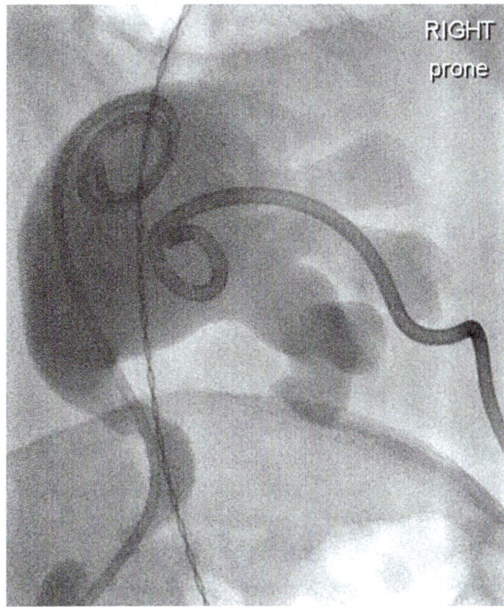

Fig. 9.9 Procedural x-ray showing position of ureteric stent and percutaneous nephrostomy

Malignant ureteric obstruction may be due to extrinsic tumour compression, retroperitoneal lymphadenopathy or direct tumour invasion [2]. Commonly involved malignancies include gastrointestinal, urologic and gynaecologic origin and can be unilateral or bilateral [2, 57].

When retrograde ureteric stenting is unsuccessful or not feasible, then percutaneous dilatation of the stricture can be performed in antegrade fashion via the PCN [2]. Following serial dilatation, an internal ureteric stent (double J or metallic) or internal-external drain catheter can usually be placed to prevent restenosis [2, 57]. Plastic stents induce less urothelial hyperplasia than metal stents and can be easily replaced, so plastic stents are preferred [2], but it has been suggested metal stents are potentially less irritating to the bladder as less stent protrudes beyond the vesicoureteric junction [57].

9.6.9.1 Percutaneous Nephrostomy

Indications: Urinary tract sepsis, pyonephritis, ureteric obstruction, malignant bladder outflow obstruction [2, 7].

Results: Safe, successful and cost-effective with reduced incidence of gram-negative septicaemia due to renal obstruction, partial recovery of renal function, correction of metabolic disturbance and reduced inpatient times [2, 57]. Effective decompression is achieved in approximately 95 %, with degree of collecting system dilatation and patient body habitus important factors that can reduce success [2].

Complications: Urine leak, bleeding, infection, catheter blockage [2, 7].

9.6.9.2 Ureteric Stent

Double J ureteric stents are traditionally used to relieve malignant ureteric obstruction, with self-expanding metal stents an effective alternative [2, 7, 57]. Both types of stent can be inserted in antegrade fashion via an existing PCN. No significant difference in quality of life or morbidity exists between PCN and ureteric stenting, when taking into account extra nursing required for management of a drainage bag with PCN and the extra surveillance for ureteric stents [57].

Indications: Malignant ureteric obstruction or stricture.

Results: Successful decompression up to 95 % in one series. Mean duration of stent patency in the order of 9 months [57].

Complications: Urine leak, ureteric perforation, infection and catheter blockage or secondary obstruction due to bladder outlet obstruction/tumour growth [2, 7, 57].

9.6.10 Vertebroplasty for Metastatic Disease Fracture

Whilst some controversy exists regarding vertebroplasty for painful osteoporotic fractures, there is considerable evidence supporting the procedure in the palliative treatment of neoplastic compression fractures, although data are more based on case series than RCTs [63–65]. The procedure is performed under fluoroscopic image guidance, with sedation or full anaesthetic support, and involves injection of a small amount of a cement product, polymethylmethacrylate (PMMA), into the vertebral body [1, 34, 63, 65]. Kyphoplasty is a variation of vertebroplasty where balloon dilatation of the vertebral body creates a cavity prior to cement injection [34, 65]. In those with multiple fracture levels, high signal on fat-saturated MR images can be a useful indicator of acute or non-healed fractures [65].

Indications: Pain from malignant vertebral fractures that is refractory to conservative treatments [34, 63, 65]. Recent evidence suggests it is still a safe treatment for patients with nerve root compression and epidural disease [63].

Contraindications: Disruption of posterior vertebral body wall (relative contraindication), local infection (discitis osteomyelitis), coagulopathy and cement allergy.

Results: The exact mechanism of pain relief is not completely understood as it does not appear to relate solely to treatment of vertebral body collapse, with cytotoxic and thermally toxic effects of PMMA on underlying tumour proposed as additional mechanisms [1, 34, 65]. However, significant reduction of pain in 80–90 % is achieved when patients are carefully selected (by ruling out other causes of the pain and that the pain is severe enough to warrant an invasive procedure), and improved mobility has also been demonstrated [2, 34, 65]. Subacute fractures demonstrate better response than chronic fractures [2].

Complications: Higher major complication rates in the cancer setting (5 %) compared with the general population (1 %) including cement leak into the spinal canal, PE (chemoembolisation to lungs via paravertebral veins), pulmonary oedema [2]. Cement leak into the epidural space or neural canal is rare but is the most important complication, being more common in the cancer setting and with pre-existing epidural involvement [64, 65]. Nerve root irritation (1–2 %), pain and tenderness at the injection site is common but usually resolves within 24 h [65].

9.7 Haematological/Vascular

9.7.1 Thrombosis

Malignancy is a well-established risk factor for venous thromboembolism due to hypercoagulable state [2, 66]. Complications from vascular thrombosis are the second leading cause of death in patients with malignancy [66].

For larger vessel venous disease, stenting is an option, such as in superior vena cava (SVC) syndrome and less commonly inferior vena cava (IVC). IVC stenting may provide symptomatic relief of lower limb oedema and prevent late stage complications of thrombus/venous congestion or secondary organ failure (renal or hepatic venous involvement) [66]. Primary and secondary IVC stent patency rates of around 80 % have been shown at 19 months in one series [66]. Stenting also provides effective palliation of tumour involvement of the IVC [18].

Catheter-directed and mechanical thrombolysis therapies are also possible for those who have failed conservative management of thrombosis and help to reduce the symptoms of venous congestion such as limb swelling and pain, with reduced risk of haemorrhagic complications of systemic thrombolysis [2, 18].

9.7.1.1 IVC Filter

Proven to be effective in preventing pulmonary embolus in patients with lower limb DVT who are not suitable for anticoagulation [2, 18]. The current devices are inserted either via jugular vein or common femoral vein, and the procedure can be performed under local anaesthetic, with majority of current filters designed to be removable if needed (Fig. 9.10) [18].

Indications: Lower limb DVT when anticoagulation is contraindicated; complication of anticoagulation has occurred; those who develop PE despite anticoagulation [2, 18].

Results: Successful filter placement in over 97 % [2] and failure rate between 2 and 7 %, with new clinically significant PE after filter placement [18].

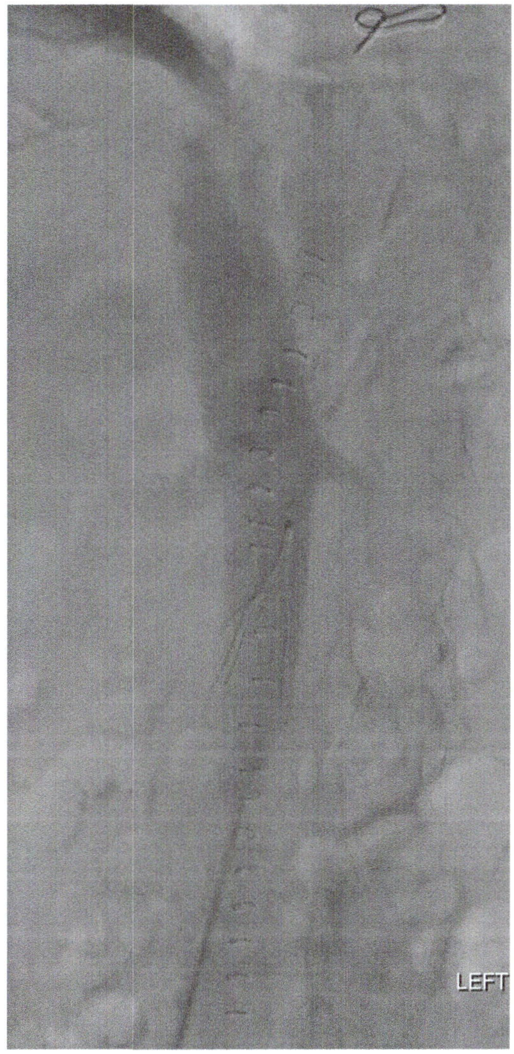

Fig. 9.10 Post-deployment cavogram showing adequate position of the IVC filter below level of renal veins

Complications: Major complication rate 0.3 % with mortality related to the procedure 0.2 % comparable for suprarenal and infra-renal filter deployment [18]. There is an associated increase in lower limb DVT in up to 20 % of patients [18]. Other uncommon complications include IVC perforation, infection, migration and inability to remove the filter (less important in the palliative setting) [18].

9.7.2 Bleeding

Haemorrhage can occur in up to 10 % of patients with advanced cancer [67]. Causes include vessel damage/tumour invasion, disseminated intravascular coagulation (DIC), platelet dysfunction, hepatic failure, systemic tumour treatments or the cancer itself [67]. The role of interventional radiology in management of bleeding lies in embolisation of a bleeding vessel, usually after active bleeding has been identified on CT angiogram [67, 68]. This is performed most commonly via a femoral artery approach, although axillary, brachial and radial artery approaches may be used depending on the target vessel [67, 68].

Although evidence of success is based mainly on case reports, embolisation is successful in nearly all situations with limiting factors being presence of underlying bleeding disorder and inability to safely access the bleeding vessel [67]. The procedure can usually be performed under local anaesthetic or mild sedation and is generally well tolerated [67, 68]. Once the bleeding vessel is accessed, agents available to the interventionalist for endovascular treatment include Gelfoam, particles, coils or vascular occlusion devices such as Amplatzer plugs [2, 18, 67].

Severe epistaxis, haemoptysis, haematemesis and lower gastrointestinal bleeding are all potentially amenable to treatment with embolisation, depending on the underlying cause, response to other available therapies and the parameters of the patient's advanced care plan. Endovascular stents can also be used in the setting of incipient or acute carotid rupture [67, 68].

Major complications of endovascular treatment of bleeding mostly relate to nontarget embolisation (with potential for organ necrosis) and catheter malposition (can cause vessel spasm, dissection or rupture), with more minor complications including bleeding at the access site and infection [68]. Post-embolisation syndrome is a well-documented self-limiting common side effect of solid organ embolisation thought to result from tissue necrosis and/or intravascular thrombosis [68]. The clinical features include pain, fever, nausea and vomiting, with symptoms lasting for up to 1–2 weeks posttreatment [18, 68].

9.7.2.1 SVC Stenting/Syndrome

SVC syndrome primary symptoms include facial and periorbital swelling, bilateral arm swelling and superficial vein distension over the chest wall [18, 66]. Primary treatment with endovascular stenting is considered a first-line option, with high technical success rates (90–100 %) and effective symptom relief (Fig. 9.11a, b) [66].

Indications: SVC stenosis or clinical symptoms of SVC syndrome.

Results: Six months primary and secondary patency rates between 70–80 and 80–90 %, respectively [66].

Complications: Range from 4 to 10 % including bleeding (due to thrombolysis), recurrent laryngeal nerve palsy, congestive heart failure, PE, valvular dysfunction and cardiac tamponade.

9.8 Palliative Therapies

Numerous image-guided treatment options exist for the palliative control of tumours including endovascular (chemoembolisation, radioembolisation) and percutaneous (thermal ablation) [18, 53]. Demonstration of the arterial tumour supply by contrast-enhanced CT or MRI facilitates planning of the endovascular treatment approach, as well as clearly defining the target tumour for percutaneous treatments. The principles of each therapy will be outlined, followed by a description of organ-/site-specific applications, with a focus on the palliative setting, although ablation techniques can have a curative result in certain instances (e.g. some renal tumours).

9.8.1 Embolisation

9.8.1.1 Endovascular Embolisation

Embolotherapy can be considered bland where agents that cause vessel occlusion alone are employed, such as Gelfoam, polyvinyl alcohol particles, microspheres and coils [2, 66]. It is termed chemoembolisation when chemotherapeutic agents are mixed with an embolic agent and delivered directly to the target tumour by selective cannulation of the feeding artery, with

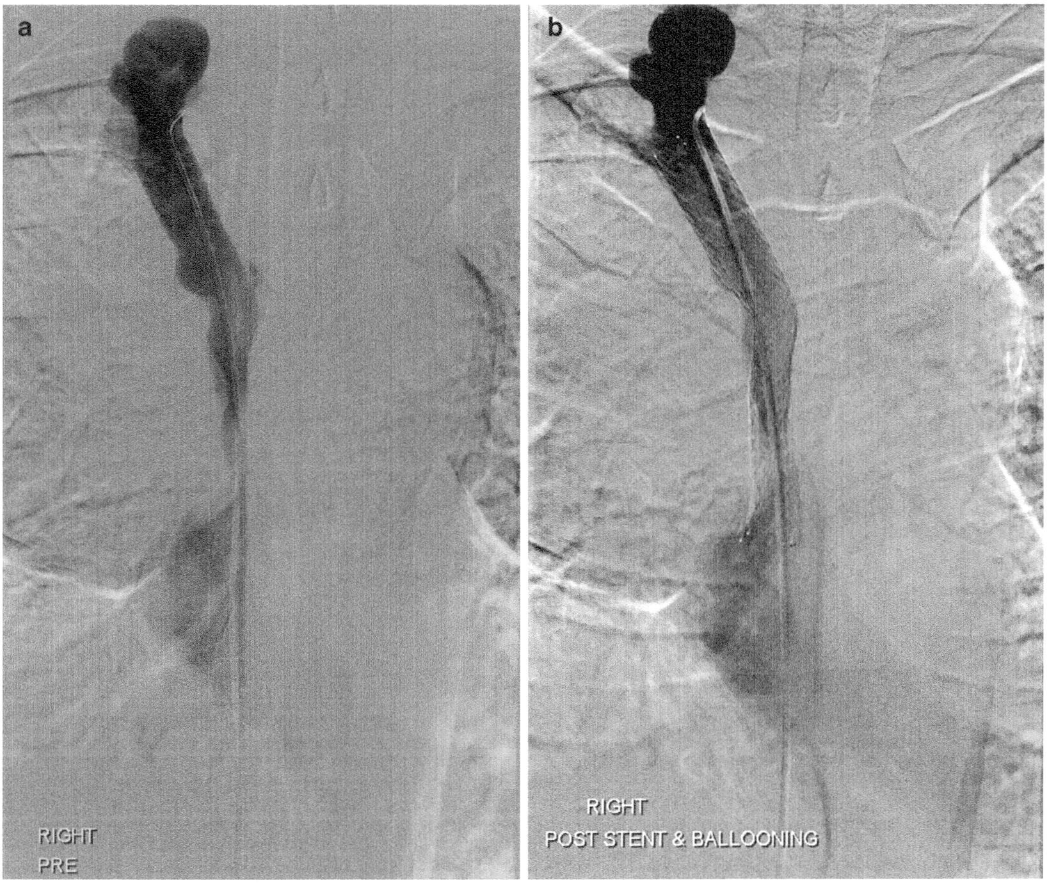

Fig. 9.11 (**a**, **b**) SVC stenosis and stenting. (**a**) DSA image shows catheter tip in right brachiocephalic vein and significant stenosis in lower SVC due to extrinsic compression from nodal disease in lymphoma. (**b**) DSA image post-deployment of self-expanding metal stent and post-balloon dilatation of the stent, with increased contrast flow through the stent and into the right atrium

an overall aim to devascularise the tumour as well as deliver concentrated chemotherapy (Fig. 9.12a, b) [1, 2, 18, 53]. This method facilitates increased chemotherapy dose to the tumour due to the concomitant occlusion of the feeding artery, as well as enabling lower systemic chemotherapy dose [2, 18, 53, 68].

Nonselective chemoembolisation is performed when the feeding vessel of a single lesion cannot be safely accessed, or if multiple lesions exist, with a downside of a nonselective treatment being increased risk of post-embolisation syndrome [68].

Chemoembolisation is a repeatable procedure, and the liver in particular is able to tolerate this due to its dual blood supply, but caution should be used in treating patients without a patent portal vein [2].

Indications: Locoregional therapy for HCC, unresectable colorectal liver metastases (CRLM), neuroendocrine liver metastases, life expectancy >12 months [18, 52, 53, 68].

Contraindications: Systemic infection, widespread extrahepatic disease, with relative contraindications uncorrectable coagulopathy and renal failure [18].

Results: Safe and effective treatment in HCC with survival benefit demonstrated in prospective RCTs [1, 18, 68–70]. Increased survival has been seen in CRLM, even in nonresponders to systemic chemotherapy, with a few studies demonstrating less impressive outcomes (possibly a

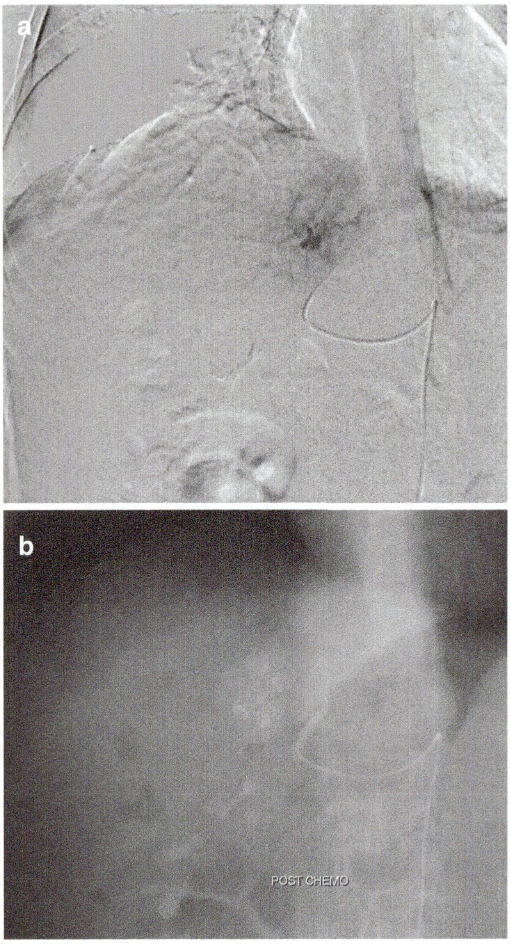

Fig. 9.12 (**a**, **b**) Transarterial chemoembolisation for HCC. (**a**) Frontal digital subtraction angiogram (DSA) images with selective microcatheter position in artery to segment 4a of the liver demonstrating abnormal vascularity in the HCC. (**b**) Frontal DSA post-chemoembolisation showing lipiodol uptake within the tumour and slow flow in the embolised vessel

result of treatment recipients having more complex or extensive disease) [52, 68]. Effective symptomatic control in carcinoid syndrome, also with improved survival [52, 68].

Complications: Acute liver failure (2.3 %), neutropenia, infection/abscess (1 %), bile duct damage (1–10 %), nontarget embolisation can result in gastrointestinal haemorrhage/ulceration (1 %) and cholecystitis [18, 52, 68]. More a side effect than complication, post-embolisation syndrome (pain, fever, nausea and fatigue) is usually self-limiting and seen in up to 90 % of patients [18, 52, 68]. Biliary damage is more common in non-cirrhotic livers [68]. Tumour crisis is a risk in neuroendocrine tumour treatment and pretreatment somatostatin administration is recommended [18].

Embolotherapy has also been described for the palliation of inoperable or haemorrhagic renal cell carcinoma, utilising permanent agents such as polyvinyl alcohol and is mostly well tolerated, although renal failure is a recognised complication [53, 68].

9.8.1.2 Radioembolisation

Radioembolisation or selective internal radiation therapy (SIRT) enables delivery of high dose brachytherapy to the liver by the selective injection of yttrium-90 microspheres, used in the setting of HCC and CRLM [1, 2]. The therapy exploits the finding that arterial supply to liver tumours is different from normal liver tissue, which is supplied by the portal vein system [1]. There is low penetration of the beta particles from yttrium-90 (about 2.5 mm in human tissues), so necrotising effects are localised [2]. Preliminary results show this to be a safe and effective therapy, with stabilisation of disease in patients with unresectable liver metastases and chemorefractive CRLM [2, 53].

Due to the risk of radiation pneumonitis if there is significant hepatopulmonary shunting, there is essential pretreatment workup with nuclear medicine lung scan and formal hepatic artery angiogram to assess degree of shunting [2, 68]. The entire treatment process is technically challenging and quite labour intensive, with embolisation of extrahepatic collateral vessels prior to final drug delivery also performed to reduce risk of gastrointestinal complications [18, 68].

Indications: Unresectable HCC, liver metastases (CRLM, neuroendocrine tumours, breast cancers), life expectancy >3 months [18, 68].

Contraindications: Significant hepatopulmonary shunting and limited hepatic reserve (due to excessive tumour involvement) [18, 68].

Results: Similar effectiveness and safety to chemoembolisation, although there are some data to support radioembolisation as better than chemoembolisation for downstaging disease to within transplant criteria in HCC and effective use in patients with portal vein thrombosis [18, 53, 71]. More RCTs are recommended to more completely evaluate the role of locoregional therapies in advanced HCC, however [71].

Complications: Less toxicity than chemoembolisation with post-radioembolisation syndrome (fatigue, nausea, abdominal pain) in up to 50 % of patients, lasting up to 2 weeks [18, 52]. Radiation-induced pneumonitis is rare, <1 % [52]. Gastrointestinal ulcerations, cholecystitis and pancreatitis due to off-target embolisation in less than 5 % [2, 52, 68]. Liver dysfunction up to 4 %, more commonly in those with pre-existing liver disease or patients previously treated with chemotherapy [52].

9.8.2 Percutaneous Ablation

Thermal ablation techniques involve placement of a specially designed probe/electrode into the centre of a lesion, usually under US +/– CT guidance [1, 2, 18]. The device is connected to an energy source able to generate extremes of temperature to cause irreversible tumour necrosis, ranging from microwave or radiofrequency ablation (RFA) in excess of 60° Celsius to cryotherapy using argon gas under pressure to create subfreezing temperatures [1, 2, 18, 72]. Chemical ablation has also been described using absolute alcohol and phenol, but thermal ablation is more commonly performed [18, 72]. Chemical ablation is effective in treating HCC, but efficacy is reduced in liver metastases, particularly in more solid adenocarcinomas [72].

9.8.2.1 Radiofrequency Ablation

RFA utilises electrical current oscillation between electrodes to generate frictional agitation of tissues near the electrode, leading to tissue heating, known as the Joule effect, with end point of coagulation necrosis [18, 72]. Although devices differ by manufacturer, the size of the effective treatment area around the tip of the electrode/probe is around 3 cm, so multiple electrodes or multiple treatment sessions are needed to treat lesions >3 cm [72]. A 0.5–1.0 cm zone of coagulation necrosis around the lesion is required to enable a tumour-free margin [18]. RFA is a described therapy for locoregional tumour control in liver, lung, adrenal, renal and skeletal malignancy [2, 72]. Because RFA relies on electrical current flow, effective tissue/tumour heating is reduced adjacent blood vessels >3 mm due to heat sink effect and loss of heat [18, 72].

Indications: HCC and CRLM in those not suitable for surgical therapy, particularly small lesions [18, 68].

Results: Efficacy demonstrated for treatment of small HCC primarily, with the exact role in the palliative setting of liver metastases not entirely clear, but evidence suggesting a survival benefit over systemic chemotherapy [18, 73]. Two RCTs have demonstrated equivalent efficacy with RFA versus surgical resection for small HCC [1, 74, 75]. Mortality rate is 0.3 % and major complication rate 2.2 % [2, 72]. In the setting of palliation of neuroendocrine tumour (NET) liver metastases, thermal ablation has been used successfully as an adjunctive therapy at the time of aggressive surgical resection and for symptomatic relief in majority of nonsurgical candidates [18, 52].

Complications: Overall complication rate less than 9 %, most commonly haemorrhage, abscess and biliary stricture [18]. Tumour lysis syndrome has been described after treatment of large tumours and consists of severe thrombocytopaenia and liver or renal failure, but is uncommon [18]. Tumour seeding has been reported in a minority of cases and incidence is reduced by thermocoagulation of the needle tract [76, 77].

9.8.2.2 Microwave Ablation

Microwave range electromagnetic energy (usually 915 MHz to 2.45 GHz for clinical applications) agitates water molecules in targeted tissue causing frictional heating, leading to coagulation necrosis and irreversible cell death (Fig. 9.13a, b) [2, 72]. This has comparable efficacy to RFA, particularly for HCC [2, 76]. Advantages over RFA include larger treatment volumes (up to 8 cm), optimal heating of cystic masses, less pain and less heat sink effect in lesions adjacent vascular structures [2, 76].

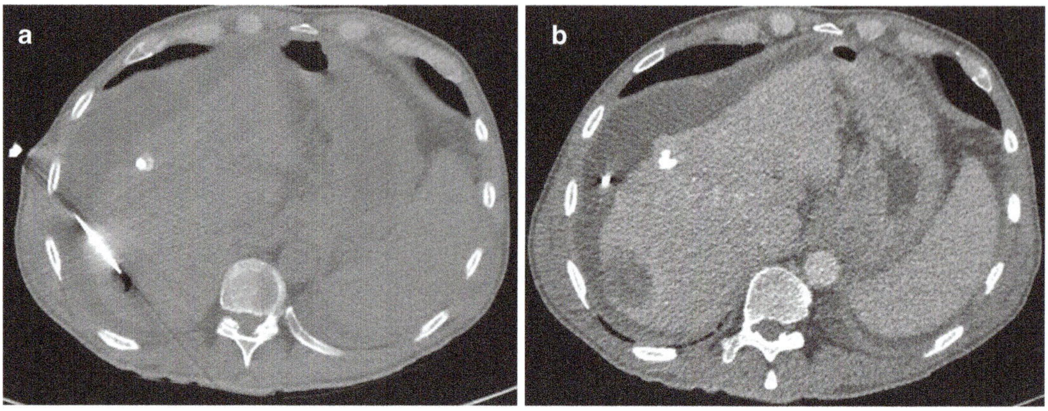

Fig. 9.13 (**a**) Microwave ablation electrode within the segment 6 lesions. (**b**) Immediate post-ablation axial CT liver demonstrating increased hypodensity in region of previously demonstrated HCC, consistent with posttreatment appearances of coagulation necrosis. Small volume ascites is present in (**a**, **b**)

Indications: Inoperable HCC, CRLM and symptomatic relief in liver metastases from NET [18, 52, 77].

Results: RCT evidence of equivalent efficacy (local tumour control and survival) and safety as RFA in HCC, but RFA has potential advantage of achieving tumour ablation in fewer sessions [2, 76, 77]. Some case series have demonstrated higher survival rates and lower recurrence rates in RFA versus microwave ablation, but this is not yet proven in RCTs [2, 77].

Complications: Similar rates and types of major and minor complications to RFA, including haemorrhage, abscess, bile duct injury, pain, fever, ascites, liver enzyme elevation, pleural effusion/empyema and diaphragmatic injury (approach dependent), skin burn and tumour seeding [76–78]. Mortality as low as 0.2 % [78].

9.8.2.3 Cryoablation

Cryoablation utilises alternating cycles of freezing (up to −140° C) and thawing to cause mechanical stress upon cell membranes, resulting in irreversible cell death [2, 72]. Associated ice formation and microvascular thrombosis help to limit procedural bleeding [2]. Similar to the heat sink effect seen in RFA, cryoablation can be affected by cold sink effect when treating lesions adjacent to blood vessels [18].

Indications: Inoperable HCC and CRLM [18, 77].

Results: Effective in locoregional control in HCC, with similar results to RFA, inducing less operative pain, but with higher complication rates and recurrence rates [18, 77]. There is less robust evidence for use in CRLM [53].

Complications: Tumour lysis syndrome in 1 % (more than in RFA) [18, 76, 77]. Haemorrhage, cold injury to adjacent organs, biliary fistula and hepatic parenchymal fracture have been described with complication rates up to 31 and 41 % in two studies and as a result have become less favoured as a treatment modality [76, 77, 79, 80].

Post-ablation CT and MRI can be used to confirm completeness of ablation and to detect residual or recurrent disease [2].

Overall, thermal ablative therapies (primarily RFA and microwave) are the preferred treatment option for small lesions, with chemoembolisation therapy preferred for larger lesions. Radioembolisation currently is considered in those who are unsuitable for chemoembolisation. Combining ablation therapies with other therapies is a focus of research in order to improve completeness of tumour destruction, investigating potential synergistic effects with chemotherapy, radiotherapy or chemoembolisation [72].

9.9 Summary

Many image-guided interventions are available to assist in the management of patients requiring palliative care. It behoves the attending clinician to consider not just the technical feasibility of a radiologic intervention procedure but whether it is justified in terms of quality of life improvement. The interventional radiologist has an important role in multidisciplinary care and is well placed to provide valuable information to guide appropriate use of the available procedures.

References

1. Requarth J. Image-guided palliative care procedures. Surg Clin North Am. 2011;91:367–402.
2. O'Neill SB, O'Connor OJ, Ryan MF, Maher MM. Interventional radiology and the care of the oncology patient. Radiol Res Pract (2011); Volume 2011;Article ID 160867: 11.
3. Chow DS, Itagaki MW. Interventional oncology research in the United States: slowing growth, limited focus, and a low level of funding. Radiology. 2010;257(2):410–7.
4. McCullough HK, Bain RM, Clark HP, Requarth J. The interventional radiologist as a palliative care sub-specialist: providing symptom relief when cure is not possible. AJR Am J Roentgenol. 2010;196: 462–7.
5. Campbell TC, Von Roenn JH. Palliative care for interventional radiology: an oncologist's perspective. Semin Intervent Radiol. 2007;24:375–81.
6. Baerlocher MO, Asch MR. Interventional radiology in palliative care. CMAJ. 2007;176(6):762–3.
7. Gervais DA, Sabharwal T, editors. Interventional procedures in biopsy and drainage. London: Springer; 2011.
8. Seldinger SI. Catheter replacement of the needle in percutaneous arteriography: a new technique. Acta Radiol. 1953;39(5):368–76. (Original article reprint 2008 Acta Radiologica Suppl).
9. Goodwin ML. The Seldinger method for PICC insertion. J Intraven Nurs. 1989;12:238–43.
10. Patel IJ, Davidson JC, Nikolic B, Salazar GM, Schwartzberg MS, Walker TG, Saad WA, for the Standards of Practice Committee, with Cardiovascular and Interventional Radiological Society of Europe (CIRSE) Endorsement. Consensus guidelines for periprocedural management of coagulation status and hemostasis risk in percutaneous image-guided interventions. Coagulation guidelines periprocedural interventional radiology. J Vasc Interv Radiol. 2012;23:727–36.
11. Gupta S, Wallace MJ, Cardella JF, Kundu S, Miller DL, Rose SC. Quality improvement guidelines for percutaneous needle biopsy. J Vasc Interv Radiol. 2010;21(7):969–75.
12. Hainsworth JD, Greco FA. Treatment of patients with cancer of an unknown primary site. N Engl J Med. 1993;329(4):257–63.
13. Arellano RS, Maher M, Gervais DA, Hahn PF, Mueller PR. The difficult biopsy: let's make it easier. Curr Probl Diagn Radiol. 2003;32(5):218–26.
14. Solomon SB, Silverman SG. Imaging in interventional oncology. Radiology. 2010;257(3):624–40.
15. Hakime A, Deschamps F, de Carvalho EGM, Teriitehau C, Auperin A, de Baere T. Clinical evaluation of spatial accuracy of a fusion imaging technique combining previously acquired computed tomography and real-time ultrasound for imaging of liver metastases. Cardiovasc Intervent Radiol. 2011;34(2): 338–44.
16. Rabindranath KS, Kumar E, Shail R, Vaux EC. Ultrasound use for the placement of haemodialysis catheters. Cochrane Database Syst Rev 2011:(11):CD005279.
17. Dariushnia SR, Wallace MJ, Siddiqi NH, et al. Quality improvement guidelines for central venous access. J Vasc Interv Radiol. 2010;21(7):976–81.
18. Valji K. The practice of interventional radiology: with online cases and videos. Philadelphia: Saunders; 2012.
19. Verso M, Agnelli G. Venous thromboembolism associated with long-term use of central venous catheters in cancer patients. J Clin Oncol. 2003;21(19):3665–75.
20. Akl EA, Kamath G, Yosuico V, et al. Thromboprophylaxis for patients with cancer and central venous catheters: a systematic review and meta-analysis. Cancer. 2008;112(11):2483–92.
21. Timsit JF, Farkas JC, Boyer JM, et al. Central vein catheter-related thrombosis in intensive care patients: incidence, risk factors, and relationship with catheter related sepsis. Chest. 1998;114(1):207–13.
22. O'Neill JP, Shaha AR. Nutrition management of patients with malignancies of the head and neck. Surg Clin North Am. 2011;91:631–9.
23. Copeland III EM, Pimiento JM, Dudrick SJ. Total parenteral nutrition and cancer: from the beginning. Surg Clin North Am. 2011;91:727–36.
24. Ryu J, Nam B, Jung Y. Clinical outcomes comparing parenteral and nasogastric tube nutrition after laryngeal and pharyngeal cancer surgery. Dysphagia. 2009;24(4):378–86.
25. Lowe AS, Laasch HU, Stephenson S, Butterfield C, Goodwin M, et al. Multicentre survey of radiologically inserted gastrostomy feeding tube (RIG) in the UK. Clin Radiol. 2012;67(9):843–54.
26. Barkmeier JM, Trerotola SO, Wiebke EA, et al. Percutaneous radiologic, surgical endoscopic, and percutaneous endoscopic gastrostomy/gastrojejunostomy: comparative study and cost analysis. Cardiovasc Intervent Radiol. 1998;21:324–8.
27. Blondet A, Lebigot J, Nicolas G, et al. Radiologic versus endoscopic placement of percutaneous

gastrostomy in amyotrophic lateral sclerosis: multivariate analysis of tolerance, efficacy, and survival. J Vasc Interv Radiol. 2010;21:527–33.
28. Ho C, Yeung E. Percutaneous gastrostomy and transgastric jejunostomy. AJR Am J Roentgenol. 1992;158(2):251–7.
29. Kim CY, Patel MB, Miller MJ, et al. Gastrostomy-to-gastrojejunostomy tube conversion: impact of the method of original gastrostomy tube placement. J Vasc Interv Radiol. 2010;21:1031–7.
30. Joshi M, Chambers WA. Pain relief in palliative care: a focus on interventional pain management. Expert Rev Neurother. 2010;10(5):747–56.
31. Tam A, Ahrar K. Palliative interventions for pain in cancer patients. Semin Intervent Radiol. 2007;24:419–29.
32. Twycross R, Harcourt J, Bergl S. A survey of pain in patients with advanced cancer. J Pain Symptom Manage. 1996;12:273–82.
33. World Health Organization. Cancer pain relief: with a guide to opioid availability. 2nd ed. Geneva: World Health Organization; 1996.
34. de Courcy JG. Interventional techniques for cancer pain management. Clin Oncol. 2011;23:407–17.
35. Cope DK, Zhao Z. Interventional management for cancer pain. Curr Pain Headache Rep. 2011;15:237–43.
36. Bahn BM, Erdek MA. Celiac plexus block and neurolysis for pancreatic cancer. Curr Pain Headache Rep. 2013;17:310.
37. Eisenberg E, Carr DB, Chalmers TC. Neurolytic celiac plexus block for treatment of cancer pain: a meta-analysis. Anesth Analg. 1995;80:290–5.
38. Scott-Warren JT, Hill V, Rajasekaran A. Ganglion impar blockade: a review. Curr Pain Headache Rep. 2013;17:306.
39. Rathmell JP, Manion SC. The role of image guidance in improving the safety of pain treatment. Curr Pain Headache Rep. 2012;16:9–18.
40. Yu H. Management of pleural effusion, empyema and lung abscess. Semin Intervent Radiol. 2011;28:75–86.
41. Stokes LS. Percutaneous management of malignant fluid collections. Semin Intervent Radiol. 2007;24:398–408.
42. Musani AI. Treatment options for malignant pleural effusion. Curr Opin Pulm Med. 2009;15(4):380–7.
43. Tremblay A, Michaud G. Single centre experience with 250 tunneled pleural catheter insertions for malignant pleural effusion. Chest. 2006;129(2):362–8.
44. Lee YC, Baumann MH, Maskell NA, et al. Pleurodesis practice for malignant pleural effusions in five English-speaking countries: survey of pulmonologists. Chest. 2003;124(6):2229–38.
45. Putnam Jr JB, Light RW, Rodriguez RM, et al. A randomized comparison of indwelling pleural catheter and doxycycline pleurodesis in the management of malignant pleural effusions. Cancer. 1999;86(10):1992–9.
46. Shaw P, Agarwal R. Pleurodesis for malignant pleural effusions. Cochrane Database Syst Rev. 2004;1, CD002916.
47. Campbell C. Controlling malignant ascites. Eur J Palliat Care. 2001;8:187–9.
48. Ringenberg QS, Doll DC, Loy TS, et al. Malignant ascites of unknown origin. Cancer. 1989;64:753–5.
49. Spratt JS, Edwards M, Kubota T, et al. Peritoneal carcinomatosis: anatomy, physiology, diagnosis, management. Curr Probl Cancer. 1986;10:558–84.
50. Yeh T-S, Jan Y-Y, Jeng L-B, Hwang T-L, Chao T-C, Chien R-N, Chen M-F. Pyogenic liver abscess in patients with malignant disease: a report of 52 cases treated at a single institution. Arch Surg. 1998;133: 242–5.
51. Clark HP, Carson WF, Kavanagh PV, Ho CPH, Shen P, Zagoria RJ. Staging and current treatment of hepatocellular carcinoma. Radiographics. 2005;25:S3–23.
52. Mahnken AH, Pereira PL, de Baere T. Interventional oncologic approaches to liver metastases. Radiology. 2013;266(2):407–30.
53. Lewandowski RJ, Geschwind J-F, Liapi E, Salem R. Transcatheter intraarterial therapies: rationale and overview. Radiology. 2011;259(3):641–57.
54. Maher MM, Gervais DA, Kalra MK, Lucey B, Sahani DV, Arellano R, Hahn PF, Mueller PR. The inaccessible or undrainagble abscess: how to drain it. Radiographics. 2004;24(3):717–35.
55. Gervais DA, Ho CH, O'Neill MJ, Arellano RA, Hahn PF, Mueller PR. Recurrent abdominal and pelvic abscesses: incidence, results of repeated percutaneous drainage, and underlying causes in 956 drainages. AJR Am J Roentgenol. 2004;182(2):463–6.
56. Harisinghani MG, Gervais DA, Hahn PF, Cho CH, Jhaveri K, Varghese J, Mueller PR. CT-guided transgluteal drainage of deep pelvic abscesses: indications, technique, procedure-related complications, and clinical outcome. Radiographics. 2002;22(6):1353–67.
57. Sato KT, Takehana C. Palliative nonvascular interventions. Semin Intervent Radiol. 2007;24:391–7.
58. Rossi P, Bezzi M, Rossi M, et al. Metallic stents in malignant biliary obstruction: results of a multicenter European study of 240 patients. J Vasc Interv Radiol. 1994;5(2):279–85.
59. Becker CD, Glattli R, Maibach R, Baer HU. Percutaneous palliation of malignant obstructive jaundice with the Wallstent endoprosthesis: follow-up and reintervention in patients with hilar and non-hilar obstruction. J Vasc Interv Radiol. 1993;4(5):597–604.
60. Carrasco CH, Zornoza J, Bechtel WJ. Malignant biliary obstruction: complications of percutaneous drainage. Radiology. 1984;152(2):343–6.
61. Sagar J. Colorectal stents for the management of malignant colonic obstructions. Cochrane Database Syst Rev 2011;(1):CD007378.
62. Freeman RK, Ascioti AJ, Mahidhara RJ. Palliative therapy for patients with unresectable esophageal carcinoma. Surg Clin North Am. 2012;92:1337–51.
63. Baelocher MO, Munk PL, Liu DM, Tomlinson G, Badii M, Kee ST, Loh CT, Hardy BW, Murphy KJ. Clinical utility of vertebroplasty: need for better evidence. Radiology. 2010;255:669–74.
64. Sailou G, Kocheida EM, Lehmann P, Depriester C, Paradot G, Le Gars D, Balut A, Deramond H. Percutaneous vertebroplasty for pain management in

malignant fractures of the spine with epidural involvement. Radiology. 2010;254(3):882–90.
65. Shaibani A, Ali S, Bhatt H. Vertebroplasty and kyphoplasty for the palliation of pain. Semin Intervent Radiol. 2007;24:409–18.
66. Desai KR, Chen RI. Endovascular therapy for palliative care of cancer patients. Semin Intervent Radiol. 2007;24:382–90.
67. Pereira J, Phan T. Management of bleeding in patients with advanced cancer. Oncologist. 2004;9:561–70.
68. Kessel DO, Ray CE, editors. Transcatheter embolization and therapy. London: Springer; 2010.
69. Lo CM, Ngan H, Tso WK, et al. Randomised controlled trial of transarterial lipiodol chemoembolization for unresectable hepatocellular carcinoma. Hepatology. 2002;35(5):1164–71.
70. Llovet J, Real MI, Montana X, et al. Arterial embolization or chemoembolization versus symptomatic treatment in patients with unresectable hepatocellular carcinoma: a randomized control trial. Lancet. 2002;359(9319):1734–9.
71. Lencioni R, Crocetti L. Local-regional treatment of hepatocellular carcinoma. Radiology. 2012;262(1): 43–58.
72. Ahmed M, Brace CL, Lee Jr FT, Goldberg SN. Principles of and advances in percutaneous ablation. Radiology. 2011;258(2):351–69.
73. Saldanha DF, Khiatani VL, Carillo TC, et al. Current tumour ablation technologies: basic science and device review. Semin Intervent Radiol. 2010;27:247–54.
74. Chen MS, Li QJ, Zheng Y, et al. A prospective randomized trial comparing percutaneous local ablative therapy and partial hepatectomy for small hepatocellular carcinoma. Ann Surg. 2006;243: 321–8.
75. Lu MD, Kuang M, Liang LJ, et al. Surgical resection versus percutaneous thermal ablation for early stage hepatocellular carcinoma: a randomized control trial. Zhonghua Yi Xue Za Zhi. 2006;86:801–5 [in Chinese].
76. Seinstra BA, van Delden OM, van Erpecum KJ, van Hillegersberg R, Mali WP, van den Bosch MA. Minimally invasive image-guided therapy for inoperable hepatocellular carcinoma: what is the evidence today? Insights Imaging. 2010;1:167–81.
77. McWilliams JP, Yamamoto S, Raman SS, Loh CT, Lee EW, Liu DM, Kee ST. Percutaneous ablation of hepatocellular carcinoma: current status. J Vasc Interv Radiol. 2010;21:S204–13.
78. Liang P, Wang Y, Yu XL, Dong B. Malignant liver tumours: treatment with percutaneous microwave ablation- complications among cohort of 1136 patients. Radiology. 2009;251(3):933–40.
79. Xu KC, Niu LZ, Zhu Q, et al. Sequential use of transarterial chemoembolization and percutaneous cryosurgery for hepatocellular carcinoma. World J Gastroenterol. 2009;15:3664–9.
80. Pearson AS, Izzo F, Fleming RY, et al. Intraoperative radiofrequency ablation or cryoablation for hepatic malignancies. Am J Surg. 1999;178:592–9.

Part III

Palliative Surgery: The Domains

The majority of patients with oesophageal cancer present with advanced and incurable disease [6, 7]. This is reflected by declining rates of surgical resection. In the Western population, resection rates are declining and have decreased from 25 % to around 20 % in the last 5 years [7–12]. Whilst palliative surgery for oesophageal cancer may be less glamorous, it forms the bulk of an oesophago-gastric surgeon's work. Palliative strategies are therefore essential to lengthen survival and lessen symptoms whilst maintaining or improving quality of life as long as possible until death.

Whilst chemotherapy is the most effective treatment for advanced metastatic oesophageal cancer, multimodal techniques are often needed to treat other symptoms such as dysphagia, odynophagia and gastrointestinal haemorrhage. This may include surgical, endoscopic, radiotherapeutic and other palliative approaches.

This chapter focuses on appropriate patient selection for palliative surgery, palliative strategies utilised in the treatment of advanced oesophageal cancer, methods for maintaining adequate nutrition, controlling pain and nausea, preserving adequate swallow and managing gastrointestinal haemorrhage.

10.2 Selection for Palliative Care

Patient preclusion from potentially curative treatment is broadly based on the extent of regional disease, presence of metastatic disease, patient co-morbidities and of course patient choice. Thorough staging investigations are mandatory to decide if treatment is directed at curative or palliative intent. No single modality is perfect, but a multimodal approach including endoscopy and biopsy; computerised tomography (CT) of the chest, abdomen and pelvis; endoscopic ultrasound (EUS); and positron emission tomography (PET CT) can accurately stage oesophageal disease with a false-negative rate of 1–2 % [13]. This means that a small proportion of patients still undergo surgery to assess resectability.

When deciding on palliative strategies, prognostic factors for survival are important. The SEER cancer statistics database has one of the largest population cohorts on which to base epidemiology and survival data [14]. Despite recent improvements in treatment and modest survival gains, overall 5-year survival for oesophageal cancer remains disappointing at around 17 %. Patients with inoperable local disease fared even worse with less than 3 % of patients with metastatic disease surviving 5 years. It is clearly inappropriate to subject a patient to potentially toxic therapy with a life expectancy measured in weeks. The World Health Organization (WHO) performance score, serum lactate dehydrogenase and extent of local disease have all been implicated as poor prognostic markers [15, 16].

10.2.1 Staging Investigations

Upper gastrointestinal endoscopy with biopsy and a CT of the chest, abdomen and pelvis remain mandatory staging investigations. PET and EUS have been valued additions to the staging algorithm over the last decade. The staging investigations may reveal characteristics of the tumour not amenable to curative therapies (metastatic disease, extra regional nodal involvement, long high-volume proximal tumour, local invasion) and patient factors (significant cardiorespiratory co-morbidities, concurrent terminal illness and of course patient wishes). An algorithm for selecting those for palliative treatment is shown in Fig. 10.1.

10.2.2 Multidisciplinary Team and Specialist Centres

All cases of oesophageal cancer are routinely discussed at a local oesophago-gastric multidisciplinary team (MDT) meeting, which is now regarded as the standard of care [17]. Clinical policy is generally agreed through a local cancer network. MDT members invariably comprise a lead clinician (generally the lead surgeon), medical gastroenterologist, consultant histopathologist, radiologist, radiation and medical oncologist, specialist cancer nurse, dietician and palliative care physician [18]. Patients managed by the MDT are more likely to have appropriate and timely

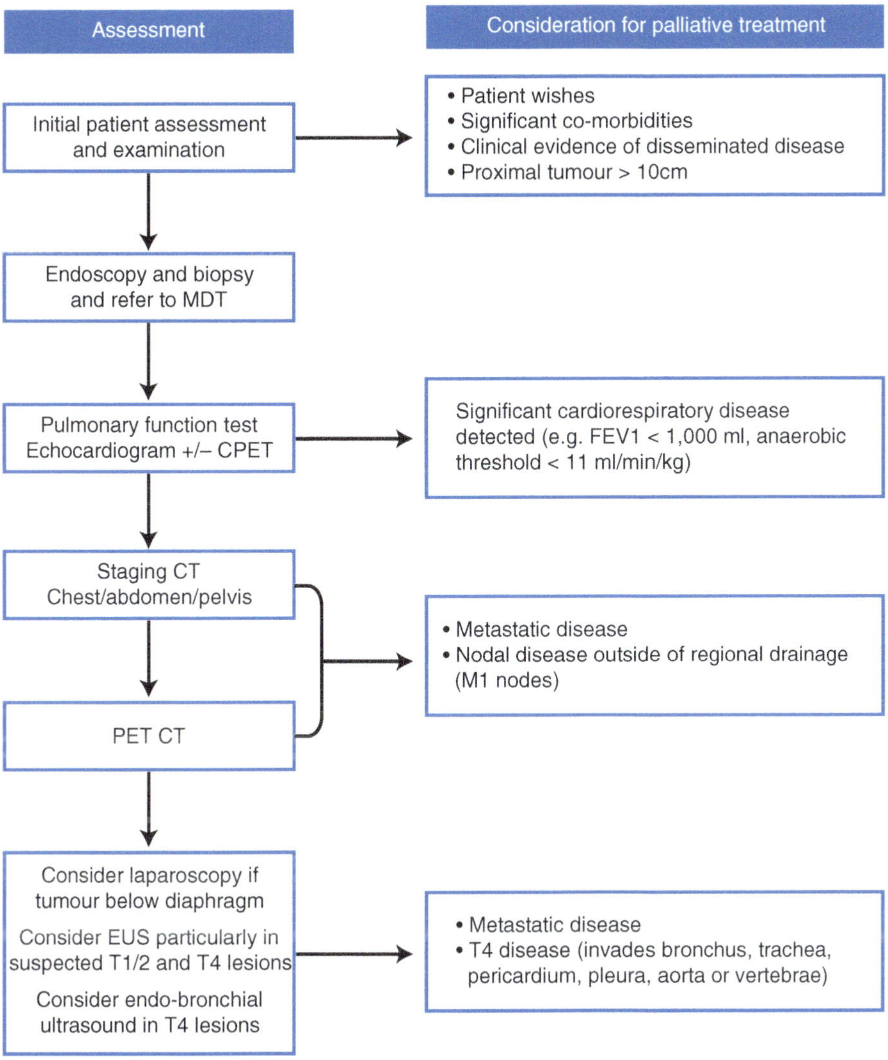

Fig. 10.1 Algorithm to aid patient selection for palliative care. *MDT* multidisplinary team, *CPET* cardiopulmonary exercise test, *FEV1* force expiratory volume in one second, *PET* positron emission tomography

treatment and better trial recruitment and cancer outcomes, and it is recommended that all patients should be assessed at an MDT [12, 19–21].

Benefits of the MDT included increased provision for evidence-based medicine, individualised treatment options, psychosocial support, education and audit and streamlined referral pathway and may help decide on the best form of palliation. In the UK, it has been recommended that all upper gastrointestinal cancers be discussed at an MDT meeting since the year 2000; it has been recommended but is not mandatory in North America or Australia [22, 23].

10.2.3 Tumour Burden Precluding Curative Treatment

Patients presenting with distant metastasis, nodal disease outside of the operative field and locally invasive tumours (T4b) are obviously not candidates for curative surgery. Liver resections of oesophageal metastasis have been undertaken; however, survival remains dismal even with the addition of chemotherapy [24, 25]. Tumour-free resection margins are crucial as a positive circumferential resection margin (CRM) is associated with an extremely poor prognosis. Reid et al. [26]

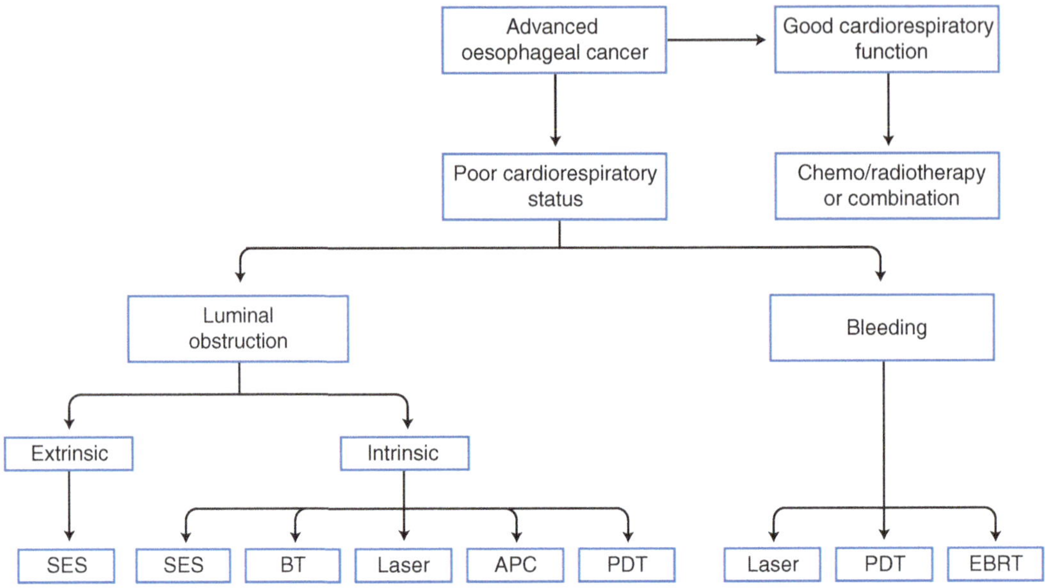

Fig. 10.2 Palliative treatment algorithm for unresectable advance oesophageal cancer. *SES* self expanding stent, *BT* brachytherapy, *APC* Argon plasma coagulation, *PDT* photodyanamic therapy, *EBRT* external beam radiotherapy

showed that in all patient groups, median survival for those with a positive CRM vs. those with a negative CRM was 19 vs. 63 months.

Tumour length and volume is an important prognostic indicator and is associated with a worse disease-free survival [27, 28]. PET CT is now routinely used to assess tumour volume and response to chemotherapy [29].

10.3 Palliative Treatments for Cancer of the Oesophagus

As discussed elsewhere in this book, palliative treatments in any cancer have to be very carefully balanced against prolonging life which is of poor quality. A wide variety of techniques are available for the palliation of advanced oesophageal cancer, and the majority of these techniques focus on alleviating the most troublesome symptoms, namely, dysphagia and bleeding. Modalities used in the palliation of oesophageal cancer must carry a low side effect profile and be achieved with minimal intervention.

This section will concentrate on the strategies available to palliate advanced oesophageal cancer focusing on endoscopic methods for relieving luminal obstruction; modalities for treating chromic bleeding; the role of chemotherapy, radiotherapy and chemoradiotherapy; and of course palliative oesophageal surgery.

An algorithm to aid decision-making in selecting the best palliative management strategy is shown in Fig. 10.2.

10.3.1 Endoluminal Therapies

Endoluminal therapies provide rapid relief of dysphagia and control of bleeding with minimal side effects. They are less likely to result in the deterioration of physical well-being, fatigue and dyspnoea associated with oesophagectomy [30].

Oesophageal stenting is the most commonly employed technique currently and will form much of the discussion in this chapter. Other techniques include brachytherapy (BT), external beam radiotherapy (EBRT) laser recannulation, argon plasma coagulation (APC), cryotherapy (CT) and intratumoural injections, and they will also be discussed.

Randomised trials conducted this century comparing various endoluminal techniques for palliation are illustrated in Table 10.1.

Table 10.1 Randomised trials comparing endoluminal palliative techniques (since year 2000)

Authors	*N*	Group 1	Group 2	Outcome	Relief of dysphagia	HRQL	Survival
Javed et al. (2012) [31]	84	SEMS: Ultraflex ($n=42$)	SEMS: Ultraflex + EBRT ($n=42$)	No difference in complications	SEMS + EBRT > SEMS	SEMS > SEMS + EBRT	SEMS + EBRT > SEMS
Rupinski et al. (2011) [32]	82	APC ($n=28$)	APC + BT 12 Gy ($n=28$) or APC + PDT ($n=26$)	More complications with PDT	APC + BT > APC + PDT > APC	APC + BT better	No difference
Rosenblatt et al. (2010) [33]	219	BT 8 Gy ($n=109$)	BT 8 Gy + external beam EBRT 30 Gy ($n=110$)	No difference in morbidity	Improved with addition of external beam EBRT	N/a	No difference
Blomberg et al. (2010) [34]	65	SEMS: Anti-reflux Z-stent ($n=28$)	SEMS: Gianturco Z-stent/Ultraflex/ Wallstent ($n=37$)	More reflux in anti-reflux group No difference in complications	No difference	No difference	No difference
Kim et al. (2009) [35]	37	SEMS: Double-layer Niti-S ($n=17$)	SEMS: covered Niti-S ($n=19$)	More complications and stent migration in covered Niti-S stent	No difference	N/a	No difference
Shenfine et al. (2009) [36]	215	SEMS: 18 mm Z-stent ($n=54$)	SEMS: 24 mm Z-stent ($n=54$) or plastic stent ($n=57$) or non-stent treatment ($n=50$)	Complications equal No difference with stent diameter QALY equal	Worse in plastic stent group	Reduced in all groups but worse with SEMS (due to pain)	Better in non-stent group
Verschuur et al. (2008) [37]	125	SEMS: Ultraflex ($n=42$)	SEPS: Polyflex ($n=41$) or SEMS:double-layer Niti-S ($n=42$)	Greater stent migration with Polyflex	No difference initially Recurrent dysphagia with Ultraflex due to tissue ingrowth	N/a	No difference
Sabharwal (2008) [38]	49	SEMS: FerX-ella with ARV ($n=22$)	SEMS: Ultraflex ($n=26$) + PPI	No difference	No difference	N/a	No difference
Conio et al. (2007) [39]	101	SEPS: Polyflex ($n=46$)	SEMS: Ultraflex ($n=54$)	More complications and stent migration in Polyflex group	No difference	N/a	No difference
Power et al. (2007) [40]	49	SEMS: Hanarostent with ARV ($n=24$)	SEMS: Ultraflex ($n=25$)	Less reflux with ARV	No difference	No difference	No difference
Wenger et al. (2006) [41]	41	SEMS: Z-stent with ARV ($n=19$)	SEMS: Z-stent ($n=22$)	No difference	No difference	N/a	No difference

(continued)

Table 10.1 (continued)

Authors	*N*	Group 1	Group 2	Outcome	Relief of dysphagia	HRQL	Survival
Bergquist et al. (2005) [42]	52	SEMS: Ultraflex stent ($n=28$)	BT 7 Gy×3 ($n=24$)	No difference in complications	Stent > BT at 1 month BT effect more prolonged	BT > stent at 3 months	No difference
Shenfine et al. (2005) [43]	217	SEMS: either 18 or 24 mm stent ($n=108$)	Plastic stent or no stent ($n=109$)	18 and 24 mm SEMS equally effective More complications with plastic stent Bipolar and ethanol tumour necrosis poor palliative modalities	Worse with plastic stent	Better with 18 mm stents (less pain)	Survival advantage in no stent group
Homs et al. (2004) [44]	209	12 Gy BT ($n=101$)	SEMS: Ultraflex ($n=108$)	More complications in Stent group	Stent > BT at 1 month BT effect more prolonged	BT > stent (mostly at long term due to less pain)	N/a
Homs et al. (2004) [45]	30	SEMS: FerX-Ella ARS($n=15$)	SEMS: FerX-Ella ($n=15$)	More reflux in anti-reflux (Ns)	No difference	N/a	No difference
Sabharwal et al. (2003) [46]	53	SEMS: Ultraflex ($n=31$)	SEMS: Wallstent ($n=22$)	No difference	No difference	N/a	N/a
O Donnell et al. (2002) [47]	50	Rigid plastic stent ($n=50$)	SEMS: Wallstent/ Ultraflex ($n=50$)	No difference in complications	No difference but a trend to favour SEMS	No difference	SEMS > rigid stent
Siersema et al. (2001) [48]	100	SEMS: covered Wallstent ($n=33$)	SEMS: Covered Ultraflex ($n=34$) or Gianturco Z-stent ($n=33$)	No difference	No difference	N/a	No difference
Vakil et al. (2001) [49]	62	SEMS: covered ($n=32$)	SEMS: Uncovered ($n=30$)	More reinterventions in uncovered SEMS	No difference	N/a	No difference
Dallal et al. (2001) [50]	65	Thermal ablative therapy (Nd:YAG laser/argon diode laser/argon plasma coagulation)($n=34$)	SEMS: Ultraflex ($n=31$)	No difference in complications No improvement in dysphagia	No difference	Thermal ablative therapy >stent	Thermal ablative therapy > SEMS
Konigsrainer et al. (2000) [51]	39	SEMS + EBRT ($n=18$)	Nd:YAG laser + EBRT ($n=21$)	Higher re-stenosis with laser	No difference	N/a	No difference

SEMS self-expanding metal stent, *SEPS* self-expanding plastic stent, *BT* brachytherapy, *APC* argon plasma coagulation, *Nd:YAG* neodymium:yttrium-aluminium garnet laser, *QALY* quality-adjusted life year, *ARV* anti-reflux valve

Box 10.1 Commonly utilised SES

Wallflex®	Partially or fully covered nitinol stents (Boston Scientific, USA)
Evolution®	Partially or fully covered nitinol stents (Cook Endoscopy, USA)
Z-stent®	Partially covered stainless steel (Cook Endoscopy, USA)
Ultraflex™	Partially or fully covered nitinol stents (Boston Scientific, USA)
Niti-S Stent	Fully covered nitinol, single or double layer (Taewoong Medical, Korea)
Polyflex®	Fully covered polyester stent (Boston Scientific, USA)
Hanarostent ®	Partially or fully covered (option of S shape ARV) tri-weave Nitinol mesh (M. I. tech, Seoul, Korea)

10.3.1.1 Oesophageal Stents

Intraluminal stenting of the oesophagus for relief of malignant dysphagia is not a new concept and was first described in the British Medical Journal in the late nineteenth century [52]. Rigid stents made from ivory or silver are no longer used, but rigid plastic stents have been used widely until recently. Stent technology has advanced significantly over the last decade; self-expanding stents (SES) have superseded rigid prostheses, and they are associated with less morbidity, improved dysphagia scores and less reintervention and are therefore recommended over rigid prostheses [36, 43, 47, 53]. Although commonly used to palliate intraluminal obstruction, they can also be used to alleviate extrinsic compression and fistula formation [54]. Examples of SES are illustrated in Fig. 10.3. Commonly used SESs are listed in Box 10.1.

A comprehensive Cochrane review in 2009 involving over 2,500 patients concluded that SES and BT provide good palliation of dysphagia and were recommended over endoscopic ablative therapies [56]. BT provides a less instant relief of dysphagia than SES but is associated with a better quality of life (QOL) and survival.

SES

The 1990s saw the development of SES. Initial manufacturing focused on self-expanding metal stents (SEMS), and this quickly gained favour. However, technology with self-expanding plastic stents (SEPS) is rapidly progressing, and newer designs are entering the market place. Compared to their rigid counterparts, SES can be placed endoscopically often without the need for oesophageal dilatation. They are associated with less pain, are less prone to stent migration and have superseded their rigid counterparts [43, 47].

SEMS

SEMS are made from several tiny metallic wires arranged in braided, cross hatched or interconnecting rows to produce an expandable mesh tube. Stent sizes commonly used are between 10 and 15 cm long with an internal diameter of 18–23 mm. SEMS were traditionally made from stainless steel but are now more commonly made from nitinol (an alloy of titanium and nickel). Nitinol has superelastic properties with "shape" or "form memory." This allows it to be compressed to 30 % of its original diameter, ideal for a slimline delivery catheter.

SEMS have revolutionised the treatment of malignant dysphagia due to their ease of placement with low perioperative risk. However, complications do occur and late complications may be as high as 40 % [57]. Complications of SEMS include tumour ingrowth, food bolus obstruction, stent migration and fistula formation [57–59].

SEPS

SEPS are commonly made from braided polyesters with a silicone or polyurethane outer membrane. They have excellent uniform radial force and flared ends to "grip" the oesophagus and minimise stent migration. They can be used as a temporising measure as they maintain the ability to be extracted if the stent is no longer required. This is a rare occurrence in the palliative setting but extremely useful when dealing with an anastomotic leak, iatrogenic oesophageal perforation or benign strictures. They are compatible with CT and magnetic resonance imaging (MRI) and are considerably cheaper to manufacture (typically \$2,100 vs. \$1,100) [39].

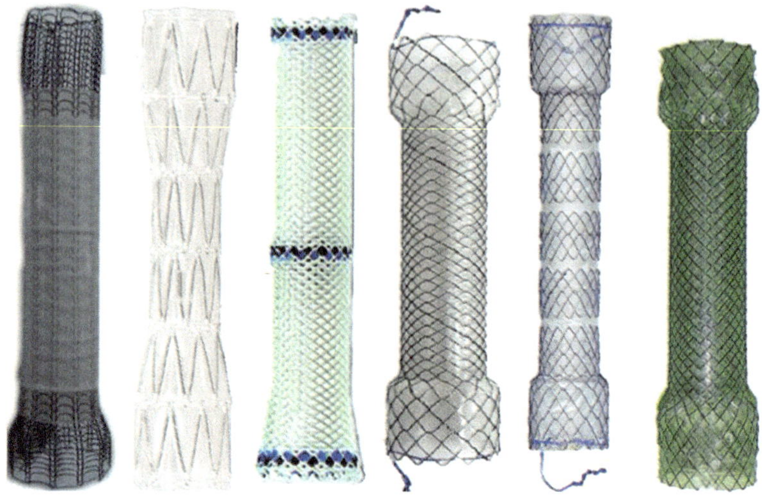

Fig. 10.3 Illustration of popular SES. From *left* to *right*: Ultraflex™ (Boston Scientific, USA), Z-stent® (Cook Endoscopy, USA), Polyflex® (Boston Scientific, USA), Niti-S stent (Taewoong Medical, Korea), Choostent® (M. I. Tech, Korea) and Bonastent® (Standard Sci-Tech, Korea) (Reprinted with permission from Shim [55])

SES Design

Recent advances in stent design have focused on two key areas; preventing gastro-oesophageal reflux and improved anti-migration properties.

Anti-reflux valves (ARV) have been incorporated into SEMS with varying degrees of success. Several designs including polyurethane "windsock" valves (Dua stent, Wilson-Cook) and S-type valves (Bonastent®, Standard Sci-Tech) have been utilised, and their efficacy has been shown in non-randomised trials [60] (Fig. 10.4).

Power et al. [40] randomised 49 patients to either an anti-reflux stent (Hanarostent®, M.I. Tech) or a traditional non-reflux valve stent (Ultraflex™, Boston Scientific). Reflux was significantly less in those with the anti-reflux valve, and dysphagia scores were equal. However, other randomised trials have failed to show any significant improvement in reflux with ARVs and in some cases a nonsignificant trend to more complications and more reflux [34, 41, 45]. This may in part be due to the ARV causing a degree of intraluminal obstruction and oesophageal stasis with regurgitation. Moreover, reflux that does occur after stent insertion is often controllable with a low-dose proton pump inhibitor (PPI) [38]. Along with guidelines from the British Society of Gastroenterology, a meta-analysis has failed to show any significant benefit for ARVs and is therefore not currently recommended [21, 61].

To combat stent migration, the Flamingo Wallstent™ (Boston Scientific) has an altered braid angle between the proximal and distal portions of the stent which allows the distal part of the stent to stretch with oesophageal peristalsis. Many stents are now "partially covered" which allow the normal oesophageal mucosa to grip the proximal and distal ends of the stent along with "flared" ends (Ultraflex™, Boston Scientific) or conical design (Flamingo Wallstent) to act as anchor points. The Alimaxx-E™ (Alveolus) covered stent has 20 "anti-migration struts" on the outside of the stent; however, initial results have failed to show any significant advantage [62].

SES Insertion

SES can be placed endoscopically or radiologically. We prefer to place our own stents under direct endoscopic vision. Our technique is to perform a gastroscopy to assess tumour length, tortuosity of the oesophagus and the degree of stenosis. The proximal extent of the tumour is then marked by injecting a small volume of submucosal radioopaque solution (usually Ultravist®, Bayer Healthcare or Omnipaque™, GE Healthcare) in two separate areas diametrically opposite. Marking can also be performed by placing metal clips on the patient's chest, but we feel this is a less precise technique. A flexible guidewire (Savary-Gilliard, Cook Medical) is then placed under direct vision into the second part of the duodenum and the endoscope is withdrawn. An appropriately sized stent is chosen. The length should cover 2 cm proximal and distal

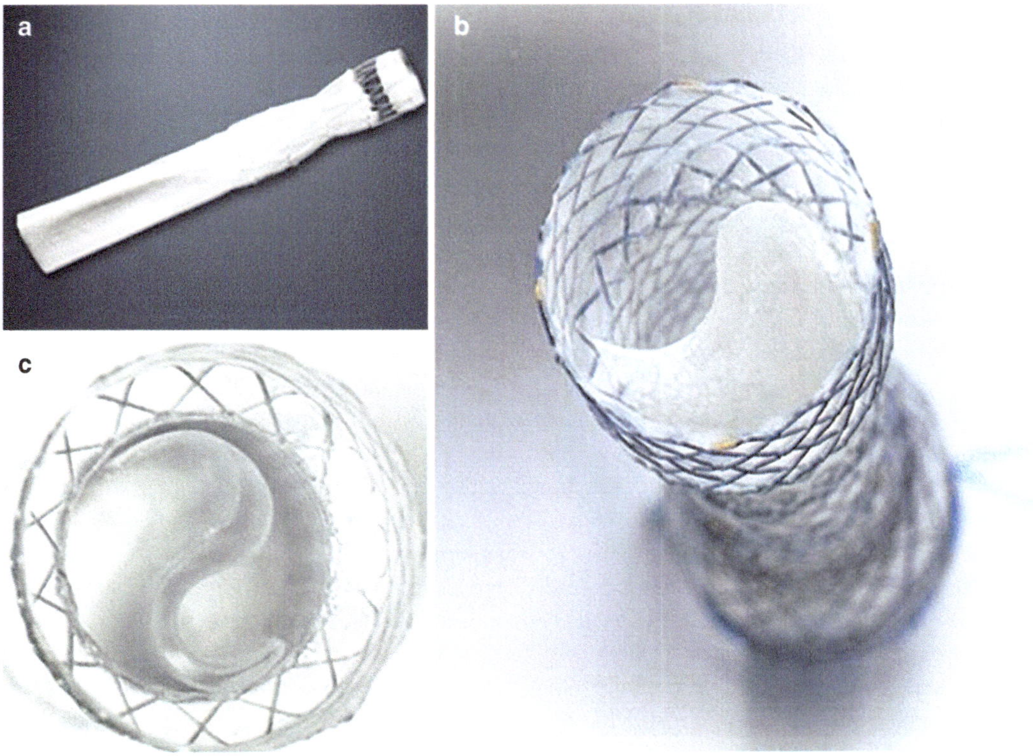

Fig. 10.4 Illustration of types of SES with ARVs. A: Dua Z-stent® (Wilson-Cook Medical, USA) with the windsock-type valve. B: S-type valve in the Choostent® (M. I. Tech, Korea). C: Bonastent® (Standard Sci-Tech, Korea) with the S-type valve (Reprinted with permission from Shim [55])

to the tumour and be approximately 18 mm in diameter (there is no evidence to favour a larger internal diameter) [36]. Under fluoroscopic guidance, the stent is fed down the guidewire and deployed with a 2 cm margin above the proximal extent of the tumour. Care must be taken in the final stages of deployment as some stents are prone to migrate distally (Ultraflex, Boston Scientific). A check endoscopy is then performed to check the position of the stent and that it has deployed correctly.

Particular issues arise when placing SEMS across the gastro-oesophageal junction (GOJ). Abutment of the distal end of the stent into the gastric wall (often the greater curve) may lead to a functional obstruction [63]. This risk can be minimised by ensuring that when placing the stent, a long length of distal stent does not protrude into the stomach.

Stent insertion is limited proximally to within 2 cm of the cricopharyngeus as the patient will experience pain and globus; therefore, SES are often not suitable for proximal oesophageal tumours.

Procedural Care

SEMS can be placed under intravenous sedation with midazolam and good opioid analgesia. However, some endoscopists prefer anaesthetic support and use intravenous propofol as sedation or perform insertion under general anaesthesia. This is our preferred approach as it provides airway protection and permits time to deal with any unforeseen complications during stent deployment, should they arise.

Postoperatively, patients are nursed upright to avoid aspiration risk and monitored by experienced nursing staff until the patient is alert and fully conscious. Patients are allowed liquids on day 1 and a low residue diet for the first week. We routinely recommend to our patients that they should remain on a soft diet and avoid foods which require excessive mastication, as food bolus obstruction can occur.

Patients may also experience retro sternal chest pain and should be counselled prior to the procedure. Antispasmodics, paracetamol and low-dose opioid analgesia (codeine phosphate) usually suffice to alleviate pain.

Uncovered Versus Partially Covered Versus Covered SEMS

Initial SEMS were uncovered, and whilst having excellent anti-migratory properties, early tumour ingrowth occurred. Fully covered stents negated this problem but often underwent migration [35]. This in part has been overcome with a change in design with proximal and distal flared ends or conical form.

Most SEMS in use now are partially covered with a 1–2 cm uncovered proximal and distal end and covered central section (usually silicone or polyurethane) to prevent migration and tumour ingrowth. Fully covered stents are still the first choice for dealing with oesophageal perforations and leaks. Partially covered stents still may suffer from tumour ingrowth, but this can usually be treated with argon plasma coagulation (APC) or photodynamic therapy (PDT) [64].

Few published randomised trials comparing covered vs. uncovered SEMS exist. Vakil et al. [49] randomised 62 patient with malignant oesophageal obstruction to covered or noncovered SEMS. Primary endpoints were the relief of dysphagia and stent migration. Initial palliation of dysphagia was similar but tumour ingrowth and the need for reintervention as a consequence were significantly greater in the uncovered stent group. There was a nonsignificant trend to more stent migration in the covered group.

Currently, the majority of physicians opt for partially covered stents as they appear to offer the positive benefits of both covered and uncovered stents.

SEMS Versus SEPS

It appears that both SEMS and SEPS are equally effective at palliating dysphagia. However, in two RCTs, SEPS are associated with increased stent migration [37, 39].

A group from Italy randomised 101 patients to Polyflex® (Boston Scientific) or partially covered Ultraflex stents [39]. Successful placement was achieved in 100 % of the Ultraflex and 98 % of the Polyflex group. Whilst control of dysphagia was equivalent, significantly more complications including late migration occurred in the Polyflex group.

Veschuur et al. [37] randomised 125 patients with malignant dysphagia into a trial of Polyflex, Ultraflex or Niti-S stent (Taewoong Medical). Again, all three stents effectively palliated dysphagia, with a higher rate of stent migration in the Polyflex group and tumour ingrowth with the Ultraflex stent.

Meta-analysis has shown that SEMS are superior to SEPS with regard to a lower periprocedural mortality and morbidity, stent migration and quality of palliation [65].

Does the Type of Stent Really Matter?

Some of the evidence regarding this issue is confounding and subject to bias. At present, there is no high-level evidence to suggest one stent is superior to another. It appears more important that an appropriately sized stent is placed and that the operator is comfortable and familiar with the delivery device and can manage any immediate complications.

Siersema et al. [48] randomised 100 patients to a covered Flamingo Wallstent or Ultraflex stent or Gianturco Z-stent (Wilson-Cook, Denmark). There was no significant difference in complications between either of the stents and offered the same palliation of dysphagia. Stent migration was reduced with an increase in stent diameter. These findings were replicated in a later randomised controlled trial (RCT) of 53 patients using two of the same stents [46].

Does Size Really Matter?

Debate continues around the optimum diameter stent. Some hold the view that the largest diameter possible should be used to avoid stent migration, food bolus obstruction and recurrent dysphagia at the risk of increased chest pain and odynophagia. Our experience, however, suggests "bigger" may not be "better."

Shenfine et al. [36] published the long-term clinical outcomes from their original cost analysis study and found significantly worse dysphagia scores in the rigid stent group at 6 weeks. Global quality of life scores fell across all groups but the non-stent treatments return to baseline quicker mainly due to less pain when compared to SEMS. In terms of relief of dysphagia and rates of early and late complications, there was no advantage using 24 mm stent over the smaller 18 mm stent, and the latter was recommended. Results from this trial have been adopted into our practice.

SEMS and Multimodal Therapy

There is some evidence for using SEMS as multimodal therapy. In a RCT from India, 84 patients were randomised to SEMS (Ultraflex) or SEMS (Ultraflex) + 30 Gy of external beam radiotherapy (EBRT) [31]. The addition of EBRT prolonged the dysphagia-free survival and overall survival with the expense of a transient decline in QOL immediately after the EBRT.

In a retrospective analysis of 437 patients, the outcomes of patients deemed palliative at MDT were analysed in four subgroups: SEMS, chemotherapy, radiotherapy and chemoradiotherapy (CRT) [66]. Radiotherapy was administered in 40–60 Gy, those without metastatic disease receiving the higher doses. The survival in the CRT arm was significantly better than the SEMS group and not significantly better than a single modality treatment, and it was therefore recommended as the palliative treatment of choice in those medically fit.

Cost Analysis

In one of the largest and most comprehensively designed RCTs conducted in the UK, 217 patients with malignant oesophageal obstruction were randomised on an intention to treat basis [43]. Patients were divided into experimental and control arms. Each arm was then subdivided into two further arms; the experimental arm was randomised to either 18 or 24 mm SEMS and the control arm was randomised to rigid endoprosthesis or non-stent therapy (EBRT or APC). If the non-stent therapy failed, there was a second randomisation to any of the three stent options to avoid clinical bias.

Although SEMS initial cost was considerably more than the plastic endoprostheses (£1,200 vs. £350), there was no overall cost difference as the majority of cost incurred was from hospital length of stay. Rigid endoprostheses were associated with increased morbidity and worse dysphagia scores requiring more frequent hospital admission.

Complications and Contraindications of SES

Recognised complications of stent insertion are listed in Box 10.2.

Box 10.2 Recognised complications of SES

Early complications
- Severe pain
- Technical failure
- Stent malposition
- Early stent migration
- Aspiration pneumonia
- Incomplete stent expansion
- Perforation

Late complications
- Stent migration
- Tumour overgrowth
- Haemorrhage
- Gastro-oesophageal reflux
- Fistula formation
- Stent disruption/collapse

Whether it is due directly to the SEMS or whether it is a consequence of dealing with an advanced disease in its final stages, further procedures following SEMS insertion are common and occur in up to 50 % of patients [36]. Most early complications can be overcome endoscopically. Stents can be repositioned early if misplaced or early migration occurs. Incomplete stent expansion can be overcome with balloon dilation.

Oesophageal perforation is the most serious complication and occurs in 3–5 % of SEMS insertion [36, 39]. Fully covered SEPS have shown successful occlusion of the perforation in 90–95 %

of cases and may be an option if the perforation is recognised early [67]. Patients should be managed nil by mouth and be prescribed high-dose acid suppression and broad-spectrum antibiotics, and the clinician should have a low threshold for pleural/mediastinal drainage if sepsis ensues. Depending on prognosis, distal enteral feeding with a surgical jejunostomy or percutaneous gastrostomy should be considered.

Although perforated oesophageal tumours can be treated with subtotal oesophagectomy, they are generally considered incurable with high perioperative mortality [68–70]. Therefore, in the context of palliative measures from the onset, there is little role for oesophagectomy if iatrogenic perforation occurs.

Food bolus obstruction can often be cleared endoscopically, and late tumour ingrowth can be treated with APC or laser recanalisation, but often requires frequent sessions. A further stent can be "rail roaded" to provide extra proximal or distal cover, but in our experience, this gives a poor functional result and should be avoided if possible.

Contraindications to SES placement include tumours which require the SES to be placed within 2 cm of the upper oesophageal sphincter due to high rates of stent migration, globus sensation and severe pain. Tortuous oesophagus and near luminal obstruction makes SES placement difficult but not impossible. We have also found that patients do badly with tumours requiring stents greater than12 cm in length.

10.3.1.2 Brachytherapy

BT has been successfully used to palliate oesophageal malignancy for over 40 years. The attractiveness of BT is that it allows targeted delivery of radiotherapy to the tumour with potential sparing of surrounding healthy tissue. Its effectiveness has been proven with response rates of up to 70 % [71]. The optimal dose is unknown, but 8–20 Gy in single or double doses is common.

Berquist et al. [42] randomised 65 patients with advanced oesophageal cancer to undergo SEMS insertion or BT (7 Gy × 3 fractions). The stent group showed improved dysphagia scores at 1 month compared to BT but worse functioning and symptom scale health-related quality of life scores (HRQL). BT offered similar improvements of dysphagia at 3 months and more stable HRQL scores. Recommendations from the study were that BT should be the treatment of choice for those with a life expectancy of greater than 3 months.

In the SIREC study from the Netherlands, 209 patients with dysphagia were randomised to SEMS or BT (12 Gy) [44, 72]. The primary outcome measure of this study was dysphagia score with HRQL and cost as a secondary outcome measures. The authors concluded that despite an initial slow improvement in dysphagia, BT offered a more sustained relief of dysphagia and was associated with fewer complications. There was no significant difference in HRQL, overall cost or survival [72, 73]. As such, the authors recommended BT as first-line treatment for the palliation of malignant dysphagia.

A further publication from the same group devised a prognostic model to help chose palliative strategies. The score was based on tumour length, age, presence of metastasis and WHO performance score. Interestingly, it was shown that those in a "poor prognosis" group (Score >5) actually had 23 more days dysphagia-free survival with SEMS compared to those in the BT group [74].

Finally, Rupinski et al. [32] compared three palliative regimes for dysphagia including BT, PDT and APC. All patients received APC and were then randomised to BT, PDT or no further treatment. They showed that all therapies were effective at relieving dysphagia compared to controls. The addition of PDT or BT doubled the return time to dysphagia with fewer complications in the BT group.

High-quality randomised evidence exists supporting the use of high-dose response brachytherapy, which should be recommended as first-line treatment especially in those with a prognosis of >3 months.

10.3.1.3 Photodynamic Therapy

Photodynamic therapy (PDT) is a relatively simple technique with rapid onset of action. It is also one of the few options in relieving dysphagia with high cervical oesophageal lesions and is also highly effective for controlling tumour haemorrhage [75]. In spite of this, it is not commonly used as first-line therapy due to high initial costs of equipment and side effects of the photosensitising agent. In spite of counselling patients to avoid direct sunlight for 6 weeks, skin hypersensitivity rash still occurs in up to 10 % of patients [76]. This naturally hinders patient willingness to undergo the treatment. Stricture formation, chest pain, odynophagia, candidiasis, pleural effusions and perforations also occur, especially in patients who have undergone prior chemoradiotherapy [75, 77].

In one comprehensive review of 215 patients spanning 6 years, PDT was successful in palliating dysphagia in 85 % of patients with a mean dysphagia-free period of 66 days. PDT was required in 19 % of patients and 16 % required SEMS for recurrent dysphagia [77].

Lightdale et al. [78] randomised 236 patients to neodymium:yttrium-aluminium-garnet (Nd:YAG) laser ablation or PDT. PDT was superior to laser at controlling dysphagia at 1 month with an overall better tumour response with PDT. There were more perforations in the laser group and not surprisingly more photosensitive reactions in the PDT group. There were significantly more adverse events leading to cessation of treatment in the laser group.

In spite of this, the lack of randomised trials in the last 15 years comparing PDT against other modalities for palliative oesophageal cancer speaks volumes, and at present there are no good data to support its first-line use. It may, however, remain useful in treating those with high oesophageal lesions, controlling tumour bleeding and for stent tumour overgrowth. Newer shorter acting photosensitisers may make the treatment more acceptable.

Argon Plasma Coagulation

APC is also technically straightforward and improves dysphagia in 95 % of patients with improved HRQL when compared to SEMS [50, 79]. The equipment is relatively inexpensive and is readily available in most endoscopy suites. Repeated treatments are often needed, and the most common reported complication is bleeding [79, 80]. It is, however, extremely useful for tackling tumour overgrowth after SEMS insertion.

In one of the largest RCTs using APC in combination therapy, patients were randomised to APC with BT, APC and PDT or APC alone as a per protocol analysis [32]. There was a significant difference in dysphagia-free period with APC + BT superior to APC + PDT, which was in turn superior to APC alone. There was no significant difference in palliation of dysphagia between the APC + BT and APC + PDT. Also, HRQL was significantly better in the APC + BT group.

There is thus good evidence to support the role of APC and this, along with its relative inexpense, high operator confidence and low perforation risk, means that APC has largely superseded laser therapy for the debulking of oesophageal neoplasms in spite of the need for repeated treatments [80, 81].

Laser Recanalisation

Nd:YAG laser has been traditionally used for rapid relief of dysphagia secondary to obstructing oesophageal malignancy especially in the cervical oesophagus. Despite its effectiveness its use is dwindling mainly due to high initial setup cost of the laser, difficulty in treating long obstructing tumours and the need for multiple treatment sessions to restore intraluminal patency when compared to SEMS [51].

In a randomised trial by Dallal et al. [50], 65 patients were randomised to undergo thermal ablative therapy (Nd:YAG, APC or Argon diode laser) or SEMS. Ablative therapy was associated with significantly longer hospital stay and cost. Palliation of dysphagia was equal as were serious complications. HRQL scores deteriorated across the board but were worse in the stent group.

In randomised trials, multimodal treatment with the addition of radiotherapy has shown promise with doubling of the effective dysphagia-free time [82, 83].

Alcohol Injections

Endoscopic alcohol injection is a more traditional method and involves the injection of intratumoural 98 % ethanol. A sclerotherapy needle is used to deliver the alcohol into several locations, normally the most protuberant areas of the tumour. Up to 32 ml has been used but mean volumes of 20 ml are typical [84]. Endoscopic dilatations with Savary-Gilliard dilators may be required prior to injection.

It is an inexpensive therapy with the equipment readily available in most endoscopy suites. It does, however, often require repeat treatments and is not as efficacious as other modalities and complications including fistula formation, chest pain and mediastinitis do occur [85].

One randomised trial showed it successfully palliated dysphagia in 78 % of patients, but its action was short lived (30 days) and it was not as effective as Nd:YAG laser [86]. There is little evidence for its first-line use.

Intratumoural Chemotherapy Injections

A less mainstream option for palliation of malignant dysphagia is the injection of intratumoural chemotherapy. Cisplatin-epinephrine gel has been used with limited success. The gel and epinephrine combination is aimed at keeping the chemotherapeutic agent in the targeted location and resists diffusion into peripheral tissues.

In a study of 24 patients, one third reported an improvement in swallowing function with only one serious adverse event [87]. Although the technique is simple and equipment is readily available, there is no evidence for its first-line use.

Other Endoluminal Modalities

Bipolar electrocoagulation (BiCAP) can be used to deliver 2–3 mm of electrocautery to a tumour surface. Repeated sessions are needed, and the effects are short lived with a higher rate of perioperative mortality compared to other modalities [88]. Its role has been superseded by APC, and it is rarely used today.

Cryotherapy uses supercooling to induce tumour necrosis and cell death and has been used in the treatment of Barrett's mucosa since 2005 [89]. Low-pressure liquid nitrogen is instilled to the target tissue in 20-s bursts via an endoscopy catheter and a period of time is allowed for tissue thawing between cycles. Complete luminal response rates of 61 % with no serious adverse events have been reported [90, 91].

Oesophageal dilatation still has a role in treating malignant dysphagia especially when used as a bridge to more definitive treatment with either SEMS or chemoradiotherapy. Although there is the risk of perforation particularly during radiotherapy treatment, we have found this to be extremely low if performed over three sessions using sequential Savary-Gilliard dilators.

10.3.2 Chemotherapy, Radiotherapy and Chemoradiotherapy

Chemotherapy, radiotherapy and chemoradiotherapy are widely used in the adjuvant and neoadjuvant setting and as definitive or palliative treatments for oesophageal cancer. There is a comprehensive array of various combinations and permutations of treatment published in the literature. Yet, there is still no internationally agreed consensus on the "gold standard" for definitive treatment let alone in the palliative setting.

It is difficult to know what exactly palliative treatment entails. Some treatments may begin with the intent of being definitive and end up palliative due to disease progression or patient co-morbidities. There may be an argument that chemotherapy and radiotherapy never intend to cure so in some respects are by nature, palliative.

Discussing in detail the evidence and practical application of each modality is outside the scope of this chapter. However, considering medical and radiation oncology is integral in the treatment of oesophageal cancer, key peer review evidence has been referenced here for the interest of the reader [33, 66, 92–94].

10.3.3 The Role of Surgery in the Palliative Setting

The majority of symptoms from advanced oesophageal cancer can now be palliated with non-surgical techniques and as such palliative surgery in the form of resection or bypass is rarely if ever performed, despite its technical feasibility [95]. Furthermore, the recovery period from an oesophagectomy will delay potentially beneficial oncological therapy in those with metastatic disease. Appropriate patient selection is crucial; patients must be fit enough to withstand the rigors of surgery with a predicted life expectancy long enough to reap the benefits.

10.3.3.1 Patient Selection for Surgery

Assessing fitness for surgical treatment is essential as embarking on a treatment which may do more harm than good is unacceptable (*Primum non nocere*). Cardiorespiratory reserve is routinely assessed with pulmonary function testing (PFT) and echocardiography despite often poor correlation with functional capacity [96]. A more sophisticated method for assessing cardiorespiratory reserve is with shuttle walk testing and cardiopulmonary exercise testing (CPET) [97–99].

Currently, CPET is not widely established in oesophageal surgery as studies have been non-randomised, with small numbers. However, early data have shown that reduced peak oxygen consumption correlates with increased cardiorespiratory complications following oesophagectomy [100, 101].

10.3.3.2 Nutritional Support

One of the main indications for any form of palliative surgery is to aid nutrition. Malnutrition is common with advanced oesophageal cancer due to malignant dysphagia and the catabolic state. Percutaneous gastrostomies (PEG) and radiologically inserted gastrostomies (RIG) are easily placed and permit bolus feeding which patients often prefer. They are not suitable if there is gastric involvement of the tumour due to tumour infiltration. Gastrostomies are well tolerated by patients with minimal morbidity. Occasionally if the oesophageal lumen is completely occluded, a surgical gastrostomy or feeding jejunostomy can be placed either openly through a small left upper abdominal incision or laparoscopically.

10.3.3.3 Salvage Oesophagectomy

Salvage oesophagectomy following chemoradiotherapy is to be embarked upon with great caution due to operative challenges and increased perioperative risk [102–104]. However, it does offer the only potential cure in those patients with locoregional failure following chemoradiotherapy, and 5-year survival of 25–35 % can be achieved [105].

The effect of radiotherapy induces fibrosis within tissue planes and makes anatomical dissection difficult and sometimes impossible. Risks include damage to the thoracic duct, recurrent laryngeal nerve and major airway along with a higher incidence of anastomotic leak [104–106]. Pulmonary complications are common too with a higher incidence of pneumonia and acute respiratory distress syndrome [107–109]. Tumour-free resection margins are technically more challenging to achieve and positive margins are more likely [102, 103].

Until recently, almost all studies involved squamous cell carcinoma (SCC). However, of late Marks et al. [106] case matched 65 patients undergoing salvage oesophagectomy following CRT with 521 patients with oesophageal adenocarcinoma (AC) who underwent planned oesophagectomy after neoadjuvant CRT. Despite a higher anastomotic leak rate in the salvage group, the major perioperative events, 30-day mortality and 3-year survival were similar in both groups. Interestingly, they also found that the timing of salvage surgery post-CRT had no impact on outcome in a multivariate analysis.

Meticulous preoperative staging is paramount, and decision-making should be made in the context of the MDT; up-to-date PET and CT imaging is crucial to assess any sign of disease outside of the operative field, and CPET is recommended to assess physiological fitness which often declines after cytotoxic agents.

Although careful selection of patients is obviously paramount, it does appear that salvage oesophagectomy has a definite role to play in patients who might otherwise be considered for palliative treatment.

10.3.3.4 Palliative Oesophagectomy

Despite advances in perioperative care, surgical techniques and meticulous patient selection, planned curative oesophagectomy still remains a morbid procedure with a mortality rates up to 6 % and morbidity over 50 % [110]. Notwithstanding minimally invasive surgical techniques, average length of hospital stay ranges from 14 to 17 days and return to base line physiological function and activities of daily living taking up to 6 months [110, 111]. Fatigue and dyspnoea may even continue for longer [112]. Furthermore, patients with advanced oesophageal cancer have a limited life expectancy, and a substantial proportion of their remaining life span may be spent in hospital [42, 113].

Palliative bypass operations have been performed since the 1920s; however, in-hospital mortality rates of 32 % and median survival of less than 4 months have been reported [95]. Palliative oesophagectomy has a limited use as relief of dysphagia can now be overcome with much less invasive techniques. In short today, palliative oesophagectomy is not a realistic option.

References

1. Melhado R, Alderson D, Tucker O. The changing face of esophageal cancer. Cancer. 2010;2(1379):404.
2. Ferlay J, Shin H R, Bray F, Forman D, Mathers CD, Parkin D. GLOBCAN. Cancer incidence and mortality worldwide. International Journal of Cancer 2010;127(12):2893–2917.
3. Holmes RS, Vaughan TL. Epidemiology and pathogenesis of esophageal cancer. Semin Radiat Oncol. 2007;17(1):2–9.
4. Howlader N, Noone AM, Krapcho M, Neyman N, Aminou R, Altekruse SF. SEER cancer statistics review, 1975–2009 (Vintage 2009 populations). Bethesda: National Cancer Institute; 2009.
5. Whiteman DC, Sadeghi S, Pandeya N, Smithers BM, Gotley DC, Bain CJ, et al. Combined effects of obesity, acid reflux and smoking on the risk of adenocarcinomas of the oesophagus. Gut. 2008;57(2):173–80.
6. Frenken M. Best palliation in esophageal cancer: surgery, stenting, radiation, or what? Dis Esophagus. 2001;14(2):120–3.
7. Dikken JL, van Sandick JW, Allum WH, Johansson J, Jensen LS, Putter H, et al. Differences in outcomes of oesophageal and gastric cancer surgery across Europe. Br J Surg. 2013;100(1):83–94.
8. Rouvelas I, Zeng W, Lindblad M, Viklund P, Ye W, Lagergren J. Survival after surgery for oesophageal cancer: a population-based study. Lancet Oncol. 2005;6(11):864–70.
9. Al-Sarira AA, David G, Willmott S, Slavin JP, Deakin M, Corless DJ. Oesophagectomy practice and outcomes in england. Br J Surg. 2007;94(5):585–91.
10. Stavrou EP, Ward R, Pearson SA. Oesophagectomy rates and post-resection outcomes in patients with cancer of the oesophagus and gastro-oesophageal junction: a population-based study using linked health administrative linked data. BMC Health Serv Res. 2012;12:384.
11. Coupland VH, Lagergren J, Luchtenborg M, Jack RH, Allum W, Holmberg L, et al. Hospital volume, proportion resected and mortality from oesophageal and gastric cancer: a population-based study in England, 2004–2008. Gut. 2013;62(7):961–6.
12. Palser T, Cromwell D, J. Van der Meulen. The National Oesophago-Gastric Cancer Audit. An audit of the care received by people with oesophago-gastric cancer in England and Wales. First annual report 2008. London: NHS Information Centre; 2008.
13. Noble F, Bailey D, Panel SUGT, Tung K, Byrne JP. Impact of integrated PET/CT in the staging of oesophageal cancer: a UK population-based cohort study. Clin Radiol. 2009;64(7):699–705.
14. Howlader N, Noone AM, Krapcho M, Neyman N, Aminou R, Altekruse SF, et al. SEER cancer statistics review, 1975–2009 (vintage 2009 populations). Bethesda: National Cancer Institute. Available from: http://seer.cancer.gov/statfacts/html/esoph.html. Last accessed 10 Dec 2012.
15. Polee MB, Hop WC, Kok TC, Eskens FA, van der Burg ME, Splinter TA, et al. Prognostic factors for survival in patients with advanced oesophageal cancer treated with cisplatin-based combination chemotherapy. Br J Cancer. 2003;89(11):2045–50.
16. Dreilich M, Bergstrom S, Wagenius G, Brattstrom D, Bergqvist M. A retrospective study focusing on clinical predictive factors in 126 patients with oesophageal carcinoma. Anticancer Res. 2004;24(3b):1915–20.
17. NCCN Clinical Practice Guidelines in Oncology. Esophageal and esophagogastric junction cancers. Version 1. 2013; Available from: http://www.nccn.org/professionals/physician_gls/f_guidelines.asp#esophageal. Last accessed 21 Feb 2013.
18. Jalil R, Lamb B, Russ S, Sevdalis N, Green JS. The cancer multi-disciplinary team from the coordinators' perspective: results from a national survey in the UK. BMC Health Serv Res. 2012;12:457.
19. Health Do. Guidance on commissioning cancer services. Improving outcomes in upper GI cancer. The manual. NHS Executive. 2011; Available from: http://www.dh.gov.uk/en/Publicationsandstatistics/Publications/PublicationsPolicyAndGuidance/DH_127785. Last Accessed 01 Dec 2012.
20. Allum WH, Griffin SM, Watson A, Colin-Jones D, Association of Upper Gastrointestinal Surgeons of Great B, Ireland, et al. Guidelines for the management of oesophageal and gastric cancer. Gut. 2002;50 Suppl 5:v1–23.
21. Allum WH, Blazeby JM, Griffin SM, Cunningham D, Jankowski JA, Wong R, et al. Guidelines for the management of oesophageal and gastric cancer. Gut. 2011;60(11):1449–72.
22. South Australian Upper Gastrointestinal Cancer Care Pathway. Upper GI Working Party of the Statewide Cancer Clinical, South Australia Network. 2010

23. The NHS Cancer Plan. Department of Health, London. 2000. Available from: www.dh.gov.uk/prod_consum_dh/groups/dh.../dh_4014513.pdf.
24. Hanazaki K, Kuroda T, Wakabayashi M, Sodeyama H, Yokoyama S, Kusama J. Hepatic metastasis from esophageal cancer treated by surgical resection and hepatic arterial infusion chemotherapy. Hepatogastroenterology. 1998;45(19):201–5.
25. Yamamoto T, Tachibana M, Kinugasa S, Yoshimura H, Nagasue N. Esophagectomy and hepatic arterial chemotherapy following hepatic resection for esophageal cancer with liver metastasis. J Gastroenterol. 2001;36(8):560–3.
26. Reid TD, Chan DS, Roberts SA, Crosby TD, Williams GT, Lewis WG. Prognostic significance of circumferential resection margin involvement following oesophagectomy for cancer and the predictive role of endoluminal ultrasonography. Br J Cancer. 2012;107(12):1925–31.
27. Griffiths EA, Brummell Z, Gorthi G, Pritchard SA, Welch IM. Tumor length as a prognostic factor in esophageal malignancy: univariate and multivariate survival analyses. J Surg Oncol. 2006;93(4):258–67.
28. Twine CP, Roberts SA, Lewis WG, Dave BV, Rawlinson CE, Chan D, et al. Prognostic significance of endoluminal ultrasound-defined disease length and tumor volume (EDTV) for patients with the diagnosis of esophageal cancer. Surg Endosc. 2010;24(4):870–8.
29. Lordick F, Ott K, Krause BJ, Weber WA, Becker K, Stein HJ, et al. PET to assess early metabolic response and to guide treatment of adenocarcinoma of the oesophagogastric junction: the MUNICON phase II trial. Lancet Oncol. 2007;8(9):797–805.
30. Blazeby JM, Farndon JR, Donovan J, Alderson D. A prospective longitudinal study examining the quality of life of patients with esophageal carcinoma. Cancer. 2000;88(8):1781–7.
31. Javed A, Pal S, Dash NR, Ahuja V, Mohanti BK, Vishnubhatla S, et al. Palliative stenting with or without radiotherapy for inoperable esophageal carcinoma: a randomized trial. J Gastrointest Cancer. 2012;43(1):63–9.
32. Rupinski M, Zagorowicz E, Regula J, Fijuth J, Kraszewska E, Polkowski M, et al. Randomized comparison of three palliative regimens including brachytherapy, photodynamic therapy, and APC in patients with malignant dysphagia (CONSORT 1a) (revised II). Am J Gastroenterol. 2011; 106(9):1612–20.
33. Rosenblatt E, Jones G, Sur RK, Donde B, Salvajoli JV, Ghosh-Laskar S, et al. Adding external beam to intra-luminal brachytherapy improves palliation in obstructive squamous cell oesophageal cancer: a prospective multi-centre randomized trial of the International Atomic Energy Agency. Radiother Oncol. 2010;97(3):488–94.
34. Blomberg J, Wenger U, Lagergren J, Arnelo U, Agustsson T, Johnsson E, et al. Antireflux stent versus conventional stent in the palliation of distal esophageal cancer. A randomized, multicenter clinical trial. Scand J Gastroenterol. 2010;45(2):208–16.
35. Kim ES, Jeon SW, Park SY, Cho CM, Tak WY, Kweon YO, et al. Comparison of double-layered and covered Niti-S stents for palliation of malignant dysphagia. J Gastroenterol Hepatol. 2009;24(1):114–9.
36. Shenfine J, McNamee P, Steen N, Bond J, Griffin SM. A randomized controlled clinical trial of palliative therapies for patients with inoperable esophageal cancer. Am J Gastroenterol. 2009; 104(7):1674–85.
37. Verschuur EM, Repici A, Kuipers EJ, Steyerberg EW, Siersema PD. New design esophageal stents for the palliation of dysphagia from esophageal or gastric cardia cancer: a randomized trial. Am J Gastroenterol. 2008;103(2):304–12.
38. Sabharwal T, Gulati MS, Fotiadis N, Dourado R, Botha A, Mason R, et al. Randomised comparison of the FerX Ella antireflux stent and the ultraflex stent: proton pump inhibitor combination for prevention of post-stent reflux in patients with esophageal carcinoma involving the esophago-gastric junction. J Gastroenterol Hepatol. 2008;23(5):723–8.
39. Conio M, Repici A, Battaglia G, De Pretis G, Ghezzo L, Bittinger M, et al. A randomized prospective comparison of self-expandable plastic stents and partially covered self-expandable metal stents in the palliation of malignant esophageal dysphagia. Am J Gastroenterol. 2007;102(12):2667–77.
40. Power C, Byrne PJ, Lim K, Ravi N, Moore J, Fitzgerald T, et al. Superiority of anti-reflux stent compared with conventional stents in the palliative management of patients with cancer of the lower esophagus and esophago-gastric junction: results of a randomized clinical trial. Dis Esophagus. 2007;20(6):466–70.
41. Wenger U, Johnsson E, Arnelo U, Lundell L, Lagergren J. An antireflux stent versus conventional stents for palliation of distal esophageal or cardia cancer: a randomized clinical study. Surg Endosc. 2006;20(11):1675–80.
42. Bergquist H, Wenger U, Johnsson E, Nyman J, Ejnell H, Hammerlid E, et al. Stent insertion or endoluminal brachytherapy as palliation of patients with advanced cancer of the esophagus and gastroesophageal junction. Results of a randomized, controlled clinical trial. Dis Esophagus. 2005;18(3):131–9.
43. Shenfine J, McNamee P, Steen N, Bond J, Griffin SM. A pragmatic randomised controlled trial of the cost-effectiveness of palliative therapies for patients with inoperable oesophageal cancer. Health Technol Assess. 2005;9(5):iii, 1–121.
44. Homs MY, Steyerberg EW, Eijkenboom WM, Tilanus HW, Stalpers LJ, Bartelsman JF, et al. Single-dose brachytherapy versus metal stent placement for the palliation of dysphagia from oesophageal cancer: multicentre randomised trial. Lancet. 2004;364(9444):1497–504.

45. Homs MY, Wahab PJ, Kuipers EJ, Steyerberg EW, Grool TA, Haringsma J, et al. Esophageal stents with antireflux valve for tumors of the distal esophagus and gastric cardia: a randomized trial. Gastrointest Endosc. 2004;60(5):695–702.
46. Sabharwal T, Hamady MS, Chui S, Atkinson S, Mason R, Adam A. A randomised prospective comparison of the Flamingo Wallstent and Ultraflex stent for palliation of dysphagia associated with lower third oesophageal carcinoma. Gut. 2003;52(7):922–6.
47. O'Donnell CA, Fullarton GM, Watt E, Lennon K, Murray GD, Moss JG. Randomized clinical trial comparing self-expanding metallic stents with plastic endoprostheses in the palliation of oesophageal cancer. Br J Surg. 2002;89(8):985–92.
48. Siersema PD, Hop WC, van Blankenstein M, van Tilburg AJ, Bac DJ, Homs MY, et al. A comparison of 3 types of covered metal stents for the palliation of patients with dysphagia caused by esophagogastric carcinoma: a prospective, randomized study. Gastrointest Endosc. 2001;54(2):145–53.
49. Vakil N, Morris AI, Marcon N, Segalin A, Peracchia A, Bethge N, et al. A prospective, randomized, controlled trial of covered expandable metal stents in the palliation of malignant esophageal obstruction at the gastroesophageal junction. Am J Gastroenterol. 2001;96(6):1791–6.
50. Dallal HJ, Smith GD, Grieve DC, Ghosh S, Penman ID, Palmer KR. A randomized trial of thermal ablative therapy versus expandable metal stents in the palliative treatment of patients with esophageal carcinoma. Gastrointest Endosc. 2001;54(5):549–57.
51. Konigsrainer A, Riedmann B, De Vries A, Ofner D, Spechtenhauser B, Aigner F, et al. Expandable metal stents versus laser combined with radiotherapy for palliation of unresectable esophageal cancer: a prospective randomized trial. Hepatogastroenterology. 2000;47(33):724–7.
52. Symonds CJ. The treatment of malignant stricture of the oesophagus by tubage or permanent Catheterism. Br Med J. 1887;1(1373):870–3.
53. Siersema PD, Hop WC, Dees J, Tilanus HW, van Blankenstein M. Coated self-expanding metal stents versus latex prostheses for esophagogastric cancer with special reference to prior radiation and chemotherapy: a controlled, prospective study. Gastrointest Endosc. 1998;47(2):113–20.
54. van Heel NC, Haringsma J, Spaander MC, Bruno MJ, Kuipers EJ. Esophageal stents for the relief of malignant dysphagia due to extrinsic compression. Endoscopy. 2010;42(7):536–40.
55. Shim C-S. How I do it: expandable eophageal stents." Publication of the World Endoscopy Organization http://www.worldendo.org/assets/downloads/pdf/publications/how_i_doit/2007/omed_hid_expandable_esophageal_stents.pdf
56. Sreedharan A, Harris K, Crellin A, Forman D, Everett SM. Interventions for dysphagia in oesophageal cancer. Cochrane Database Syst Rev 2009(4):CD005048.
57. Wenger U, Luo J, Lundell L, Lagergren J. A nationwide study of the use of self-expanding stents in patients with esophageal cancer in Sweden. Endoscopy. 2005;37(4):329–34.
58. Kozarek RA. Complications and lessons learned from 10 years of expandable gastrointestinal prostheses. Dig Dis. 1999;17(1):14–22.
59. Raijman I, Siddique I, Ajani J, Lynch P. Palliation of malignant dysphagia and fistulae with coated expandable metal stents: experience with 101 patients. Gastrointest Endosc. 1998;48(2):172–9.
60. Laasch HU, Marriott A, Wilbraham L, Tunnah S, England RE, Martin DF. Effectiveness of open versus antireflux stents for palliation of distal esophageal carcinoma and prevention of symptomatic gastroesophageal reflux. Radiology. 2002;225(2):359–65.
61. Sgourakis G, Gockel I, Radtke A, Dedemadi G, Goumas K, Mylona S, et al. The use of self-expanding stents in esophageal and gastroesophageal junction cancer palliation: a meta-analysis and meta-regression analysis of outcomes. Dig Dis Sci. 2010;55(11):3018–30.
62. Uitdehaag MJ, van Hooft JE, Verschuur EM, Repici A, Steyerberg EW, Fockens P, et al. A fully-covered stent (Alimaxx-E) for the palliation of malignant dysphagia: a prospective follow-up study. Gastrointest Endosc. 2009;70(6):1082–9.
63. Freeman RK, Ascioti AJ, Giannini T, Mahidhara RJ. Analysis of unsuccessful esophageal stent placements for esophageal perforation, fistula, or anastomotic leak. Ann Thorac Surg. 2012;94(3):959–64. discussion 64–5.
64. Sharma P, Kozarek R, Practice Parameters Committee of American College of G. Role of esophageal stents in benign and malignant diseases. Am J Gastroenterol. 2010;105(2):258–73. quiz 74.
65. Yakoub D, Fahmy R, Athanasiou T, Alijani A, Rao C, Darzi A, et al. Evidence-based choice of esophageal stent for the palliative management of malignant dysphagia. World J Surg. 2008;32(9):1996–2009.
66. Sgourakis G, Gockel I, Karaliotas C, Moehler M, Schimanski CC, Schmidberger H, et al. Survival after chemotherapy and/or radiotherapy versus self-expanding metal stent insertion in the setting of inoperable esophageal cancer: a case–control study. BMC Cancer. 2012;12:70.
67. Moyes LH, Mackay CK, Forshaw MJ. The use of self-expanding plastic stents in the management of oesophageal leaks and spontaneous oesophageal perforations. Diagn Ther Endosc. 2011;2011:418103.
68. Jethwa P, Lala A, Powell J, McConkey CC, Gillison EW, Spychal RT. A regional audit of iatrogenic perforation of tumours of the oesophagus and cardia. Aliment Pharmacol Ther. 2005;21(4):479–84.
69. Griffin SC, Desai J, Townsend ER, Fountain SW. Oesophageal resection after instrumental perforation. Eur J Cardiothorac Surg. 1990;4(4):211–3.

70. Adam DJ, Thompson AM, Walker WS, Cameron EW. Oesophagogastrectomy for iatrogenic perforation of oesophageal and cardia carcinoma. Br J Surg. 1996;83(10):1429–32.
71. Sur RK, Donde B, Levin VC, Mannell A. Fractionated high dose rate intraluminal brachytherapy in palliation of advanced esophageal cancer. Int J Radiat Oncol Biol Phys. 1998;40(2):447–53.
72. Homs MY, Essink-Bot ML, Borsboom GJ, Steyerberg EW, Siersema PD, Dutch SSG. Quality of life after palliative treatment for oesophageal carcinoma – a prospective comparison between stent placement and single dose brachytherapy. Eur J Cancer. 2004;40(12):1862–71.
73. Polinder S, Homs MY, Siersema PD, Steyerberg EW, Dutch SSG. Cost study of metal stent placement vs single-dose brachytherapy in the palliative treatment of oesophageal cancer. Br J Cancer. 2004;90(11):2067–72.
74. Steyerberg EW, Homs MY, Stokvis A, Essink-Bot ML, Siersema PD, Group SS. Stent placement or brachytherapy for palliation of dysphagia from esophageal cancer: a prognostic model to guide treatment selection. Gastrointest Endosc. 2005;62(3):333–40.
75. Luketich JD, Christie NA, Buenaventura PO, Weigel TL, Keenan RJ, Nguyen NT. Endoscopic photodynamic therapy for obstructing esophageal cancer: 77 cases over a 2-year period. Surg Endosc. 2000;14(7):653–7.
76. Pass HI. Photodynamic therapy in oncology: mechanisms and clinical use. J Natl Cancer Inst. 1993; 85(6):443–56.
77. Litle VR, Luketich JD, Christie NA, Buenaventura PO, Alvelo-Rivera M, McCaughan JS, et al. Photodynamic therapy as palliation for esophageal cancer: experience in 215 patients. Ann Thorac Surg. 2003;76(5):1687–92. discussion 92–3.
78. Lightdale CJ, Heier SK, Marcon NE, McCaughan Jr JS, Gerdes H, Overholt BF, et al. Photodynamic therapy with porfimer sodium versus thermal ablation therapy with Nd:YAG laser for palliation of esophageal cancer: a multicenter randomized trial. Gastrointest Endosc. 1995;42(6):507–12.
79. Eickhoff A, Jakobs R, Schilling D, Hartmann D, Weickert U, Enderle MD, et al. Prospective nonrandomized comparison of two modes of argon beamer (APC) tumor desobstruction: effectiveness of the new pulsed APC versus forced APC. Endoscopy. 2007;39(7):637–42.
80. Kofoed SC, Lundsgaard M, Ellemann AC, Svendsen LB. Low morbidity after palliation of obstructing gastro-oesophageal adenocarcinoma to restore swallowing function. Dan Med J. 2012;59(6):A4434.
81. Manner H, May A, Rabenstein T, Pech O, Nachbar L, Enderle MD, et al. Prospective evaluation of a new high-power argon plasma coagulation system (hp-APC) in therapeutic gastrointestinal endoscopy. Scand J Gastroenterol. 2007;42(3):397–405.
82. Sargeant IR, Tobias JS, Blackman G, Thorpe S, Glover JR, Bown SG. Radiotherapy enhances laser palliation of malignant dysphagia: a randomised study. Gut. 1997;40(3):362–9.
83. Spencer GM, Thorpe SM, Blackman GM, Solano J, Tobias JS, Lovat LB, et al. Laser augmented by brachytherapy versus laser alone in the palliation of adenocarcinoma of the oesophagus and cardia: a randomised study. Gut. 2002;50(2):224–7.
84. Chung SC, Leong HT, Choi CY, Leung JW, Li AK. Palliation of malignant oesophageal obstruction by endoscopic alcohol injection. Endoscopy. 1994; 26(3):275–7.
85. Moreira LS, Coelho RC, Sadala RU, Dani R. The use of ethanol injection under endoscopic control to palliate dysphagia caused by esophagogastric cancer. Endoscopy. 1994;26(3):311–4.
86. Carazzone A, Bonavina L, Segalin A, Ceriani C, Peracchia A. Endoscopic palliation of oesophageal cancer: results of a prospective comparison of Nd:YAG laser and ethanol injection. Eur J Surg. 1999;165(4):351–6.
87. Harbord M, Dawes RF, Barr H, Giovannini M, Viens P, Eysselein V, et al. Palliation of patients with dysphagia due to advanced esophageal cancer by endoscopic injection of cisplatin/epinephrine injectable gel. Gastrointest Endosc. 2002;56(5):644–51.
88. Mambrini P, Audibert P, Barthet M, Bertolino JG, Brequeville JM, Amoros F, et al. [Palliative treatment of esophageal neoplastic stenosis using bipolar electrocoagulation probe. Gastroenterol Clin Biol. 1996;20(10):844–51. Traitement palliatif des stenoses neoplasiques oesophagiennes par sonde d'electrocoagulation bipolaire (BICAP).
89. Johnston MH, Eastone JA, Horwhat JD, Cartledge J, Mathews JS, Foggy JR. Cryoablation of Barrett's esophagus: a pilot study. Gastrointest Endosc. 2005; 62(6):842–8.
90. Greenwald BD, Dumot JA, Abrams JA, Lightdale CJ, David DS, Nishioka NS, et al. Endoscopic spray cryotherapy for esophageal cancer: safety and efficacy. Gastrointest Endosc. 2010;71(4):686–93.
91. Greenwald BD, Dumot JA, Horwhat JD, Lightdale CJ, Abrams JA. Safety, tolerability, and efficacy of endoscopic low-pressure liquid nitrogen spray cryotherapy in the esophagus. Dis Esophagus. 2010; 23(1):13–9.
92. Cunningham D, Starling N, Rao S, Iveson T, Nicolson M, Coxon F, et al. Capecitabine and oxaliplatin for advanced esophagogastric cancer. N Engl J Med. 2008;358(1):36–46.
93. Grunberger B, Raderer M, Schmidinger M, Hejna M. Palliative chemotherapy for recurrent and metastatic esophageal cancer. Anticancer Res. 2007;27(4C):2705–14.
94. Homs MY, v d Gaast A, Siersema PD, Steyerberg EW, Kuipers EJ. Chemotherapy for metastatic carcinoma of the esophagus and gastro-esophageal junction. Cochrane Database Syst Rev 2006(4):CD004063.

95. Whooley BP, Law S, Murthy SC, Alexandrou A, Chu KM, Wong J. The Kirschner operation in unresectable esophageal cancer: current application. Arch Surg. 2002;137(11):1228–32.
96. Halm EA, Browner WS, Tubau JF, Tateo IM, Mangano DT. Echocardiography for assessing cardiac risk in patients having noncardiac surgery. Study of Perioperative Ischemia Research Group. Ann Intern Med. 1996;125(6):433–41.
97. Older P, Hall A, Hader R. Cardiopulmonary exercise testing as a screening test for perioperative management of major surgery in the elderly. Chest. 1999; 1116(2):355–62.
98. Murray P, Whiting P, Hutchinson SP, Ackroyd R, Stoddard CJ, Billings C. Preoperative shuttle walking testing and outcome after oesophagogastrectomy. Br J Anaesth. 2007;99(6):809–11.
99. Older P, Smith R, Hall A, French C. Preoperative cardiopulmonary risk assessment by cardiopulmonary exercise testing. Crit Care Resusc. 2000;2(3):198–208.
100. Nagamatsu Y, Shima I, Yamana H, Fujita H, Shirouzu K, Ishitake T. Preoperative evaluation of cardiopulmonary reserve with the use of expired gas analysis during exercise testing in patients with squamous cell carcinoma of the thoracic esophagus. J Thorac Cardiovasc Surg. 2001;121(6): 1064–8.
101. Forshaw MJ, Strauss DC, Davies AR, Wilson D, Lams B, Pearce A, et al. Is cardiopulmonary exercise testing a useful test before esophagectomy? Ann Thorac Surg. 2008;85(1):294–9.
102. Borghesi S, Hawkins MA, Tait D. Oesophagectomy after definitive chemoradiation in patients with locally advanced oesophageal cancer. Clin Oncol. 2008;20(3):221–6.
103. Schieman C, Wigle DA, Deschamps C, Nichols 3rd FC, Cassivi SD, Shen KR, et al. Salvage resections for recurrent or persistent cancer of the proximal esophagus after chemoradiotherapy. Ann Thorac Surg. 2013;95(2):459–63.
104. Miyata H, Yamasaki M, Takiguchi S, Nakajima K, Fujiwara Y, Nishida T, et al. Salvage esophagectomy after definitive chemoradiotherapy for thoracic esophageal cancer. J Surg Oncol. 2009;100(6): 442–6.
105. Gardner-Thorpe J, Hardwick RH, Dwerryhouse SJ. Salvage oesophagectomy after local failure of definitive chemoradiotherapy. Br J Surg. 2007; 94(9):1059–66.
106. Marks JL, Hofstetter W, Correa AM, Mehran RJ, Rice D, Roth J, et al. Salvage esophagectomy after failed definitive chemoradiation for esophageal adenocarcinoma. Ann Thorac Surg. 2012;94(4):1126–32. discussion 1132–3.
107. Tachimori Y. Role of salvage esophagectomy after definitive chemoradiotherapy. Gen Thorac Cardiovasc Surg. 2009;57(2):71–8.
108. Tachimori Y, Kanamori N, Uemura N, Hokamura N, Igaki H, Kato H. Salvage esophagectomy after high-dose chemoradiotherapy for esophageal squamous cell carcinoma. J Thorac Cardiovasc Surg. 2009;137(1):49–54. Epub 2009/01/22.
109. Yoo C, Park JH, Yoon DH, Park SI, Kim HR, Kim JH, et al. Salvage esophagectomy for locoregional failure after chemoradiotherapy in patients with advanced esophageal cancer. Ann Thorac Surg. 2012;94(6):1862–8.
110. Merritt RE, Whyte RI, D'Arcy NT, Hoang CD, Shrager JB. Morbidity and mortality after esophagectomy following neoadjuvant chemoradiation. Ann Thorac Surg. 2011;92(6):2034–40.
111. Parameswaran R, Titcomb DR, Blencowe NS, Berrisford RG, Wajed SA, Streets CG, et al. Assessment and comparison of recovery after open and minimally invasive esophagectomy for cancer: an exploratory study in two centers. Ann Surg Oncol. 2013;20(6):1970–7.
112. Scarpa M, Valente S, Alfieri R, Cagol M, Diamantis G, Ancona E, et al. Systematic review of health-related quality of life after esophagectomy for esophageal cancer. World J Gastroenterol. 2011;17(42):4660–74.
113. Cancer Research UK. CancerStats report – oesophageal cancer UK, Cancer Research UK. 2008. Available from: http://www.cancerresearchuk.org/cancer-info/cancerstats/types/oesophagus/incidence/uk-oesophageal-cancer-incidence-statistics. Last accessed 30 Nov 2012.

Stomach

11

Markus Albertsmeier, Karl-Walter Jauch, and Martin K. Angele

Contents

M. Albertsmeier, MD • K.-W. Jauch, MD, FACS
M.K. Angele, MD, FACS (✉)
Department of General, Visceral, Transplantation, Vascular and Thoracic Surgery, Ludwig Maximilians University, Munich 81377, Germany
e-mail: markus.albertsmeier@med.uni-muenchen.de; karl-walter.jauch@med.uni-muenchen.de; martin.angele@med.uni-muenchen.de

Although progress in systemic therapy has changed the surgical approach to advanced gastric carcinoma, allowing gastrectomy with or without metastasectomy in selected cases, the goal of therapy remains non-curative and directed towards symptom control for most patients. This chapter focuses on quality of life and the treatment of complications in advanced gastric carcinoma. The role of palliative surgery in the management of bleeding, obstruction, and perforation is discussed and weighed against nonsurgical alternatives such as endoscopy, radiotherapy, and interventional radiology. Sections on peritoneal carcinosis and chemotherapy-refractory ascites are also included.

11.1 Introduction

Gastric carcinoma represents the second leading cause of cancer-related death worldwide. Despite improvements in overall survival, the majority (60–70 %) of patients diagnosed with gastric cancer present with advanced stages, i.e., metastatic disease or recurrence after primary resection. Innovations in systemic therapy have changed the surgical approach to advanced gastric cancer, allowing gastrectomy with or without metastasectomy in selected patients. For most patients, however, the goal of therapy is frequently non-curative and directed towards symptom control.

Bleeding is the most important adverse event caused by locally advanced gastric cancer. Other major complications are gastric outlet obstruction and malnutrition. Rarely, patients

M. Wichmann, G. Maddern (eds.), *Palliative Surgery*,
DOI 10.1007/978-3-642-53709-7_11, © Springer-Verlag Berlin Heidelberg 2014

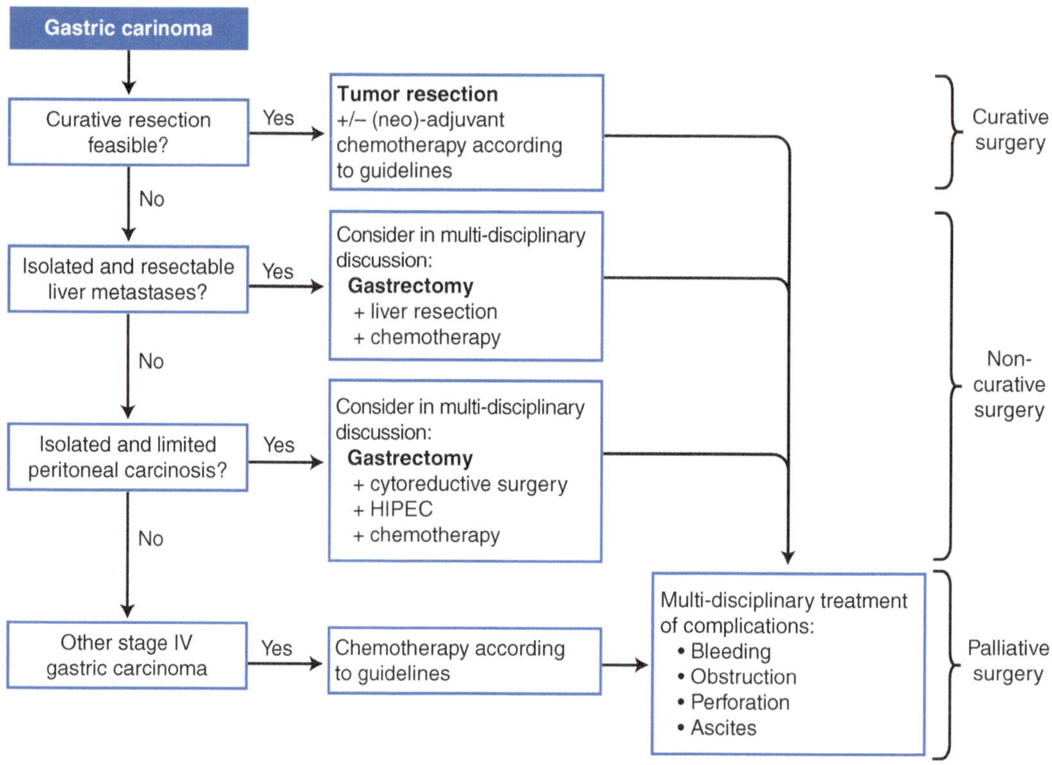

Fig. 11.1 Role of surgery in the curative, non-curative, and palliative treatment of gastric carcinoma

will develop gastric perforation due to the primary tumor, resulting in severe abdominal sepsis. While bleeding and obstruction may often be controlled endoscopically or with radiotherapy, perforation almost always requires surgical intervention. Nonetheless, when considering palliative interventions in a patient with advanced gastric cancer, surgeons need to take into account the overall prognosis of the patient avoiding excessive morbidity and mortality or lengthy hospital stays in those with a limited life span.

While cytotoxic chemotherapy is the most effective treatment modality for patients with metastatic disease, it is less effective for the control of symptoms associated with a locally advanced or recurrent primary tumor. This book chapter will focus on palliative surgical options for patients with advanced gastric cancer as part of the multidisciplinary approach required in this situation (Fig. 11.1). Due to the lack of properly designed prospective trials as a basis, this book chapter, to a large extent, relies on retrospective studies and personal experience.

11.2 Goal of Treatment in Palliative Gastric Surgery

The aims of palliative surgery for gastric cancer are to relieve symptoms, i.e., pain, nausea, vomiting, and weight loss, and hereby improve the patient's quality of life or to control an emergency situation, i.e., bleeding or infection due to gastric perforation. In the literature, the term "palliative surgery" is often applied to any type of non-curative surgery, which is not correct. Surgical palliation should be consistently defined as a procedure intended to control symptoms or improve quality of life. Palliative surgery is not intended to prolong life or prevent tumor-associated death. Thus, palliative surgery requires the presence of symptoms. Symptom control rather than overall survival should be the endpoint for any analysis of palliative surgery.

11.3 Quality of Life

Specific questionnaires for patients with gastric cancer have been developed to measure quality of life. The EORTC QLQ-OG25, e.g., considers dysphagia, eating restrictions, reflux, odynophagia, pain, and anxiety in addition to standard measurements of quality of life. In particular, eating restriction and consecutive cachexia limit life quality of patients with advanced gastric cancer. Most studies evaluating the quality of life following palliative surgery used hospital-free survival as a surrogate marker for quality of life. Moreover, prospective studies dealing with life quality and palliative surgery are not available. Thus, the effect of palliative surgery in patients with advanced gastric cancer on quality of life is unknown. Studies in the field of quality of life require changes to improve the decision-making process for these patients.

11.4 Non-Curative Surgery

It is important to emphasize that palliative surgery is not equal to non-curative resections in gastric cancer. The term non-curative surgery includes procedures performed with the intention to prolong survival that almost achieve the goal of complete resection of all gross and microscopic disease. Therefore, non-curative resections may or may not be considered palliative. The exact definition, however, is important for the interpretation of studies dealing with stage IV gastric cancer.

Non-curative resections have been shown to prolong survival in patients with distant lymph node metastases, liver metastasis, and locally advanced late-stage gastric cancer but not when peritoneal dissemination or multiorgan metastases are present [1]. Nonetheless, non-curative resection in patients with advanced gastric cancer does not represent the standard of care and should be performed only in selected patients according to an interdisciplinary tumor board decision. Currently, two prospective randomized controlled trials are comparing overall survival in patients with stage IV gastric cancer treated systemically with or without resection of the primary tumor. The results of these studies may change the strategy (Fig. 11.1) in the future.

11.5 Peritoneal Carcinosis and HIPEC

In recent years, the therapeutic approach combining cytoreductive surgery with hyperthermic intraperitoneal chemoperfusion (HIPEC) for peritoneal carcinosis has been evaluated with promising results. The rationale, here, is to surgically resect all gross tumor masses and to treat any remaining microscopic disease with high intraperitoneal concentrations of cytotoxic agents. Prospective randomized controlled trials are still needed, but first results may justify this approach in selected patients with limited and resectable peritoneal carcinosis and without other organ metastases [2]. Patients need to be carefully selected for cytoreductive surgery and HIPEC: "Limited" peritoneal carcinosis means the peritoneal cancer index according to Sugarbaker et al. should be less than 19.[1] Moreover, patients should have a good or excellent performance status (ECOG 0 or 1). Finally, HIPEC should only be performed as part of a multimodal therapeutic approach.

Complications due to peritoneal carcinomatosis, i.e., stenosis, bleeding, or perforation, have to be treated considering tumor mass, distribution and localization, performance status, nutritional status, and overall prognosis. Potential surgical therapeutic approaches include small bowel resections, ileostomies or colostomies, bypass surgery, or percutaneous endoscopic gastrostomy (PEG) placement to drain gastric and small bowel fluid.

[1] The peritoneal cancer index divides the abdomen into 13 regions. A lesion size score of 0–3 is assigned to each region, resulting in a maximum overall score of 39.

11.6 Chemotherapy-Refractory Ascites

The development of ascites requiring repeated paracenteses massively impairs patients' quality of life. For these patients, intraperitoneal administration of the trifunctional antibody catumaxomab can be considered. Catumaxomab binds T cells and the epithelial adhesion molecule EpCAM which is expressed by tumor cells but not healthy peritoneum. Application of catumaxomab has been shown to increase puncture-free survival from 11 to 46 days, which is associated with an improved quality of life [3]. Fever and a rise in C-reactive protein (CRP) are common side effects of this treatment. Alternatively, laparoscopic HIPEC without previous cytoreduction can be a palliative treatment option for refractory malignant ascites due to unresectable peritoneal carcinosis of gastric origin although this approach has to be considered experimental [4].

11.7 Treatment of Complications

Gastric cancer may be complicated by bleeding, obstruction, or perforation. As most cases of bleeding and obstruction can be managed endoscopically and do not require surgery, prophylactic gastrectomy with the intention to avoid these complications is not indicated. Moreover, a relevant number of patients develop problems related to metastases and not to the primary tumor. In summary, complications should be treated as they occur.

11.7.1 Bleeding

Patients bleeding from gastric cancer often present with large tumors, and they are often cachectic due to the long course of the disease. Endoscopy, given its high success rates (70–90 %) and rare complications, is the best treatment method and should be performed whenever possible (Fig. 11.2). Hemorrhage from gastric cancer should preferably be treated by mechanical methods that avoid the risk of perforation. Injection of diluted epinephrine is effective for the initial control of bleeding and thus enables the identification of the bleeding vessel. The use of clips achieves long-lasting hemostasis and should, therefore, be the method of choice for spurting arterial bleeds and non-bleeding visible vessels. Fibrin glue is effective for bleeds from ulcerous lesions and may, like epinephrine, be combined with clip application. Argon plasma coagulation can also be used, especially for diffuse and superficial bleeding.

When plasmatic coagulation is insufficient, coagulation factors should be substituted according to local standards.

If bleeding is significant but cannot be controlled endoscopically, or if bleeding recurs more than once following endoscopic treatment, two options remain. First, angiography and selective embolization of the bleeding vessel should be attempted. The chance of success is limited by the fact that angiography is only capable to visualize bleedings of approximately 1 ml/min or more. Moreover, the stomach is perfused via five different arteries limiting the success of angiography-based procedures for bleeding control.

Second, if angiography is not possible or unsuccessful, palliative gastrectomy must be considered, taking into account the overall prognosis of the patient in advanced stages of the disease. If the decision for gastrectomy is made in an emergency situation, the priority is not to perform a complete oncological resection but to stop the bleeding and to avoid unnecessary perioperative morbidity. The operative procedure may be limited to a partial resection of the stomach, and no lymph node dissection should be performed.

For chronic and diffuse bleeding, palliative radiotherapy may be an alternative option, while there is no place for radiotherapy as a first-line treatment.

11.7.2 Gastric Obstruction

Tumor stenosis results in obstructive complications such as dysphagia, weight loss, nausea, vomiting, and discomfort. For these patients, the

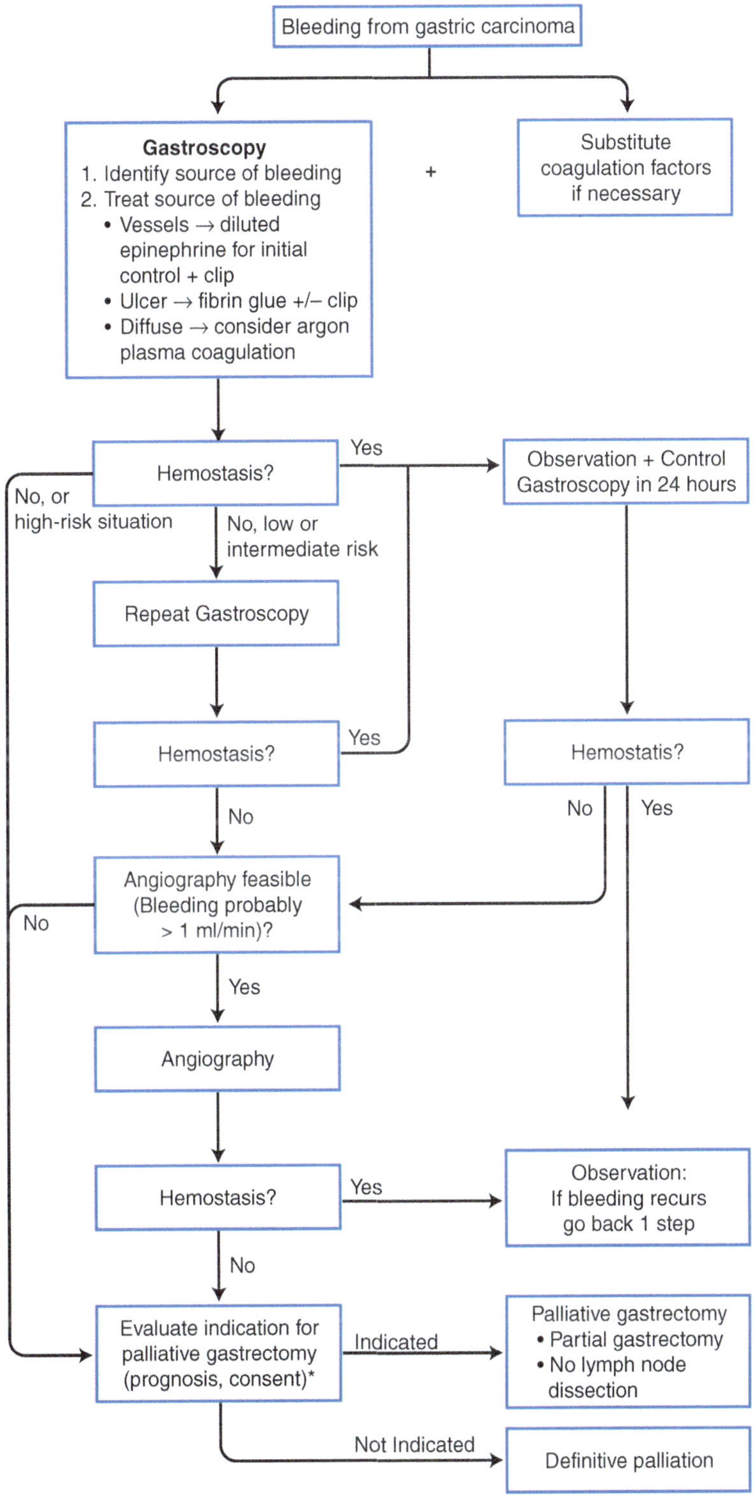

Fig. 11.2 Algorithm for the management of bleeding in advanced gastric carcinoma

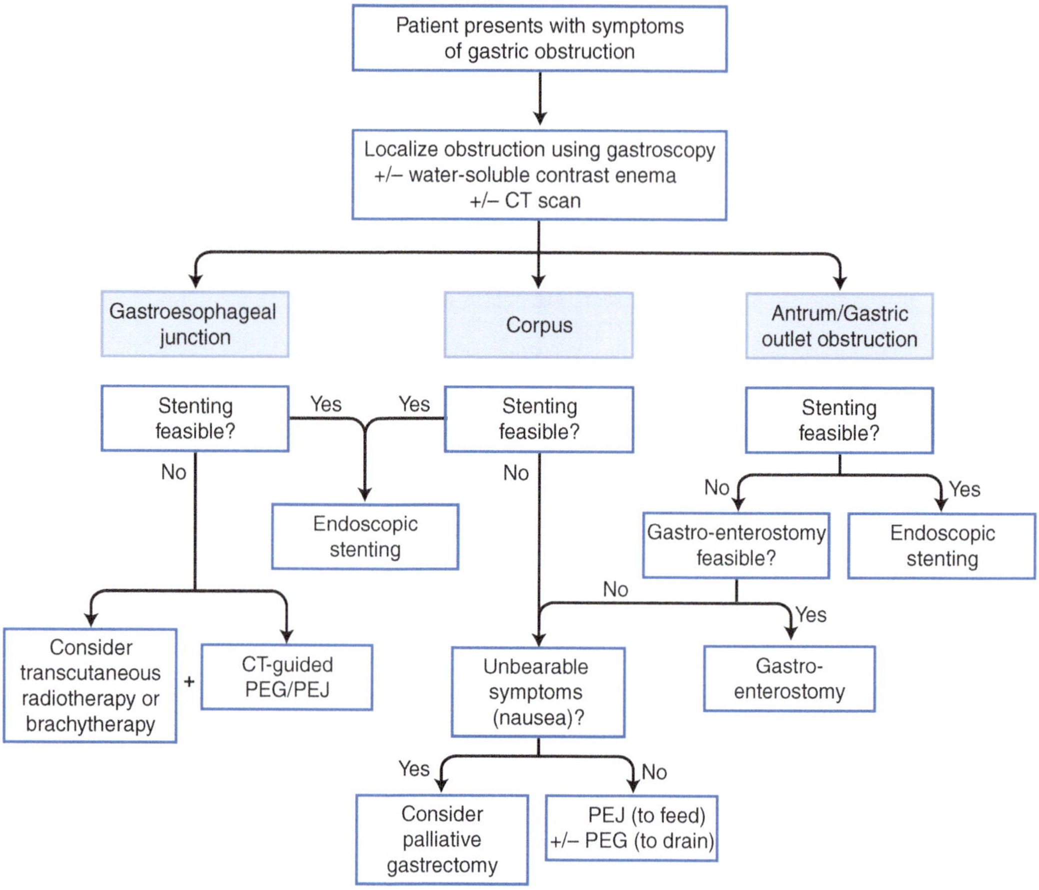

Fig. 11.3 Algorithm for the management of obstruction in advanced gastric carcinoma

therapeutic strategy is based on tumor location and tumor size as well as on the severity of symptoms (Fig. 11.3). In most locations, symptomatic stenosis of the stomach occurs in locally advanced stages of the disease. Rapid symptom relief is therefore of utmost importance and can usually be achieved by endoscopic interventions, surgical intervention, or radiotherapy.

Gastroscopy should be performed to evaluate the degree of stenosis and the involvement of the stomach. X-ray using water-soluble contrast media can be helpful in localizing the obstruction and to exclude any suspected perforation.

When the tumor is localized in the stomach (as opposed to the gastroesophageal junction), therapeutic options include endoscopic stent implantation, surgical gastroenterostomy, or placement of a jejunal feeding tube, while evidence for palliative radiation therapy is scarce. In a meta-analysis comparing endoscopic stenting to gastroenterostomy, stenting was found to be associated with higher clinical success, a shorter time to starting oral intake, reduced morbidity, a lower incidence of delayed gastric emptying, and a shorter hospital stay, while there was no significant difference between the two methods for severe complications or 30-day mortality [5]. Surgical gastroenterostomy, however, appears to allow for longer symptom-free survival. Both methods have specific limitations: For a gastroenterostomy to function, the tumor should be located in the antrum region of the stomach. In particular, when the corpus is affected, gastroenterostomy will not be successful. Endoscopic stenting requires advancing a guide wire through the stenosis for stent placement.

In some patients, introducing a jejunal feeding tube (percutaneous endoscopic jejunostomy, PEJ) is the only possibility to preserve enteral patient nutrition. These tubes, however, do not solve the problem of nausea and are associated with a poor quality of life for some patients. In patients with an otherwise untreatable gastric outlet obstruction, palliative placement of a percutaneous endoscopic gastrostomy (PEG) is indicated to drain gastric fluid.

Palliative (partial) gastrectomy may prolong survival by as much as 3 months but only at the cost of higher morbidity, longer hospital stays, and possibly reduced quality of life when compared to simple gastroenterostomy [6]. Palliative resection for obstruction should, therefore, only be performed in selected cases.

For patients with stenosis near the gastroesophageal junction, endoscopic stenting relieves symptoms faster than radiotherapy and should be the preferred method although the therapeutic effect of transcutaneous radiotherapy or endoluminal brachytherapy may last longer. Enteral nutrition may be maintained with PEG placement in patients with proximal tumor stenosis when stenting is not possible. In these patients, PEG insertion can be performed under CT guidance. Palliative resections of the distal esophagus and/or cardia should not be performed due to high morbidity and mortality rates.

11.7.3 Perforation

Perforation of the stomach is a surgical emergency that requires immediate laparotomy whatever the underlying pathology may be. At the time of the event, the cause of perforation is often not known, and even relatively small, potentially curable tumors may perforate. Tumor perforation, therefore, does not by itself mean that the situation is palliative. The surgeon encountering a perforated stomach in an emergency laparotomy will, in most situations, nonetheless decide against an oncological resection for three reasons: First, the histopathological diagnosis, even if suspected, cannot be often established in the emergency situation. Second, local inflammation often leads to intraoperative overestimation of tumor size and lymph node invasion. Third, the systemic inflammatory response syndrome caused by peritonitis requires rapid stabilization of the patient and precludes lengthy operative procedures. In the emergency situation, the operative strategy should, therefore, focus on the perforation and inflammation by performing a local resection and avoiding any unnecessary procedures. If the diagnosis of gastric cancer is confirmed, staging may be completed postoperatively and an oncological resection, if indicated, be performed in a second step [7].

References

1. Chen S, et al. Significance of palliative gastrectomy for late-stage gastric cancer patients. J Surg Oncol. 2012;106(7):862–71.
2. Glehen O, et al. Peritoneal carcinomatosis from gastric cancer: a multi-institutional study of 159 patients treated by cytoreductive surgery combined with perioperative intraperitoneal chemotherapy. Ann Surg Oncol. 2010;17(9):2370–7.
3. Heiss MM, et al. The trifunctional antibody catumaxomab for the treatment of malignant ascites due to epithelial cancer: results of a prospective randomized phase II/III trial. Int J Cancer. 2010;127(9):2209–21.
4. Valle M, Van der Speeten K, Garofalo A. Laparoscopic hyperthermic intraperitoneal peroperative chemotherapy (HIPEC) in the management of refractory malignant ascites: a multi-institutional retrospective analysis in 52 patients. J Surg Oncol. 2009;100(4):331–4.
5. Hosono S, et al. Endoscopic stenting versus surgical gastroenterostomy for palliation of malignant gastroduodenal obstruction: a meta-analysis. J Gastroenterol. 2007;42(4):283–90.
6. Hartgrink HH, et al. Value of palliative resection in gastric cancer. Br J Surg. 2002;89(11):1438–43.
7. Lehnert T, et al. Two-stage radical gastrectomy for perforated gastric cancer. Eur J Surg Oncol. 2000;26(8):780–4.

12 Pancreas

Andrea Wirsching, Mickaël Lesurtel, and Pierre-Alain Clavien

Contents

A. Wirsching, MD • M. Lesurtel, MD, PhD (✉)
P.-A. Clavien, MD, PhD, FACS, FRCS
Department of Surgery, Swiss Hepato-Pancreato-Biliary Center, University Hospital Zurich, Zurich 8091, Switzerland
e-mail: andrea.vuck@usz.ch; mickael.lesurtel@usz.ch; clavien@access.uzh.ch

About 80 % of newly diagnosed patients with pancreatic adenocarcinoma cannot benefit from a curative strategy. Palliative approaches of unresectable pancreatic cancer should be adjusted to the expected survival with the aim of preserving the quality of life of these patients. When the diagnosis of unresectable disease is made, nonsurgical endoscopic approaches should be prioritized in order to keep hospital stay as short as possible without delaying systemic chemotherapy. If an unresectable disease is diagnosed at laparotomy, an appropriate palliative surgical treatment should be considered to prevent biliary and enteral obstruction, as well as pain exacerbation due to tumour invasion. Surgical bypass procedures allow significantly more lasting palliation than endoscopic procedures in distinct situations. Since morbidity and mortality of pancreatoduodenectomy have significantly decreased in the last decades, a more aggressive approach towards palliative resection could be justified in specific circumstances. Pain control should not be neglected and is optimized when pharmacotherapy and chemical neurolysis are associated. Since palliative treatment of unresectable pancreatic cancer is not trivial, the choice of the best approach should be discussed by a multidisciplinary team including surgeons, gastroenterologists, radiologists, oncologists and physicians in charge of palliative care.

M. Wichmann, G. Maddern (eds.), *Palliative Surgery*,
DOI 10.1007/978-3-642-53709-7_12, © Springer-Verlag Berlin Heidelberg 2014

Abbreviations

CCD Cholecystoduodenostomy
CCJ Cholecystojejunostomy
CDD Choledochoduodenostomy
CDJ Choledochojejunostomy
CT Computed tomography
GOO Gastric outlet obstruction
RCT Randomized controlled trial
RFA Radiofrequency ablation

12.1 Introduction

Pancreatic cancer is known for its unfavourable prognosis. Only 20 % of newly diagnosed patients with pancreatic adenocarcinoma can be treated with a curative intent [1]. Accordingly, improvement of symptoms and preservation of quality of life constitute the main treatment goals in palliative patients.

Obstructive jaundice, gastric outlet obstruction (GOO) and pain are the common symptoms arising with disease progression. There are different surgical and nonsurgical treatment modalities to compose an individual therapy for patients in the palliative setting. When making a choice between a surgical or less aggressive palliation, the patient's general condition and the stage of disease should be considered. Patients with metastatic pancreatic cancer expect an overall survival of 3–6 months, whereas patients considered for palliation because of locally advanced disease could live from 6 to 12 months [2]. Based on the development of endoscopic stenting in the 1980s, a period during which surgical procedures were associated with significant morbidity and mortality rates, patients received most palliative therapies from the gastroenterologists [3]. During the last 10 years, however, morbidity and mortality rates of pancreatic surgery have dropped considerably, also with the advent of the laparoscopic approach, and thereby have regained interest [4]. Finally, despite remarkably improved radiologic diagnostics, some patients are still diagnosed with unresectable disease at laparotomy. In this latter situation, knowledge of palliative procedures and their indication is paramount to offer the best palliation to the patients.

The main goal of this chapter is to present different surgical treatment options in the palliative setting and to discuss their roles in the multidisciplinary palliative treatment of patients with unresectable pancreatic cancer.

12.2 Survival Scores

Knowledge of survival expectancy is key to decide on the appropriate palliative approaches. Several survival scores have been described in order to estimate survival expectancy in patients with unresectable pancreatic cancer. In a single centre from 1994 to 2006, 397 patients who underwent palliative bypass surgery (double bypass 59 %, biliary bypass 9 %, duodenal bypass 29 %) were analysed [5]. Four factors were independently associated with early mortality: metastatic disease, poor tumour differentiation, severe preoperative nausea and vomiting and lack of previous biliary stent placement. Each variable could be added to get a prognostic score (0–4 points). Six-month survival significantly decreased with each score point. Patients with a score of 0 have a predicted 6-month survival rate of 80 % compared to 30 % in the higher score group (≥3).

In another score, ASA score, pain, presence of liver metastasis, CEA level ≥10 units and CA 19–9 level ≥100 units were associated with a poor prognosis [6]. The reported overall survival was 14.5 months for patients with 0 or 1 risk factor and 3.5 months for patients with 4–5 risk factors, respectively.

Tumour size (>4 cm) and the presence of distant metastasis have been reported as predictors of poor survival [7]. In a retrospective analysis, a significant decline in survival was documented for any additional cm in tumour diameter [7].

In order to create a more practical and ready-to-use tool, Jamal et al. developed a symptom-based score, which can be assessed during the first interview [8]. They reported four symptoms, which independently predicted poor survival: weight loss >10 %, pain, jaundice and smoking. In order to build the McGill-Brisbane Symptom Score, the authors weighted each symptom according to its impact on survival (Table 12.1). In their cohort, the McGill-Brisbane Symptom Score had even a better predictive value than the presence or absence of distant metastasis [8].

12.3 Obstructive Jaundice

Jaundice is often the first sign of pancreatic head cancer. Biliary stasis leads to a variety of secondary complications like disabling pruritus, relapsing cholangitis, anorexia, malnutrition due to malabsorption and coagulation disorders. Palliative drainage of the biliary system can be achieved by either surgical (bilio-digestive anastomosis) or nonsurgical means (endoscopic or percutaneous stent placement). For many years, stent placement has been preferred to surgical biliary diversion due to high morbidity and mortality rates associated to surgery reaching 56 and 33 %, respectively [9, 10]. During the last 20 years, improved surgical skills and facilities led to reduced postoperative complications following biliary diversion approaching the rate of established stenting procedures. Recent publications report 20 % morbidity and 4 % mortality rates after palliative biliary bypass surgery [6, 11, 12] (Table 12.2). Based on the actual data, there is still an ongoing debate concerning the best palliative treatment for malignant biliary obstruction.

Table 12.1 McGill-Brisbane Symptom Score (MBSS) predicting survival in patients with unresectable pancreatic cancer

Symptom	Points
Weight loss >10 %	8
Pain	5
Jaundice	4
Smoking	4
Total possible	21
Low MBSS: A	**0–9**
High MBSS: B	**12–21**

Used with permission from Jamal et al. [8]
Overall median survival A = 14.6 months, B = 6.3 months

12.3.1 Nonsurgical Biliary Drainage

12.3.1.1 Percutaneous and Endoscopic Biliary Drainage

Beside numerous retrospective studies, which failed to show any difference in procedure effectiveness [19–21] between percutaneous and endoscopic biliary drainage, there are only two randomized controlled trials (RCTs) comparing the two procedures [22, 23]. One RCT [10] showed better jaundice resolution rates after endoscopic stent placement compared to percutaneous drainage (81 % vs. 61 %, respectively, $p=0.017$). Moreover endoscopic drainage showed a favourable 30-day mortality rate of 15 % vs. 33 %, respectively ($p=0.016$) [22]. In contrast, the second RCT documented better outcomes for biliary drainage by percutaneous stenting resolving jaundice in 71 % vs. 42 %, respectively ($p=0.03$ %) [23]. In routine clinical practice, endoscopic stenting is primarily performed in conjunction with endoscopic

Table 12.2 Morbidity and mortality of palliative bypass procedures for unresectable pancreatic adenocarcinoma in recent studies (after 2000)

Authors	Patients	Mortality (%)	Morbidity (%)	Length of hospital stay (days)	Median survival (months)
Isla et al. (2000) [18]	56	0	35	14	6
Stumpf et al. (2001) [17]	107	3.7	24	–	6.7
Urbach et al. (2003) [16]	1,919	11.8	–	–	5.3
Mortenson et al. (2005) [15]	84	–	25	12.3	6.2[a]
Lesurtel et al. (2006) [12]	83	4.8	26.5	16	9
Mukherjee et al. (2007) [14]	108	6.5	15.7	11	6
Muller et al. (2008) [6]	136	3	15	11	8.3
Hwang et al. (2009) [13]	38	2.2	15.5	19	8

[a]Mean survival

ultrasound (EUS) staging and biopsy. Endoscopic stenting offers some advantages for the patient as there is no external catheter to handle and thus less infectious risk. Percutaneous drainage constitutes an alternative, if endoscopic stenting is not feasible, but there is an increased risk of complications like biliary leakage and bleeding.

Plastic vs. Metal Stents

The incidence of recurrent jaundice following biliary stenting is highly dependent on the type of stent inserted [24]. There are two types of stents, plastic stents (polyethylene) and self-expandable metal stents. Plastic stents show a median patency rate of approximately 2–4 months [25], with early occlusion due to biofilm formation with aggregation of bacteria, protein and bilirubin. Self-expandable metal stents offer a superior median patency rate of 4–9 months [25], with intraluminal obstruction mostly due to tumour invasion. A RCT comparing plastic stent vs. metal stent placement for malignant biliary obstruction found recurrent jaundice in 43 % of patients after a median of 1 month following plastic stent insertion. In contrast, recurrent biliary obstruction after metal stent placement was reported in 18 % of cases after a median of 3.5 months [26]. Stent selection should be based on estimated overall patient survival to minimize re-interventions and hospital readmissions in the palliative setting. Additional costs for metal vs. plastic stents are balanced for patients surviving more than 6 months [27, 28].

Covered vs. Uncovered Stents

In order to reduce stent occlusion in the long term, several authors proposed during the 1990s a number of covered stents to prevent tumour invasion and intraluminal debris aggregation [29]. The advantages are referred to the anti-adherent whole wall cover of Gore-Tex, silicon and polyurethane materials. The initial results of patency rates and risk profile were encouraging, although not significantly superior compared to uncovered wallstents [30]. The efficacy of covered wallstents in the setting of unresectable malignant biliary obstruction has been assessed [31]. The reported 3-, 6- and 12-month patency rates comprised 90, 82 and 78 %, respectively [31]. A meta-analysis showed a significantly longer duration of patency for covered compared to uncovered stents [32]. To sum up, uncovered stents have a trend towards increased obstruction, when compared to their covered counterparts.

12.3.2 Surgical Drainage

12.3.2.1 Surgical Diversion Techniques

Recent publications mainly discuss four different bilio-digestive derivation techniques in the palliative setting: cholecystoduodenostomy (CCD), cholecystojejunostomy (CCJ), choledochoduodenostomy (CDD) and choledochojejunostomy (CDJ). CCD and CCJ can be easily performed laparoscopically using a linear staple device. However, compared with an anastomosis to the main hepatic duct, they are associated with higher rates of failure and recurrent jaundice [16, 33]. A direct comparison between CCJ or CCD and CDD showed superior drainage and a significantly lower recurrence rate of biliary obstruction (<8 %) for choledochal anastomosis [34, 35]. These results were explained by a tumour invasion of the hepatocystic confluence in 50 % of the cases [36]. Similarly, current literature suggests a threefold higher rate of re-interventions for CCJ compared to an anastomosis to the main hepatic duct [16]. Considering these results, diversion techniques with an anastomosis to the main hepatic duct should be preferred [34, 37]. Furthermore, CDJ or hepaticojejunostomy with a Roux-en-Y reconstruction offers an effective biliary drainage and a favourable recurrence rate (<13 %) [38].

Finally, a CDJ is recommendable, if there is any risk for duodenal tumour obstruction or if mobilization of the duodenum does not seem feasible. Nevertheless, a classic CDD could also be performed in most cases (Fig. 12.1a–c).

12.3.3 Surgical Bypass vs. Stent Drainage

There are only three RCTs comparing the efficacy of surgical vs. plastic endoscopic drainage for obstructive jaundice [39–41]. Plastic stents were

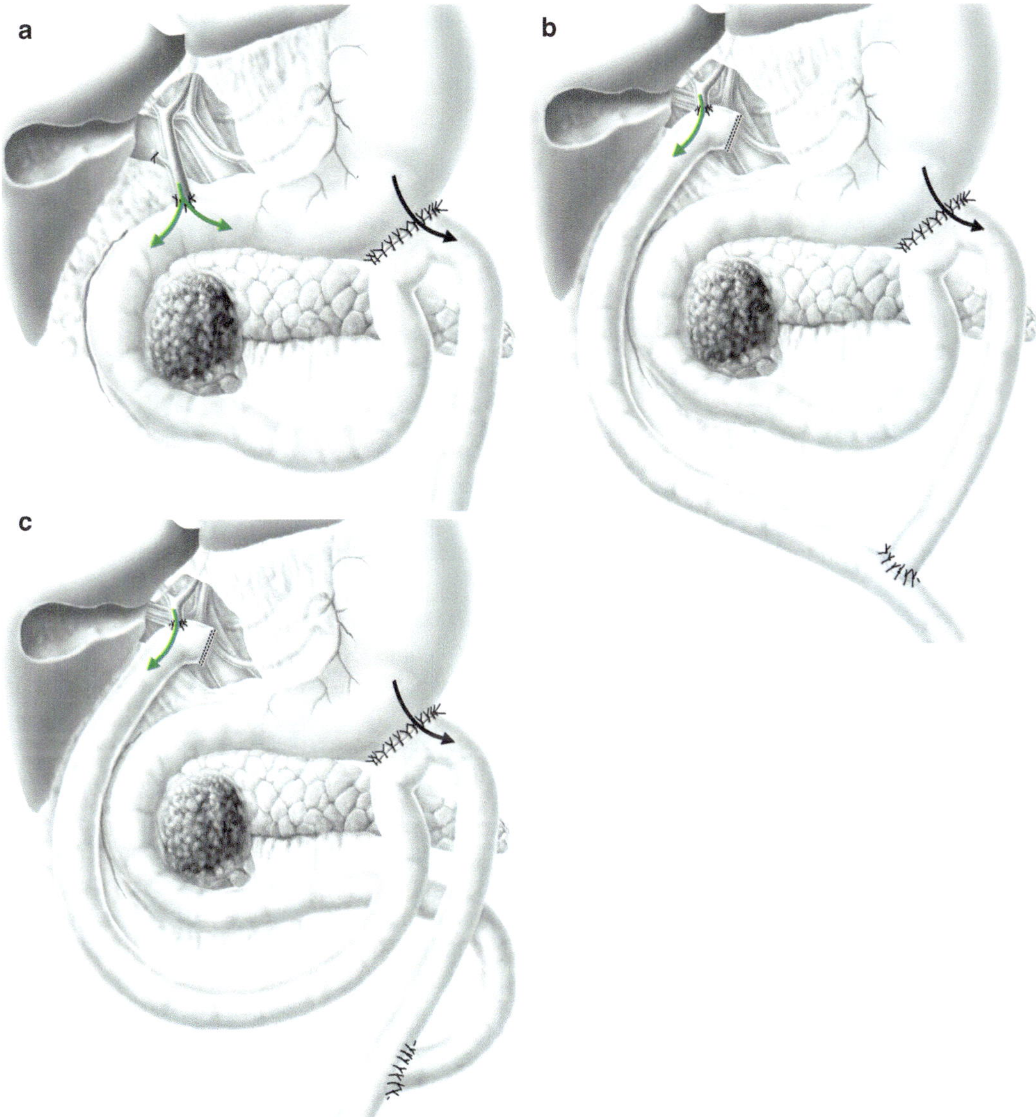

Fig. 12.1 (**a–c**) The 3 main double bypasses performed for unresectable pancreatic head cancer described in the literature. (**a**) Choledochoduodenostomy (the duodenum needs to be mobile) + gastrojejunostomy 30 cm after Treitz's angle. (**b**) Roux-en-Y hepaticojejunostomy + gastrojejunostomy 30 cm after Treitz's angle. (**c**) Hepaticojejunostomy and gastrojejunostomy on the same Roux-en-Y limb (*green arrow*, bile flow; *black arrow*, food passage) (The authors of this chapter would like to thank Stefan Schwyter for his help with these drawings)

used in all the trials (Table 12.3) [39–41]. Initial successful drainage was achieved in 95 % of the cases with both methods. Only one study found a lower mortality rate after endoscopic stenting compared to surgical bypass (3 % vs. 14 %, respectively, $p=0.006$) [39], although post-interventional complication rates were higher after surgery compared to endoscopic stenting (29 % vs.11 %, respectively, $p=0.02$) [39]. Finally, re-interventions for recurrent jaundice were up to seven times [39] more frequent after endoscopy compared to surgery [39, 40, 42].

Two retrospective analyses and one RCT compared surgical drainage with metal stent placement for obstructive jaundice [38, 43, 44]. Immediate success of biliary drainage between

Table 12.3 Randomized controlled trials comparing endoscopic plastic stent placement with surgical derivation for obstructive jaundice in the setting of unresectable pancreatic adenocarcinoma

	Sheperd et al. (1988) [40]		Andersen et al. (1989) [41]		Smith et al. (1994) [39]	
	Surgery	Stent	Surgery	Stent	Surgery	Stent
Patients	25	23	19	25	101	100
Successful drainage (%)	92	91	76	96	94	95
Median length of hospital stay	13	8	27	26	26	19
Morbidity (%)	40	22	26	36	29	11*
Recurrent jaundice (%)	0	43**	16	28	2	36
30-day mortality (%)	20	9	31	20	15	8
Median survival (weeks)	18	22	14	12	26	21

*$p=0.02$; **$p=0.01$

the two techniques was similar, ranging from 95 to 100 % [41]. Nevertheless, a tendency towards an increased early complication rate was found in the case of a surgical approach ($p=0.1$) [43]. Furthermore, surgery led to a prolonged mean hospital stay (32 ± 4 days and 12 ± 1 days, respectively, $p=0.002$). In contrast, late complications, including recurrence of jaundice, were more common after metal stent placement (42 and 10 %, respectively, $p=0.04$) [43]. One retrospective study failed to show any significant difference in terms of complication rates but highlights a higher rate of hospital readmissions after stenting compared to surgical approach (40 % vs. 13 %, $p<0.05$) [38]. Of note, total length of hospital stay ultimately favoured the surgical approach over stenting procedures (mean 34 vs. 10 days, $p>0.05$) [38]. A RCT assigned patients with biliary obstruction due to metastatic pancreatic cancer either to endoscopic metal stent or to surgical bilio-jejunostomy ($n=15$ in each group) [44]. Of note, no sample size calculation was performed. There was no difference between the two groups regarding complication rates, readmissions for complications and duration of survival. In this specific population with metastatic disease, they found that the overall total cost of care that included initial care and subsequent interventions and hospitalizations until death was lower in the endoscopy group, when compared with the surgical group (USD 4,271 ± 2,411 vs. 8,321 ± 1,821, $p=0.0013$). In addition, the quality of life scores were better in the endoscopy group at 30 days ($p=0.04$) and 60 days ($p=0.05$) [44].

In 2006, a meta-analysis of 21 studies summarizing 1,454 patients was published [24]. Similar to the previously discussed RCTs, they found an increased complication rate (RR = 0.6, $p<0.0007$) and an 18-fold reduction of re-interventions (RR = 18.9, $p<0.00001$) after surgical drainage, when compared to endoscopic stent placement. The authors concluded that endoscopic placement of a metal stent has the most favourable risk-outcome profile. Recurrent obstruction and the subsequent need of re-interventions were significantly reduced at 4 months and before death after surgical bypass compared to endoscopic stent placement (RR = 0.44 and RR = 0.52, respectively).

In summary, patients with an estimated survival of less than 6 months benefit more from interventional stent placement in terms of morbidity and length of hospital stay. On the other hand, patients whose life expectancy exceeds 6 months may benefit from a more lasting solution with a decrease need for re-interventions over time. In such a case, a surgical bypass procedure can be recommended, especially if the diagnosis of unresectability of the tumour is diagnosed at laparotomy.

12.4 Malignant Gastric Outlet Obstruction

12.4.1 Palliative Gastroenterostomy

Gastric outlet obstruction (GOO) is a common complication of advanced pancreatic cancer. Surgical management of duodenal or gastric

Table 12.4 Prospective studies comparing double bypass with single bilioenteric bypass for unresectable pancreatic cancer

First author (year)	Study design	Patients		Morbidity (%)		GOO (%)		Survival (months)	
		Double bypass	Single bypass	Double bypass	Single bypass	Double bypass	Single bypass	Double bypass	Single bypass
Lillemoe et al. (1999) [49]	RCT monocentre	44	43	32	33	0*	19	8.3	8.3
Shyr et al. (2000) [50]	Prospective cohort trial	44	22	11	14	nd	32	5	8
Van Heek et al. (2003) [46]	RCT multicentre	36	29	11	8	6*	41	7.2	8.4

GOO gastric outlet obstruction
$^*p<0.05$

tumour obstruction implies the creation of a gastrojejunostomy. However, the indication for preventive surgical treatment in the palliative setting is controversial, as not every patient develops GOO with disease progression. While only 20 % of patients initially present with symptoms of GOO, 30–50 % develop GOO during the course of their disease [3, 45]. If unresectability of the tumour is diagnosed at laparotomy, patients benefit from double bypass procedures in the long term, as this approach may reduce the incidence of GOO and obstructive jaundice [12]. Of note, a double bypass procedure including a gastrojejunostomy does not increase postoperative morbidity compared to biliary bypass alone [12, 46]. In contrast, a gastrojejunostomy performed in a second step with arising symptoms of GOO has a postoperative mortality risk of up to 22 % [47, 48].

Two RCTs and one prospective cohort study aimed at answering the question whether a prophylactic gastroenterostomy should be performed in asymptomatic palliative patients (Table 12.4) [46, 49, 50]. Lillemoe et al. [49] randomized 87 patients with unresectable periampullary cancers diagnosed upon laparotomy without impending risk of GOO to either retro-colic gastrojejunostomy ($n=44$) or no gastrojejunostomy ($n=43$). They reported no postoperative mortality and a median survival of 8.3 months in both groups [49]. Within the group without prophylactic gastrojejunostomy, 8 patients (19 %) developed late GOO requiring a therapeutic intervention compared to none in the prophylactic treatment arm. Postoperative morbidity (32 % vs. 33 %) and length of hospital stay (8.5 vs. 8 days) did not differ significantly between the two groups [49]. Similarly, 65 patients were randomized to receive either a single bypass (29 patients with bilio-digestive anastomosis) or a double bypass (36 patients with both bilio-digestive and gastroenteric anastomoses) at the time of intraoperative diagnosis of unresectable periampullary cancer [46]. To be included in the study, patients were required to present neither signs of GOO nor any endoscopic treatment for more than 3 months. Late GOO developed in two patients in the double bypass group (5.5 %) compared to 12 patients, who received a single bypass (41.4 %), $p=0.001$ [46]. There was no significant difference in postoperative morbidity including delayed gastric emptying (17 % vs. 3 %, $p=0.12$), median length of stay (11 vs. 9 days, $p=0.06$), quality of life and median survival (7.2 vs. 8.4 months, $p=0.15$) [46]. Finally, 66 patients with unresectable periampullary adenocarcinoma were prospectively enrolled to receive either a single bilio-digestive bypass ($n=22$) or, in the presence of GOO, a double bypass ($n=44$) [50]. The authors did not report any difference in postoperative morbidity and mortality. Of note, seven patients in the single bypass group (31 %) developed late GOO within 6 months after the bypass [50].

Finally, a recent meta-analysis including the aforementioned studies summarized 218 patients in total [51]. The results confirmed a significant lower risk of late GOO after prophylactic double bypass compared with bilioenteric bypass only [51]. Again double bypass surgery did not add morbidity or mortality, when compared with single bypass or no bypass procedures. The authors did not find any increased rate of delayed gastric emptying after gastrojejunostomy, which is of special concern in this group of patients. They conclude that there is sufficient evidence to recommend prophylactic double bypass surgery for patients found to have unresectable periampullary malignancy diagnosed at laparotomy and who need a bilioenteric diversion [51].

Former gastroenteric diversion techniques for malignant GOO aimed at placing the anastomosis as far as possible from the actual tumour site. Therefore, gastrojejunostomy was usually performed mainly in an ante-colic fashion. However, there is now evidence that retro-colic gastrojejunostomy is associated with a lower rate of postoperative delayed gastric emptying [52]. Surgeons at the Johns Hopkins Hospital assessed the rate of postoperative delayed gastric emptying following gastrojejunostomy in the palliative setting [2, 53]. The first retrospective study compared complications of ante- vs. retro-colic gastrojejunostomies. The authors reported delayed gastric emptying in 6 % of the patients operated in a retro-colic fashion compared to 17 % in the group with ante-colic gastrojejunostomy [53]. Similarly a subsequent study evaluated 180 patients, who received a retro-colic gastrojejunostomy and showed a 9 % rate of delayed gastric emptying [2]. Finally, a RCT documented a 2 % rate of delayed gastric emptying in patients receiving a prophylactic retro-colic gastrojejunostomy after being diagnosed with unresectable disease upon laparotomy [49].

The outcome of three different types of gastrojejunostomies in patients with malignant GOO was compared in a RCT [54]. A total of 45 patients were enrolled. One-third received a gastrojejunostomy with an anastomosis located 20 cm distal to the Treitz's ligament. The second group received the same intervention associated with duodenal partition with a linear stapler 1 cm distal to the pylorus. A reconstruction with a Roux-en-Y limb located 60 cm distal to the bilioenteric anastomosis was performed in the third group. Patients within the first group were more frequently symptomatic and showed prolonged postoperative gastric emptying [54]. "Food reentry" was documented by upper gastrointestinal imaging in 21 % of the patients within the first group. Therefore, the authors proposed duodenal partition as an easy procedure to improve outcome after gastrojejunostomy 20 cm distal to the Treitz's ligament [54].

12.4.2 Duodenal Endoscopic Stenting

At the beginning of the 1990s, after oesophageal stenting has been established, the first duodenal stents were placed for malignant outlet obstruction. First outcome reports of the new technique were encouraging. Obvious benefits comprised reduced invasiveness and faster recovery to oral intake [55]. Nevertheless, subsequent studies including a longer follow-up period reported stent-specific complications counterbalancing the initially appraised advantages [56].

Three RCTs compared duodenal stent placement with surgical gastrojejunostomy for malignant GOO (Table 12.5) [57–59]. These studies shared one shortcoming, which is a relatively small number of patients ($n = 18$, 27 and 39, respectively). Two RCTs ($n = 18$ and 27) favoured duodenal stenting over surgery because of a shorter length of hospital stay, shorter time to oral intake and decreased pain scores associated with stenting [57, 58]. A systematic review summarized two of the three RCTs with additional prospective and retrospective studies in order to compare endoscopic stenting with gastrojejunostomy [56]. The review evaluated 1,046 patients after a duodenal stenting procedure and 297 patients who underwent a gastrojejunostomy in the palliative setting [56]. A significant shorter time to oral intake and a shorter length of hospital stay favoured duodenal stenting compared to the surgery group (mean hospital stay 7 vs. 13 days, respectively) [56]. There was neither any difference between groups in terms of persistence of obstruction nor early and late major complications. Stent migration and stent obstruction by tumour ingrowth or food were

Table 12.5 RCTs comparing duodenal stent and gastrojejunostomy for malignant outlet obstruction in patients with unresectable pancreatic cancer

First author (year)	Intervention	Patients	Success of intervention (%)	Resolution of GOO (%)	Length of hospital stay (days)	Morbidity (%)	Follow-up (months)	30-day mortality (%)
Fiori et al. (2004) [57]	oGJ	9	100	89	10	22	3	–
	Stent	9	100	100	3.1*	22	3	–
Mehta et al. (2006) [58]	lapGJ	14	93	–	11	62*	–	23
	Stent	13	77	–	5*	0	–	20
Jeurnink et al. (2009) [59]	GJ	18	–	77	–	28	Monthly till death	–
	Stent	21	–	62	–	38		–

oGJ open gastrojejunostomy, *lapGJ* laparoscopic gastrojejunostomy, *GJ* composed of 16 oGJ and 2 lapGJ
*$p<0.05$

frequent complications in the stenting group, whereas complications after gastrojejunostomy included anastomotic leakage and dysfunction. However, the re-intervention rate was significantly higher following duodenal stenting compared to surgery (18 % vs. 1 %, respectively). In conclusion, the authors recommended duodenal stenting in patients with a short life expectancy, because of the advantages in early time points, but they supported surgery for patients expected to live more than 2 months in order to avoid frequent re-interventions.

The largest RCT so far was published 2 years after the systematic review and outlined a cost analysis comparing duodenal stenting with surgery ($n=39$) [59]. Total costs per patient turned out to be higher in the surgery group, when compared with the stenting procedure (12,433€ vs. 8,819€, respectively). Higher costs were mainly due to the initial procedure with higher personnel and hospital costs after surgery (8,315€ vs. 4,820€, $p<0.001$). However, 25 % of stented patients suffered from recurrent GOO vs. only one case of GOO among the 18 patients receiving a gastrojejunostomy [59]. The authors concluded that a surgical approach can still be recommended for patients with a life expectancy exceeding 2 months [59].

In summary endoscopic duodenal stenting proves to be beneficial in the early postoperative course. However, recurrent GOO makes surgery more favourable, if survival exceeds 2 months.

12.5 Palliative Pancreatoduodenectomy

Despite ongoing progress in the field of preoperative staging, surgeons are still confronted with unresectable or "borderline resectable" disease upon laparotomy. This situation urges the decision whether to risk a resection with the possibility of positive resection margins or to restrict the procedure to a biliary and intestinal diversion. Histopathologic assessment after resection of pancreatic head adenocarcinoma reveals, altogether, a microscopic incomplete resection ranging between 14 and 60 % [60, 61]. In the decision-making process, morbidity, mortality and worse quality of life associated with this extensive procedure have to be balanced. High surgical morbidity rates can preclude patients from receiving palliative chemo- or radiation therapy, which have been shown to increase survival even in the palliative setting [62]. Before the 1990s, pancreatoduodenectomy was a procedure with high morbidity and mortality rates reaching 40 and 25 %, respectively [48]. In this context, the indication to perform a resection for pancreatic carcinoma was restricted to patients, in whom curative intent appears feasible. The current mortality rates for pancreatic resection decreased under the benchmark of 3 %, challenging the indication of pancreatic resection in locally advanced disease [63]. A large retrospective study comparing outcome of palliative pancreatectomy (R1 resection) with palliative bypass procedure, adjusted for age and local organ invasion in the absence of

Table 12.6 Retrospective studies comparing palliative resection and bypass procedures for locally advanced pancreatic cancer

First author (year)	Patients		Length of hospital stay		Morbidity (%)		Median survival (months)	
	Palliative resection	Bypass	Palliative resection	Bypass	Palliative resection	Bypass	Palliative resection	Bypass
Reinders et al. (1995) [65]	36	24	18	25*	44	33	10.2	7.8*
Lillemoe et al. (1996) [62]	64	62	15	18*	42	32	12	9*
Kuhlmann et al. (2006) [66]	80	90	16	10*	41	31	15.8	9.5*
Fusai et al. (2008) [61]	40	32	13	11	30	31	18	9*
Lavu et al. (2009) [60]	37	24	7	5.5*	48	33	15.6	6.5*
Wellner et al. (2012) [67]	71	117	15	13	34	54	18	10*

*$p<0.05$

distant metastasis, showed a significant survival benefit in favour of the resection group [64].

12.5.1 Microscopically Incomplete Resection (R1)

Six retrospective studies compared outcome after microscopically incomplete (R1) resection with palliative bypass surgery for locally advanced disease without distant metastasis (Table 12.6) [60–62, 65–67]. Postoperative morbidity rates did not differ between groups. Two studies [60, 66] showed a prolonged length of hospital stay in patients receiving pancreatic resection, whereas others [62, 65] found the opposite. Every single study found a significant benefit in terms of overall survival in favour of pancreatic resection. Limitations of data interpretation comprise retrospective data collection and a rather incomplete documentation of additional therapies like chemotherapy. The unknown extent of local invasion and lymph node involvement in the bypass group adds further bias.

At this point, these studies represent the best available evidence, as a RCT comparing palliative pancreatoduodenectomy with palliative bypass surgery might be difficult to justify ethically.

12.5.2 Macroscopically Incomplete Resection (R2)

Macroscopic incomplete resection (R2) of pancreatic cancer still has a dismal prognosis and has no apparent survival benefit compared to bypass surgery [67]. Significant increased morbidity and surgery-related mortality rates after R2 resection have been reported when compared to bypass surgery [68]. There is also a negative impact on quality of life [69]. In summary, current literature does not show any benefit of R2 resection; therefore it should be avoided.

12.5.3 Hepatic Metastases

Hepatic metastases constitute a contraindication for resection of pancreatic adenocarcinoma. Some retrospective reports of concomitant pancreatoduodenectomy and hepatectomy for metastatic disease included less than ten patients for the most part [70]. While in selected, otherwise fit patients, an extensive resection is feasible without additional morbidity [70], studies have failed to show any survival benefit after resection of metastatic disease.

12.5.4 Radiofrequency Ablation

A group from Italy published their experience with radiofrequency ablation (RFA) of locally advanced pancreatic head tumours without distant metastatic disease [71]. Their first report included 50 patients with concomitant bypass surgery in 31 cases (19 double bypasses, 8 gastroenterostomies, 3 biliary bypass, 1 pancreaticojejunostomy) [71]. Because of the vicinity of the duodenum, heat production was reduced from 105 to 92 °C and a cold solution was flushed into the duodenum. Sticking to the aforementioned precautions, they found acceptable mortality and morbidity rates of 2 and 24 %, respectively. The same group recently published their experience about 100 consecutive patients [72]. In their cohort, 48 patients were treated with RFA up front, while 52 patients received different combinations of radiochemotherapy and RFA. The authors observed an impressive overall survival of 20 months, though survival did not differ according to treatment sequence. The idea of tumour downstaging after RFA did not, however, prove to be feasible. Of note, they reported a negative impact of radiotherapy prior to RFA, presumably because of local scarring. Therefore, radiotherapy, if applied, should be planned after and not before RFA [72]. Few, but severe, adverse effects occurred following RFA including portal vein thrombosis in five patients and severe duodenal injury in three others [72].

In summary, the authors concluded that RFA can be promoted as a palliative treatment to stabilize disease progression in conjunction with chemoradiation.

12.6 Role of Laparoscopy in Palliative Treatment of Pancreatic Cancer

Laparoscopy with or without ultrasonography has been suggested by some authors as a useful diagnostic tool to determine resectability along with staging computed tomography (CT) and EUS [73]. The idea of laparoscopy first is to prevent a futile laparotomy in patients suffering from advanced disease and thereby to improve palliative care.

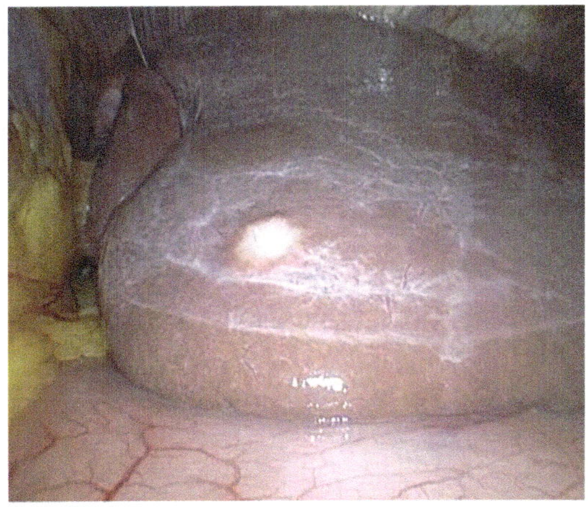

Fig. 12.2 Typical subcapsular liver metastasis in a patient with pancreatic adenocarcinoma discovered at laparoscopy and not detectable by CT scan

Laparoscopy allows a good assessment of the intraperitoneal surfaces like the peritoneal lining or subcapsular liver metastases (Fig. 12.2), but there are certain limitations concerning the assessment of deep liver metastasis or local vascular invasion. A meta-analysis assessed the benefits of diagnostic laparoscopy associated with laparoscopic ultrasound [74]. The authors concluded that laparoscopic ultrasound may be beneficial in situations where extensive disease is assumed and CT scan fails to prove it. Additionally, defenders of laparoscopic ultrasound point out the refined diagnostics including an opportunity to get an intraoperative biopsy [75]. Some authors report approximately 31 % of otherwise futile laparotomies, which can be avoided, thanks to laparoscopy associated with laparoscopic ultrasound [76].

Recently, several groups tried to find appropriate parameters to predict advanced disease in order to select proper candidates for laparoscopy. They found different predictors of bad outcomes like tumour size above 3 cm [77], CA 19–9 level >1,000 UI/mL [78, 79], daily pancreatic pain, increased leucocyte counts, hypoalbuminaemia and elevated serum levels of CEA [6]. However, none of these parameters has been broadly confirmed so far.

12.6.1 Peritoneal Cytology in Staging of Pancreatic Adenocarcinoma

Another advantage of laparoscopy is that peritoneal washing cytology can be readily performed. Different authors aimed at finding the significance of positive peritoneal lavage cytology in the absence of further metastatic disease [78, 80, 81]. The prevalence of isolated positive peritoneal cytology is low (5–9 %) [82]. Although some groups found that survival after pancreatoduodenectomy did not differ significantly between patients with positive and negative peritoneal cytology [83, 84], others showed a poorer overall survival similar to stage IV disease [82].

The impact of positive cytology on therapy and outcome remains unclear, and in practice, peritoneal cytology is not very useful since definitive results need 24 h leading to a two-step operative approach.

12.7 Pain Management

At diagnosis, approximately one third of pancreatic cancer patients complain of pain, and 90 % of them experience severe pain at the end-stage disease [85]. Therefore, any good palliation must focus on pain management in order to improve quality of life. Pain origin in pancreatic cancer is most likely due to the local infiltration of adjacent structures like the coeliac and the retropancreatic nerve plexus [86].

Pain may be controlled through either pharmacotherapy or interventional methods, some of which have been especially developed for pancreatic cancer patients. Although pharmacotherapy is central for pain control, its application is limited because of side effects especially with increased opioid dosages [86]. Stepwise escalation of painkillers is based on the three-step approach published by the World Health Organization [87].

12.7.1 Chemical Neurolysis

Chemical neurolysis can be performed by para-aortic injection of 10 mL of 95 % alcohol or 6 % of phenol on both sides to the coeliac axis. Recent publications also reported a combination of alcohol and local anaesthetics [88]. In 1993, Lillemoe et al. showed that para-aortic alcohol injection is able to reduce pain significantly compared to placebo (saline) [89]. Mean duration of pain reduction was 3.3 months after alcohol injection compared to 0.8 months with placebo [89]. Laparoscopic neurolysis merits attention, especially since its combination with staging laparoscopy is appealing. Recent literature shows equal efficacy and reasonable feasibility of laparoscopic neurolysis [77].

Beside the transperitoneal surgical access, the coeliac plexus can be percutaneously reached with the patient in prone position. Needle insertion can be followed using CT scan or fluoroscopy images [79]. A meta-analysis including 1,145 patients reported that pain relief after percutaneous neurolysis could be reached in 89 % of cases during the first 15 days and may last after 3 months in 90 % of the cases [90]. A RCT showed that pain relief exceeded 24 weeks after 95 % alcohol injection compared to placebo [91]. The authors found significantly more efficient pain reduction in patients who received chemical neurolysis compared to those treated with opioids alone. However, opioid usage and subsequent adverse effects did not vary between groups [91]. In contrast, other studies including a recent systematic review reported a significantly decreased opioid consumption [79, 92, 93].

The development of endoscopic ultrasounds led to a precise anatomical visualization of the coeliac plexus by endoscopic routes making it a useful tool for interventional neurolysis. Moreover, endoscopy may also combine stenting procedure and/or ultrasound-guided tumour biopsy. A recent meta-analysis of 8 studies, summarizing 283 patients, assessed outcomes after endoscopic neurolysis. A favourable pain control after endoscopic procedure was reached in 80 % of patients [94]. Furthermore, bilateral neurolysis proved to be more efficient than the unilateral approach with pain reduction in 84.5 and 48 % of the cases, respectively [94]. In contrast, a RCT compared endosonography-guided injection of a bupivacaine/alcohol solution at one or two sides of the coeliac trunk. They included 50 patients and did not find any significant difference in pain reduction between the two groups [14]. Therefore the authors favoured the one-application approach in order to reduce risks. After 3 months, 79–88 % of patients reported sustained pain reduction [88, 95].

In summary, chemical neurolysis improves pain control when used in association with pharmacotherapy, thereby reducing opioid consumption and opioid adverse effects and contributing to improve quality of life.

12.7.2 Splanchnicectomy

Transhiatal bilateral splanchnicectomy can be performed for pain control regardless of local tumour extension. Neurectomy was initially performed in the posterior and inferior mediastinal space, which can be reached by a transhiatal approach described by Dubois [96]. Pain relief could be achieved immediately after the intervention in more than 80 % of the cases and efficiently lasted after 3 months in 75 % of patients [97–99].

A minimal invasive left thoracoscopic splanchnicectomy has been proposed as an alternative to chemical neurolysis [100, 101]. Other groups insisted on bilateral splanchnicectomy, as described by Cuschieri et al., in order to reduce pain recurrence [102]. However, defenders of unilateral splanchnicectomy pointed out side effects like diarrhoea and hypotension, which significantly impact quality of life. In brief, thoracoscopic splanchnicectomy is a minimally invasive procedure with a low morbidity rate of 4–9 % and a rather short median hospital stay of 3 days [103, 104]. Extent of splanchnicectomy is, however, still the subject to ongoing debate.

The effects of percutaneous chemical neurolysis (bilateral approach) were compared with left thoracoscopic splanchnicectomy in a prospective study [105]. There was no difference in pain reduction between the two techniques. However, the authors showed a significant benefit concerning quality of life favouring the percutaneous approach. Surprisingly, a RCT initiated to clarify the role of interventional procedures in association with pharmacotherapy failed to show any difference [106]. Patients with malignancies of the pancreas or other upper gastrointestinal tract cancers ($n=65$) were randomized to receive either pharmacotherapy alone or pharmacotherapy with additional chemical neurolysis or thoracoscopic splanchnicectomy. The primary end point was pain relief 2 months after treatment. The authors explained the negative finding by a too small sample size and the absence of blind randomization [106].

According to the multidisciplinary approach of unresectable pancreatic cancer, we suggest a schematic algorithm of pain taking into account the benefits and limits discussed earlier (Fig. 12.3).

Conclusion

Palliative treatment strategies for unresectable pancreatic cancer have to be adapted to the expected survival and should focus on the quality of life of the patients. Many different therapeutic options have been introduced, but a few have reached a consensual acceptance. After a diagnosis of unresectable disease, nonsurgical approaches should be prioritized in order to keep hospital stay as short as possible and not delay systemic chemotherapy.

Despite remarkable progress of imaging and diagnostic laparoscopy, some patients are still diagnosed with unresectable disease at laparotomy. In this context, therapeutic or preventive double bypass and chemical neurolysis should be performed during laparotomy. These procedures can be performed in one step to prevent biliary and enteral obstruction as well as pain exacerbation due to tumour invasion. It is paramount that surgeons treating such patients are able to make the right

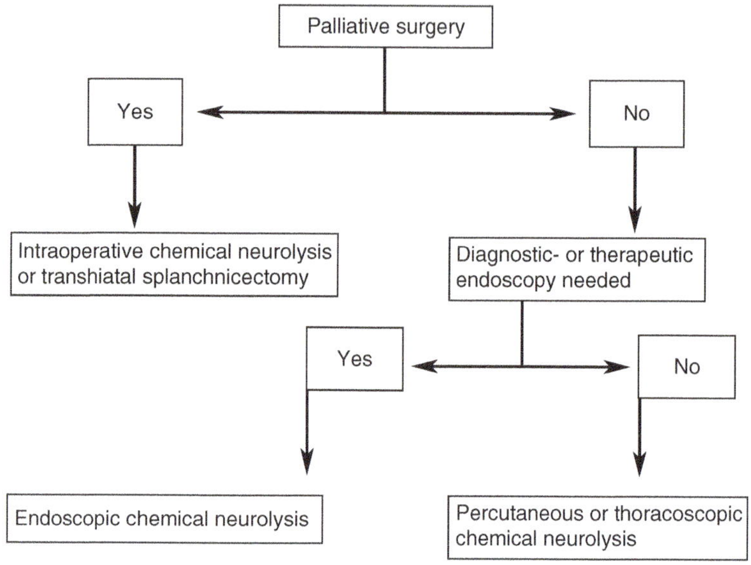

Fig. 12.3 Decision tree algorithm for pain management in unresectable pancreatic cancer patients

decision during laparotomy and to perform such palliative surgery.

Furthermore, since morbidity and mortality of pancreatoduodenectomy have dramatically decreased in the last decades, a more aggressive approach towards resection can be justified. Recent data clearly support a survival benefit in patients with R1 resection compared to double bypass procedures. It remains to be defined what is the right place of palliative resection in the therapeutic decision.

Palliation of pancreatic cancer patients is today more than ever a multidisciplinary task, which must rely on a competent interdisciplinary teamwork.

References

1. Yeo CJ. Pancreatic cancer: 1998 update. J Am Coll Surg. 1998;187(4):429–42.
2. Sohn TA, Lillemoe KD, Cameron JL, et al. Surgical palliation of unresectable periampullary adenocarcinoma in the 1990s. J Am Coll Surg. 1999;188(6):658–66; discussion 666–9.
3. Lillemoe KD. Palliative therapy for pancreatic cancer. Surg Oncol Clin N Am. 1998;7(1):199–216.
4. Eppsteiner RW, Csikesz NG, McPhee JT, et al. Surgeon volume impacts hospital mortality for pancreatic resection. Ann Surg. 2009;249(4):635–40.
5. Gray Jr PJ, Wang J, Pawlik TM, et al. Factors influencing survival in patients undergoing palliative bypass for pancreatic adenocarcinoma. J Surg Oncol. 2012;106(1):66–71.
6. Muller MW, Friess H, Koninger J, et al. Factors influencing survival after bypass procedures in patients with advanced pancreatic adenocarcinomas. Am J Surg. 2008;195(2):221–8.
7. Kuhlmann KF, de Castro SM, Wesseling JG, et al. Surgical treatment of pancreatic adenocarcinoma; actual survival and prognostic factors in 343 patients. Eur J Cancer. 2004;40(4):549–58.
8. Jamal MH, Doi SA, Simoneau E, et al. Unresectable pancreatic adenocarcinoma: do we know who survives? HPB (Oxford). 2010;12(8):561–6.
9. Huibregtse K, Katon RM, Coene PP, et al. Endoscopic palliative treatment in pancreatic cancer. Gastrointest Endosc. 1986;32(5):334–8.
10. Sarr MG, Cameron JL. Surgical palliation of unresectable carcinoma of the pancreas. World J Surg. 1984;8(6):906–18.
11. Distler M, Kersting S, Ruckert F, et al. Palliative treatment of obstructive jaundice in patients with carcinoma of the pancreatic head or distal biliary tree. Endoscopic stent placement vs. hepaticojejunostomy. JOP. 2010;11(6):568–74.
12. Lesurtel M, Dehni N, Tiret E, et al. Palliative surgery for unresectable pancreatic and periampullary cancer: a reappraisal. J Gastrointest Surg. 2006;10(2):286–91.
13. Hwang SI, Kim HO, Son BH, et al. Surgical palliation of unresectable pancreatic head cancer in elderly patients. World J Gastroenterol. 2009;15(8):978–82.
14. Mukherjee S, Kocher HM, Hutchins RR, et al. Palliative surgical bypass for pancreatic and periampullary cancers. J Gastrointest Cancer. 2007; 38(2–4):102–7.

15. Mortenson MM, Ho HS, Bold RJ. An analysis of cost and clinical outcome in palliation for advanced pancreatic cancer. Am J Surg. 2005;190(3):406–11.
16. Urbach DR, Bell CM, Swanstrom LL, et al. Cohort study of surgical bypass to the gallbladder or bile duct for the palliation of jaundice due to pancreatic cancer. Ann Surg. 2003;237(1):86–93.
17. Stumpf M, Kasperk R, Bertram P, et al. Role of surgical biliary bypass for palliation of pancreatic cancer – a retrospective study of 107 cases. Zentralbl Chir. 2001;126(11):913–6.
18. Isla AM, Worthington T, Kakkar AK, et al. A continuing role for surgical bypass in the palliative treatment of pancreatic carcinoma. Dig Surg. 2000;17(2):143–6.
19. Naggar E, Krag E, Matzen P. Endoscopically inserted biliary endoprosthesis in malignant obstructive jaundice. A survey of the literature. Liver. 1990;10(6):321–4.
20. Dowsett JF, Vaira D, Hatfield AR, et al. Endoscopic biliary therapy using the combined percutaneous and endoscopic technique. Gastroenterology. 1989;96(4):1180–6.
21. Kaufman SL. Percutaneous palliation of unresectable pancreatic cancer. Surg Clin North Am. 1995;75(5):989–99.
22. Speer AG, Cotton PB, Russell RC, et al. Randomised trial of endoscopic versus percutaneous stent insertion in malignant obstructive jaundice. Lancet. 1987;2(8550):57–62.
23. Pinol V, Castells A, Bordas JM, et al. Percutaneous self-expanding metal stents versus endoscopic polyethylene endoprostheses for treating malignant biliary obstruction: randomized clinical trial. Radiology. 2002;225(1):27–34.
24. Moss AC, Morris E, Mac Mathuna P. Palliative biliary stents for obstructing pancreatic carcinoma. Cochrane Database Syst Rev 2006;(1):CD004200.
25. Yoon WJ, Ryu JK, Yang KY, et al. A comparison of metal and plastic stents for the relief of jaundice in unresectable malignant biliary obstruction in Korea: an emphasis on cost-effectiveness in a country with a low ERCP cost. Gastrointest Endosc. 2009;70(2):284–9.
26. Soderlund C, Linder S. Covered metal versus plastic stents for malignant common bile duct stenosis: a prospective, randomized, controlled trial. Gastrointest Endosc. 2006;63(7):986–95.
27. Moss AC, Morris E, Leyden J, et al. Do the benefits of metal stents justify the costs? A systematic review and meta-analysis of trials comparing endoscopic stents for malignant biliary obstruction. Eur J Gastroenterol Hepatol. 2007;19(12):1119–24.
28. Arguedas MR, Heudebert GH, Stinnett AA, et al. Biliary stents in malignant obstructive jaundice due to pancreatic carcinoma: a cost-effectiveness analysis. Am J Gastroenterol. 2002;97(4):898–904.
29. Saito H, Sakurai Y, Takamura A, et al. Biliary endoprosthesis using Gore-Tex covered expandable metallic stents: preliminary clinical evaluation. Nippon Igaku Hoshasen Gakkai Zasshi. 1994;54(2):180–2.
30. Yoon WJ, Lee JK, Lee KH, et al. A comparison of covered and uncovered Wallstents for the management of distal malignant biliary obstruction. Gastrointest Endosc. 2006;63(7):996–1000.
31. Kahaleh M, Tokar J, Conaway MR, et al. Efficacy and complications of covered Wallstents in malignant distal biliary obstruction. Gastrointest Endosc. 2005;61(4):528–33.
32. Saleem A, Leggett CL, Murad MH, et al. Meta-analysis of randomized trials comparing the patency of covered and uncovered self-expandable metal stents for palliation of distal malignant bile duct obstruction. Gastrointest Endosc. 2011;74(2):321–7. e1–3.
33. DiFronzo LA, Egrari S, O'Connell TX. Choledochoduodenostomy for palliation in unresectable pancreatic cancer. Arch Surg. 1998;133(8):820–5.
34. Potts 3rd JR, Broughan TA, Hermann RE. Palliative operations for pancreatic carcinoma. Am J Surg. 1990;159(1):72–7; discussion 77–8.
35. Huguier M, Baumel H, Manderscheid JC, et al. Surgical palliation for unresected cancer of the exocrine pancreas. Eur J Surg Oncol. 1993;19(4):342–7.
36. Tarnasky PR, England RE, Lail LM, et al. Cystic duct patency in malignant obstructive jaundice. An ERCP-based study relevant to the role of laparoscopic cholecystojejunostomy. Ann Surg. 1995;221(3):265–71.
37. Baumel H, Huguier M. Le cancer du pancréas exocrine: diagnostic et traitement. Paris: Springer; 1991.
38. Scott EN, Garcea G, Doucas H, et al. Surgical bypass vs. endoscopic stenting for pancreatic ductal adenocarcinoma. HPB (Oxford). 2009;11(2):118–24.
39. Smith AC, Dowsett JF, Russell RC, et al. Randomised trial of endoscopic stenting versus surgical bypass in malignant low bileduct obstruction. Lancet. 1994;344(8938):1655–60.
40. Shepherd HA, Royle G, Ross AP, et al. Endoscopic biliary endoprosthesis in the palliation of malignant obstruction of the distal common bile duct: a randomized trial. Br J Surg. 1988;75(12):1166–8.
41. Andersen JR, Sorensen SM, Kruse A, et al. Randomised trial of endoscopic endoprosthesis versus operative bypass in malignant obstructive jaundice. Gut. 1989;30(8):1132–5.
42. Taylor MC, McLeod RS, Langer B. Biliary stenting versus bypass surgery for the palliation of malignant distal bile duct obstruction: a meta-analysis. Liver Transpl. 2000;6(3):302–8.
43. Maosheng D, Ohtsuka T, Ohuchida J, et al. Surgical bypass versus metallic stent for unresectable pancreatic cancer. J Hepatobiliary Pancreat Surg. 2001;8(4):367–73.
44. Artifon EL, Sakai P, Cunha JE, et al. Surgery or endoscopy for palliation of biliary obstruction due to metastatic pancreatic cancer. Am J Gastroenterol. 2006;101(9):2031–7.

45. Lyons JM, Karkar A, Correa-Gallego CC, et al. Operative procedures for unresectable pancreatic cancer: does operative bypass decrease requirements for postoperative procedures and in-hospital days? HPB (Oxford). 2012;14(7):469–75.
46. Van Heek NT, De Castro SM, van Eijck CH, et al. The need for a prophylactic gastrojejunostomy for unresectable periampullary cancer: a prospective randomized multicenter trial with special focus on assessment of quality of life. Ann Surg. 2003; 238(6):894–902; discussion 902–5.
47. Sarr MG, Cameron JL. Surgical management of unresectable carcinoma of the pancreas. Surgery. 1982;91(2):123–33.
48. Watanapa P, Williamson RC. Surgical palliation for pancreatic cancer: developments during the past two decades. Br J Surg. 1992;79(1):8–20.
49. Lillemoe KD, Cameron JL, Hardacre JM, et al. Is prophylactic gastrojejunostomy indicated for unresectable periampullary cancer? A prospective randomized trial. Ann Surg. 1999;230(3):322–8; discussion 328–30.
50. Shyr YM, Su CH, Wu CW, et al. Prospective study of gastric outlet obstruction in unresectable periampullary adenocarcinoma. World J Surg. 2000;24(1): 60–4; discussion 64–5.
51. Huser N, Michalski CW, Schuster T, et al. Systematic review and meta-analysis of prophylactic gastroenterostomy for unresectable advanced pancreatic cancer. Br J Surg. 2009;96(7):711–9.
52. House MG, Choti MA. Palliative therapy for pancreatic/biliary cancer. Surg Clin North Am. 2005;85(2): 359–71.
53. Lillemoe KD, Sauter PK, Pitt HA, et al. Current status of surgical palliation of periampullary carcinoma. Surg Gynecol Obstet. 1993;176(1):1–10.
54. Shyr YM, Su CH, King KL, et al. Randomized trial of three types of gastrojejunostomy in unresectable periampullary cancer. Surgery. 1997;121(5):506–12.
55. Nassif T, Prat F, Meduri B, et al. Endoscopic palliation of malignant gastric outlet obstruction using self-expandable metallic stents: results of a multicenter study. Endoscopy. 2003;35(6):483–9.
56. Jeurnink SM, van Eijck CH, Steyerberg EW, et al. Stent versus gastrojejunostomy for the palliation of gastric outlet obstruction: a systematic review. BMC Gastroenterol. 2007;7:18.
57. Fiori E, Lamazza A, Volpino P, et al. Palliative management of malignant antro-pyloric strictures. Gastroenterostomy vs. endoscopic stenting. A randomized prospective trial. Anticancer Res. 2004; 24(1):269–71.
58. Mehta S, Hindmarsh A, Cheong E, et al. Prospective randomized trial of laparoscopic gastrojejunostomy versus duodenal stenting for malignant gastric outflow obstruction. Surg Endosc. 2006;20(2):239–42.
59. Jeurnink SM, Polinder S, Steyerberg EW, et al. Cost comparison of gastrojejunostomy versus duodenal stent placement for malignant gastric outlet obstruction. J Gastroenterol. 2010;45(5):537–43.
60. Lavu H, Mascaro AA, Grenda DR, et al. Margin positive pancreaticoduodenectomy is superior to palliative bypass in locally advanced pancreatic ductal adenocarcinoma. J Gastrointest Surg. 2009;13(11): 1937–46; discussion 1946–7.
61. Fusai G, Warnaar N, Sabin CA, et al. Outcome of R1 resection in patients undergoing pancreatico-duodenectomy for pancreatic cancer. Eur J Surg Oncol. 2008;34(12):1309–15.
62. Lillemoe KD, Cameron JL, Yeo CJ, et al. Pancreaticoduodenectomy. Does it have a role in the palliation of pancreatic cancer? Ann Surg. 1996; 223(6):718–25.
63. DeOliveira ML, Winter JM, Schafer M, et al. Assessment of complications after pancreatic surgery: a novel grading system applied to 633 patients undergoing pancreaticoduodenectomy. Ann Surg. 2006;244(6):931–7; discussion 937–9.
64. Huguier M, Baumel H, Manderscheid JC. Cancer of the exocrine pancreas. A plea for resection. Hepatogastroenterology. 1996;43(9):721–9.
65. Reinders ME, Allema JH, van Gulik TM, et al. Outcome of microscopically nonradical, subtotal pancreaticoduodenectomy (Whipple's resection) for treatment of pancreatic head tumors. World J Surg. 1995;19(3):410–4; discussion 414–5.
66. Kuhlmann K, de Castro S, van Heek T, et al. Microscopically incomplete resection offers acceptable palliation in pancreatic cancer. Surgery. 2006; 139(2):188–96.
67. Wellner UF, Makowiec F, Bausch D, et al. Locally advanced pancreatic head cancer: margin-positive resection or bypass? ISRN Surg. 2012;2012:513241.
68. Tachezy M, Bockhorn M, Gebauer F, et al. Bypass surgery versus intentionally incomplete resection in palliation of pancreatic cancer: is resection the lesser evil? J Gastrointest Surg. 2011;15(5):829–35.
69. Walter J, Nier A, Rose T, et al. Palliative partial pancreaticoduodenectomy impairs quality of life compared to bypass surgery in patients with advanced adenocarcinoma of the pancreatic head. Eur J Surg Oncol. 2011;37(9):798–804.
70. Michalski CW, Erkan M, Huser N, et al. Resection of primary pancreatic cancer and liver metastasis: a systematic review. Dig Surg. 2008;25(6):473–80.
71. Girelli R, Frigerio I, Salvia R, et al. Feasibility and safety of radiofrequency ablation for locally advanced pancreatic cancer. Br J Surg. 2010;97(2):220–5.
72. Girelli R, Frigerio I, Giardino A, et al. Results of 100 pancreatic radiofrequency ablations in the context of a multimodal strategy for stage III ductal adenocarcinoma. Langenbecks Arch Surg. 2013;398(1): 63–9.
73. Contreras CM, Stanelle EJ, Mansour J, et al. Staging laparoscopy enhances the detection of occult metastases in patients with pancreatic adenocarcinoma. J Surg Oncol. 2009;100(8):663–9.
74. Pisters PW, Lee JE, Vauthey JN, et al. Laparoscopy in the staging of pancreatic cancer. Br J Surg. 2001; 88(3):325–37.
75. Kwon AH, Inui H, Kamiyama Y. Preoperative laparoscopic examination using surgical manipulation and ultrasonography for pancreatic lesions. Endoscopy. 2002;34(6):464–8.

76. Schachter PP, Avni Y, Shimonov M, et al. The impact of laparoscopy and laparoscopic ultrasonography on the management of pancreatic cancer. Arch Surg. 2000;135(11):1303–7.
77. Allen PJ, Chou J, Janakos M, et al. Prospective evaluation of laparoscopic celiac plexus block in patients with unresectable pancreatic adenocarcinoma. Ann Surg Oncol. 2011;18(3):636–41.
78. Schmidt J, Fraunhofer S, Fleisch M, et al. Is peritoneal cytology a predictor of unresectability in pancreatic carcinoma? Hepatogastroenterology. 2004;51(60):1827–31.
79. Arcidiacono PG, Calori G, Carrara S, et al. Celiac plexus block for pancreatic cancer pain in adults. Cochrane Database Syst Rev. 2011;3, CD007519.
80. Jimenez RE, Warshaw AL, Rattner DW, et al. Impact of laparoscopic staging in the treatment of pancreatic cancer. Arch Surg. 2000;135(4):409–14; discussion 414–5.
81. Liu RC, Traverso LW. Diagnostic laparoscopy improves staging of pancreatic cancer deemed locally unresectable by computed tomography. Surg Endosc. 2005;19(5):638–42.
82. Ferrone CR, Haas B, Tang L, et al. The influence of positive peritoneal cytology on survival in patients with pancreatic adenocarcinoma. J Gastrointest Surg. 2006;10(10):1347–53.
83. Meszoely IM, Lee JS, Watson JC, et al. Peritoneal cytology in patients with potentially resectable adenocarcinoma of the pancreas. Am Surg. 2004;70(3):208–13; discussion 213–4.
84. Yachida S, Fukushima N, Sakamoto M, et al. Implications of peritoneal washing cytology in patients with potentially resectable pancreatic cancer. Br J Surg. 2002;89(5):573–8.
85. Andren-Sandberg A, Viste A, Horn A, et al. Pain management of pancreatic cancer. Ann Oncol. 1999;10 Suppl 4:265–8.
86. Caraceni A, Portenoy RK. Pain management in patients with pancreatic carcinoma. Cancer. 1996;78(3 Suppl):639–53.
87. Zech DF, Grond S, Lynch J, et al. Validation of World Health Organization guidelines for cancer pain relief: a 10-year prospective study. Pain. 1995; 63(1):65–76.
88. LeBlanc JK, Al-Haddad M, McHenry L, et al. A prospective, randomized study of EUS-guided celiac plexus neurolysis for pancreatic cancer: one injection or two? Gastrointest Endosc. 2011;74(6):1300–7.
89. Lillemoe KD, Cameron JL, Kaufman HS, et al. Chemical splanchnicectomy in patients with unresectable pancreatic cancer. A prospective randomized trial. Ann Surg. 1993;217(5):447–55; discussion 456–7.
90. Eisenberg E, Carr DB, Chalmers TC. Neurolytic celiac plexus block for treatment of cancer pain: a meta-analysis. Anesth Analg. 1995;80(2):290–5.
91. Wong GY, Schroeder DR, Carns PE, et al. Effect of neurolytic celiac plexus block on pain relief, quality of life, and survival in patients with unresectable pancreatic cancer: a randomized controlled trial. JAMA. 2004;291(9):1092–9.
92. de Oliveira R, dos Reis MP, Prado WA. The effects of early or late neurolytic sympathetic plexus block on the management of abdominal or pelvic cancer pain. Pain. 2004;110(1–2):400–8.
93. Zhang CL, Zhang TJ, Guo YN, et al. Effect of neurolytic celiac plexus block guided by computerized tomography on pancreatic cancer pain. Dig Dis Sci. 2008;53(3):856–60.
94. Puli SR, Reddy JB, Bechtold ML, et al. EUS-guided celiac plexus neurolysis for pain due to chronic pancreatitis or pancreatic cancer pain: a meta-analysis and systematic review. Dig Dis Sci. 2009;54(11):2330–7.
95. Zou XP, Chen SY, Lv Y, et al. Endoscopic ultrasound-guided celiac plexus neurolysis for pain management in patients with pancreatic carcinoma reasons to fight a losing battle. Pancreas. 2012;41(4):655–7.
96. Dubois F. Splanchnicectomy by trans-hiatal abdominal approach. Nouv Presse Med. 1977;6(23):2069–70.
97. Sielezneff I, Sastre B, Crespy B, et al. Analgesic effect of transhiatal splanchnectomy in pain from cancer of the pancreas. Apropos of 51 operated cancers. J Chir (Paris). 1993;130(11):447–52.
98. Sastre B, Carabalona B, Crespy B, et al. Transhiatal bilateral splanchnicotomy for pain control in pancreatic cancer: basic anatomy, surgical technique, and immediate results in fifty-one cases. Surgery. 1992;111(6):640–6.
99. Bali B, Deixonne B, Rzal K, et al. Bilateral splanchnicectomy by transhiatal approach in pain of pancreatic origin. 37 Cases. Presse Med. 1995;24(20):928–32.
100. Melki J, Riviere J, Roullee N, et al. Thoracic splanchnectomy under video-thoracoscopy. Presse Med. 1993;22(23):1095–7.
101. Worsey J, Ferson PF, Keenan RJ, et al. Thoracoscopic pancreatic denervation for pain control in irresectable pancreatic cancer. Br J Surg. 1993;80(8):1051–2.
102. Cuschieri A, Shimi SM, Crosthwaite G, et al. Bilateral endoscopic splanchnicectomy through a posterior thoracoscopic approach. J R Coll Surg Edinb. 1994;39(1):44–7.
103. Pietrabissa A, Vistoli F, Carobbi A, et al. Thoracoscopic splanchnicectomy for pain relief in unresectable pancreatic cancer. Arch Surg. 2000; 135(3):332–5.
104. Saenz A, Kuriansky J, Salvador L, et al. Thoracoscopic splanchnicectomy for pain control in patients with unresectable carcinoma of the pancreas. Surg Endosc. 2000;14(8):717–20.
105. Stefaniak T, Basinski A, Vingerhoets A, et al. A comparison of two invasive techniques in the management of intractable pain due to inoperable pancreatic cancer: neurolytic celiac plexus block and videothoracoscopic splanchnicectomy. Eur J Surg Oncol. 2005;31(7):768–73.
106. Johnson CD, Berry DP, Harris S, et al. An open randomized comparison of clinical effectiveness of protocol-driven opioid analgesia, celiac plexus block or thoracoscopic splanchnicectomy for pain management in patients with pancreatic and other abdominal malignancies. J Pancreatol. 2009;9(6): 755–63.

13 Biliary Tract and Liver

Sarah Thomasset and Ashley Dennison

Contents

S. Thomasset, PhD, MRCS
A. Dennison, MD, FRCS (✉)
Department of Hepatobiliary and Pancreatic Surgery,
Leicester General Hospital,
Gwendolen Road, Leicester LE5 4PW, UK
e-mail: sarah.thomasset@uhl-tr.nhs.uk;
ashley.dennison@uhl-tr.nhs.uk

Cholestasis associated with obstruction of the biliary tract can be debilitating and significantly impacts on quality of life. Cholangiocarcinomas are the main indication for surgical palliation, in the form of a biliary-enteric bypass. These may be undertaken following failed attempts at endoscopic stenting and when unresectable disease is discovered at exploratory laparotomy. In selected patients, surgical bypass effectively palliates the symptoms of biliary tract obstruction. Neuroendocrine tumours are the predominant indication for palliative liver resection. Cytoreductive liver resections for neuroendocrine tumours can be associated with enhanced survival and can relieve symptoms caused by the mechanical effects of the tumour and hormone secretion. There is minimal evidence to support undertaking cytoreductive liver resections in other malignancies. Occasionally, when all other treatments have failed, a liver resection can be undertaken with the aim of improving tumour-related symptoms.

13.1 Biliary Tract

The main conditions involving the biliary tract that may require surgical palliation are cholangiocarcinomas and primary sclerosing cholangitis. Although both are uncommon, palliation is particularly important as cholestasis arising from biliary tract obstruction can profoundly affect both survival and quality of life. Knowledge of the surgical options for achieving biliary tract

M. Wichmann, G. Maddern (eds.), *Palliative Surgery*,
DOI 10.1007/978-3-642-53709-7_13,

decompression and the outcomes associated with these are important to ensure all appropriate approaches are considered, when either endoscopic interventions fail or unresectable disease is discovered at exploratory laparotomy for potentially operable cholangiocarcinomas.

13.1.1 Hilar Cholangiocarcinoma

Most patients with hilar cholangiocarcinomas have unresectable disease at presentation and require palliation of their symptoms, particularly pruritus and cholangitis. Studies have failed to demonstrate any significant difference in overall survival between patients with hilar cholangiocarcinomas who undergo surgical and nonsurgical procedures to relieve biliary obstruction [1, 2], and percutaneous, endoscopic and combined biliary stents should be regarded as first-line palliative treatment [3]. Palliative surgery has an important role in patients with a good estimated life expectancy (>6 months) in whom biliary stenting has failed, and it should also be considered in patients who are found to have unresectable disease at exploratory laparotomy. Although palliative surgery is associated with a greater early morbidity and mortality than biliary stenting, it palliates jaundice more effectively in the long term resulting in a lower incidence of readmission to hospital [4].

13.1.1.1 Segment III Cholangiojejunostomy

The most common surgical approach for the palliation of hilar cholangiocarcinoma is a biliary-enteric bypass to segment III. This is technically easier than a right-sided intrahepatic bypass as the left-sided ducts exhibit more constant anatomy and are more readily accessible. The segment III duct can be identified by dissection at the left base of ligamentum teres and is usually located posterosuperior to the segmental portal vein branch. An anterior hepatotomy (aided by the use of intraoperative ultrasound) to the left of the falciform ligament can enhance exposure of the duct (Fig. 13.1a) [6]. A 10 mm side-to-side Roux-en-Y biliary anastomosis is then performed (Fig. 13.1b, c).

For cholestasis to be relieved, a minimum of 30 % of the liver parenchyma, or two liver segments, should be drained [7]. It has long been recognised that unilateral hepatic drainage can successfully palliate hilar cholangiocarcinomas even when communication between the left and right ductal systems is prevented by tumour growth [8]. Relative contraindications for a segment III cholangiojejunostomy include infection in an obstructed right ductal system (commonly precipitated by previous attempts at stenting), atrophy of the left lobe arising secondary to vascular involvement, extensive metastases in the left lobe and tumour involvement of the secondary branches of the left ductal system [6, 7, 9].

Most studies reporting the outcomes for segment III cholangiojejunostomies include cohorts of patients with hilar cholangiocarcinomas and gall bladder cancers [6, 9–13]. Focusing only on hilar cholangiocarcinomas, segment III cholangiojejunostomies are associated with a morbidity rate of 17–55 % and a perioperative mortality rate of 0–33 % [6, 7, 10]. Mean survival following the procedure is 5–9 months, with a maximum survival of 19 months (Table 13.1) [7, 10].

Factors associated with significantly reduced survival following a segment III cholangiojejunostomy for cholangiocarcinoma include development of an anastomotic leak and stage IV disease [6]. Jarnagin et al. describe a subgroup of 20 patients who underwent segment III bypasses for hilar cholangiocarcinoma. Of these 20 patients, seven (35 %) were readmitted with biliary sepsis, and three (15 %) required further biliary intervention. The patency rate for segment III bypass at 1 year was 80 %.

Traynor et al. report quality of life following segment III bypasses for hilar cholangiocarcinoma in the form of a "comfort index", the duration of symptom-free survival expressed as a percentage of total survival [7]. They describe a comfort index of 91 % with a mean survival of 9.2 months. This compares with a comfort index after stenting in the region of 50 % [11]. Of the 48 patients undergoing a segment III bypass described by Traynor et al., bilirubin levels normalised in 35 patients (73 %) fell to 50 % of their preoperative value in 11 patients (23 %) but fell by less than 50 % in the remaining two patients [7].

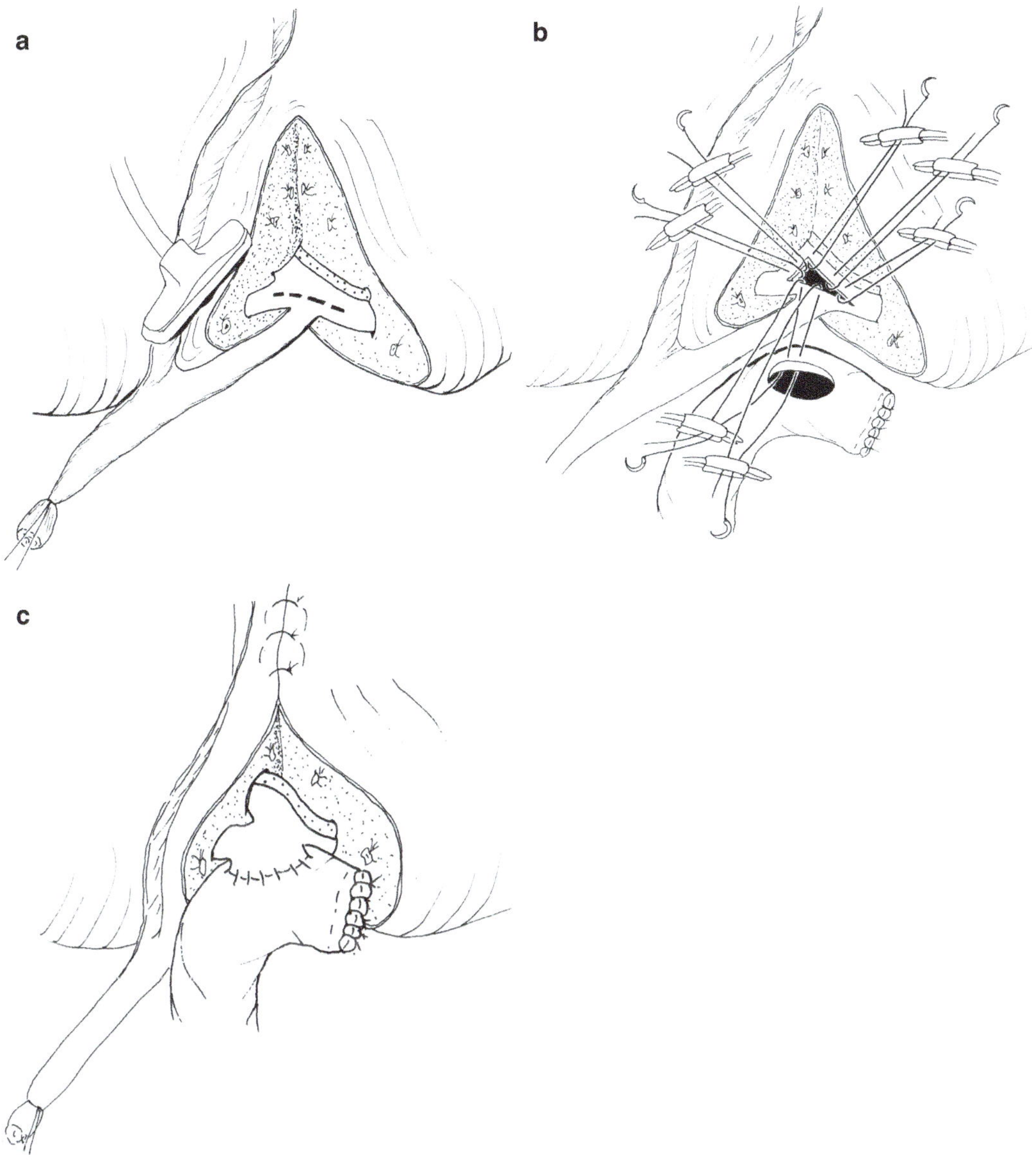

Fig. 13.1 (**a**) Position of the segment III bile duct and the use of intraoperative ultrasound to aid location. (**b**) A 2 cm bilioenteric anastomosis is constructed using an isolated Roux loop. (**c**) The finished bilioenteric anastomosis after completion of the anterior row of sutures (Reprinted with permission from Dennison and Maddern [5])

Table 13.1 Outcomes following segment III cholangiojejunostomy for hilar cholangiocarcinoma

Authors	Number of patients with hilar cholangiocarcinomas	Morbidity	Number of biliary leaks	Perioperative mortality	Survival, months
Blumgart et al. [14]	28	NR	NR	6 (21 %)	NR
Traynor et al. [7]	48	8 (17 %)	4 (8 %)	3 (6 %)	Mean, 9.2 Maximum, 19
Jarnagin et al. [6]	20	11 (55 %)	6 (30 %)	0	Median, 18.5
Launois et al. [10]	12	NR	NR	4 (33 %)	Mean, 5 Maximum, 11

NR not reported

13.1.1.2 Right-Sided Cholangiojejunostomy

For those patients in whom a segment III bypass is not feasible, a right-sided cholangiojejunostomy may be undertaken. Right-sided drainage requires identification of either the right anterior sectoral or segmental ducts, which is aided by intraoperative ultrasound following cholecystectomy (Fig. 13.2).

Division of the liver parenchyma in the base of the gall bladder fossa exposes the anterior sectoral duct that is usually utilised for right-sided intrahepatic bypasses [15]. A side-to-side biliary-enteric anastomosis is constructed using a Roux-en-Y loop of jejunum.

Jarnagin et al. report outcome data from 14 patients who underwent a right sectoral bypass for hilar cholangiocarcinoma [6]. There was a significantly higher 30-day mortality in patients undergoing a right-sided bypass than in those undergoing a segment III bypass (21.4 vs. 0 %). In addition, the rate of late bypass failure was greater for those undergoing a right sectoral bypass, and this group also required a significantly greater number of postoperative biliary interventions (55 % right sectoral vs. 15 % segment III). These observations probably reflect the greater technical challenge associated with right-sided intrahepatic bypasses and emphasise the fact that a segment III cholangiojejunostomy is preferable.

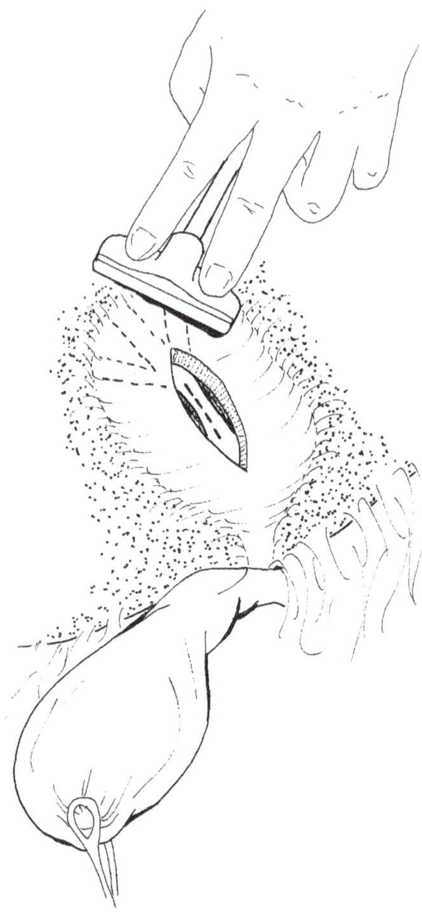

Fig. 13.2 Following a cholecystectomy, the segment V duct is located using intraoperative ultrasound. Depending on the position of the duct, a hepatotomy may be required to facilitate the anastomosis (Reprinted with permission from Dennison and Maddern [5])

13.1.2 Distal Cholangiocarcinoma

As for hilar cholangiocarcinomas, the majority of patients requiring palliative treatment for unresectable distal disease are managed with a biliary stent. Stents for distal biliary obstruction are easier to place than those for hilar obstruction and have a greater long-term patency rate [16]. A recent meta-analysis comparing stenting and surgical bypass for malignant distal biliary obstruction revealed no difference in therapeutic success rates between the procedures. A trend in 30-day mortality in favour of stenting was observed; however, the risk of recurrent biliary obstruction was significantly higher in this group [17]. These studies generally include patients with malignant distal biliary obstruction arising secondary to a number of causes, most frequently pancreatic cancer, rather than solely including patients with distal cholangiocarcinomas [18–22].

Although most patients with distal cholangiocarcinomas are managed palliatively with a biliary stent, the indications for palliative surgery are similar to those in hilar disease. Surgical bypass should be considered in patients with a distal cholangiocarcinoma in whom stenting fails or in those who are found to have unresectable disease at exploratory laparotomy. In addition, it should also be considered in occasional patients with a relatively long estimated survival [3]. A number of factors have been associated with longer survival in patients with malignant distal biliary obstruction, including the absence of metastatic disease and symptomatic gastric outlet obstruction, a favourable American Society of Anesthesiologists (ASA) score, the absence of pain and a normal C-reactive protein (CRP) and white cell count [21, 23, 24].

13.1.2.1 Hepaticojejunostomy/ choledochojejunostomy

The preferred procedure to achieve surgical palliation for patients with distal cholangiocarcinoma depends on the exact site of the tumour but is either a hepaticojejunostomy or choledochojejunostomy. It has long been recognised that these bypasses yield superior results compared to those involving the gall bladder or duodenum [25]. Concomitant gastrojejunostomy as a prophylactic measure to avoid gastric outlet obstruction is now recommended by most authors [26]. Although only 5 % of patients with malignant distal biliary obstruction exhibit gastric outlet obstruction at diagnosis, it can develop in up to 20 % of patients as the disease progresses [27]. Several recent studies including patients with malignant distal biliary obstruction, most of whom underwent combined biliary and gastric bypasses, have shown perioperative mortality rates of 0–4 % and median survival ranges from 6.4 to 8.3 months [21–23]. In the largest study of 269 patients, 9 % required further surgery, which largely reflects the fact that 23 % of patients who did not receive a gastrojejunostomy subsequently developed gastric outlet obstruction [21].

Over the last 10 years, there have been increasing reports of laparoscopic bypass procedures. The development of laparoscopic stapling devices has allowed gastrojejunostomies and cholecystojejunostomies to be conducted with relative ease. However, a significant proportion of patients are not suitable for a cholecystojejunostomy due to tumour involvement at the junction of the cystic and hepatic ducts or previous cholecystectomy [28]. Laparoscopic hepaticojejunostomies and choledochojejunostomies have been described, but they are technically challenging and not widely practised. Operating time associated with these procedures is significant, and studies to date consist of small numbers of patients.

13.1.3 Gall Bladder Cancer

Unresectable gall bladder cancer is associated with a dismal survival of approximately 2–5 months and nonsurgical methods of palliation should therefore be undertaken in the vast majority of patients. If unresectable disease is discovered at exploratory laparotomy a segment III bypass may be considered to relieve jaundice. However, mortality associated with this bypass in patients with gall bladder cancer is as high as 17 %, and few would reap any long-term benefit [6]. This group of patients should therefore be managed with postoperative endoscopic or percutaneous biliary drainage in preference to a biliary-enteric bypass.

13.1.4 Primary Sclerosing Cholangitis

Primary sclerosing cholangitis (PSC) is a progressive cholestatic liver disease of unknown aetiology that is associated with inflammatory fibrosis and strictures of the intra- and extrahepatic ducts. The prognosis of patients with PSC is poor, and the median survival from diagnosis to death or liver transplantation is only 9.6 years [29]. Dominant strictures of the extrahepatic bile ducts have been described in 10–20 % of patients with PSC and are one of the primary indications for intervention, in the form of palliative endoscopic, percutaneous or surgical techniques [30–33].

Dominant strictures of the common bile duct and common hepatic duct are defined as those reducing the diameter of the duct to ≤1.5 and ≤1.0 mm, respectively [34, 35]. Although usually asymptomatic in the early stages, progression can give rise to worsening jaundice, deteriorating liver function tests and cholangitis.

As PSC predisposes to cholangiocarcinoma, making a distinction between benign and malignant strictures clinically can be difficult. At presentation approximately 25 % of dominant strictures are malignant [36], and brush cytology at endoscopic retrograde cholangiopancreatography (ERCP) may provide a diagnosis. A recent prospective study of brush cytology obtained at ERCP revealed the sensitivity for diagnosing cholangiocarcinoma to be 80 % [37]. In terms of radiology, positron emission tomography (PET) scanning is superior to conventional investigations (CT and MRI) in differentiating between PSC and cholangiocarcinoma [38]. If diagnostic doubt regarding the nature of a dominant stricture exists despite investigation, surgical excision is indicated.

Non-cirrhotic patients with PSC who are symptomatic with cholestasis from a dominant stricture can be treated with endoscopic, percutaneous or surgical interventions. Non-operative interventions have several advantages, including lower complication rates, avoidance of a general anaesthetic and the ability to repeatedly intervene without altering biliary anatomy or compromising the possibility of a future liver transplant. They should therefore be regarded as first-line procedures for the treatment of symptomatic dominant strictures in non-cirrhotic patients with PSC. Many surgeons now advocate orthotropic liver transplantation as the only definitive form of treatment for non-cirrhotic patients with a dominant stricture; however, excision of the extrahepatic biliary tree and reconstruction using a Roux loop have been described [39–41]. Undoubtedly, cirrhotic patients with PSC are best managed with a liver transplant as other surgical treatments are associated with high operative mortality rates and poor long-term survival [42].

13.1.4.1 Biliary Resection and Bypass

In most patients with PSC, the hepatic duct bifurcation is the region most severely affected [43]. As such, resection of the extrahepatic ducts along with the hepatic bifurcation and reconstruction with a hepaticojejunostomy has been described. A number of authors have also advocated the use of long-term bilateral transhepatic biliary stents with this approach, to reduce the risk of future strictures [39–41]. A recent study described outcome data for 77 patients who underwent resection of the extrahepatic ducts and hepatic bifurcation with hepaticojejunostomies and transhepatic biliary stents. The 30-day mortality for these patients was 3.9 % with a perioperative complication rate of 38.7 %, the most frequent complications being cholangitis (24 %) and a bile leak (9.1 %). Bilirubin levels fell significantly postoperatively, and at 3 years, 57 % of patients had no PSC-related admissions. Survival rates at 5 and 10 years were 76 and 53 %, respectively [39]. When transhepatic stents are inserted, these require multiple replacements in the long term. However, of more concern is the fact that surgery involving the biliary tree can increase the morbidity and mortality associated with subsequent liver transplant [44–46].

In summary, palliative excision of the biliary tree and reconstruction using a Roux loop for PSC have been described. However, this approach has declined in popularity due to improvements in endoscopic techniques, greater access to liver transplantation and concerns regarding the potential impact on future transplantation. Although still advocated by some authors [39], most patients can now be treated symptomatically with endoscopic techniques, and these can act as a bridge to transplantation when required.

13.2 Liver

Most liver resections should be undertaken with curative intent. In the palliative setting, they are undertaken with two main aims, either to prolong survival or for symptom control. Neuroendocrine tumours are one of the most frequent indications for palliative liver resections, often yielding benefits both in terms of survival and symptom control. The morbidity associated with a liver resection is of particular concern when this is undertaken with palliative intent and the overall prognosis associated with the tumour is an important consideration (Table 13.2).

Palliative liver resections are far more appealing in those tumours that are associated with

Table 13.2 The prognosis of hepatic metastases and the site of the primary tumour

Bad prognosis associated with liver metastases	Intermediate prognosis associated with liver metastases	Better prognosis associated with liver metastases
Pancreas	Sarcoma	Kidney
Stomach	Gastrointestinal stromal tumours	Adrenal
Cutaneous melanoma	Breast	Gynaecological/ testicular tumours

a better prognosis, for example, renal tumours. Although there is very strong evidence to support the role of cytoreductive hepatic surgery in neuroendocrine tumours, evidence for its role in prolonging survival in other tumour types is far more limited. Resection may effectively palliate symptoms associated with liver tumours in a select group of patients in whom all conservative approaches fail.

13.2.1 Neuroendocrine Tumours

Neuroendocrine tumours (NETs) are a diverse group of neoplasms that are characterised by their relatively slow rate of growth along with their propensity to produce and secrete hormones and other vasoactive substances. NETs are relatively uncommon tumours; however, evidence suggests the incidence is increasing and it is currently approximately five per 100,000 [47]. Around 85 % of NETs originate from the gastrointestinal tract, and the majority of patients have liver metastases at the time of diagnosis, which substantially reduces survival. Curative (R0) surgical resection is only possible in approximately 15 % of patients with neuroendocrine liver metastases (NELM); frequently, the extent and localisation of disease means that palliation is the only treatment option [48].

13.2.1.1 Liver Resection: Rationale

The main aims of palliative liver resections for NETs are to improve symptoms (and associated quality of life) and facilitate the effect of non-operative treatments. Palliative resections for NELM can also confer a survival benefit.

Table 13.3 Clinical features associated with functional NETS

Tumour	Clinical features
Carcinoid	Flushing, diarrhoea, nausea, vomiting, abdominal pain, bronchoconstriction, fibrosis of the tricuspid and pulmonary valves
Insulinoma	Confusion, sweatiness, dizziness, loss of conscious, relief with eating
Gastrinoma	Zollinger-Ellison syndrome; severe peptic ulceration, diarrhoea
Glucagonoma	Weight loss, diabetes mellitus, stomatitis, diarrhoea, necrolytic migratory erythema
VIPoma	Verner-Morrison syndrome; profuse watery diarrhoea, hypokalaemia
Somatostatinoma	Cholelithiasis, weight loss, diarrhoea, steatorrhoea, diabetes mellitus

Symptoms from NETs that resections may palliate relate to the mass effects of the tumour and those arising from hormones and peptides secreted by functional tumours (Table 13.3).

Carcinoid syndrome, arising from the release of serotonin and other vasoactive mediators, occurs in up to 35 % of patients with NETS [49]. Symptoms include flushing, diarrhoea, abdominal pain and those arising from cardiac involvement. Pancreatic NETs are functional in approximately 40 % of cases, leading to a variety of symptoms [50] (Table 13.3). When endocrinopathies do occur, a palliative liver resection can frequently treat these symptoms very effectively. In addition to liver resections providing symptomatic relief, control of associated endocrinopathies may also improve overall survival. For example, carcinoid-related valvulopathies can lead to fatal cardiac failure, insulinomas may cause life-threatening hypoglycaemia, and gastrinomas can lead to gastrointestinal perforation or massive haemorrhage. Whilst palliative liver resections may improve survival by reducing the frequency of fatal endocrinopathies, the magnitude of this effect is difficult to determine. The main factor contributing to enhanced survival is likely to be the cytoreductive effect of liver resection.

NETs possess a number of key biological features that distinguish them from most other tumour types and justify the consideration of palliative liver resections [51]. NETs characteristically possess a relatively low proliferation index, and when distant metastases do occur, these are usually limited to the liver. Even in the presence of extensive liver metastases, the primary tumour often remains resectable. In addition, tumour volume correlates well with the severity of endocrine symptoms giving predictable effects from palliative resections. The favourable biological features of NETs manifest clinically in terms of survival. Survival from metastatic NETs far exceeds that associated with an equal tumour volume arising from a metastatic gastrointestinal adenocarcinoma. These biological and clinical features result in NELM being the predominant indication for a liver resection in the palliative setting.

Where major palliative surgery is planned with the primary aim of symptomatic relief, the morbidity and mortality associated with the procedure are of paramount importance. As palliative liver resections for NELM are also associated with prolonged survival in addition to relief of associated symptoms and liver resection is associated with low rates of mortality in high volume centres, the procedure is clearly justified.

13.2.1.2 Surgical Considerations

Most authors advocate cytoreductive hepatic surgery when at least 90 % of the bulk of the tumour can be resected which is very likely to yield a successful outcome [52, 53]. In synchronous disease, concurrent resection of the primary tumour, along with hepatic metastases, can be undertaken safely in selected patients [54–56]. In the palliative setting particularly, where patients should undergo the minimum possible number of surgical procedures, adjuncts to resection can be helpful (vide infra). Successful palliative outcomes can be obtained in those with bilobar NELM [57]. Every case must be assessed on an individual basis, considering the potential benefits from surgery, along with the patients' comorbidities and the risks involved.

Symptoms associated with functional NETs must be controlled prior to surgical intervention to reduce the risk of complications. All patients with carcinoid syndrome must receive prophylactic administration of a somatostatin analogue to prevent potential carcinoid crisis, characterised by profound flushing, bronchospasm, tachycardia and a labile blood pressure. This may be precipitated by anaesthetic induction or handling of the tumour intraoperatively. The use of short-acting octreotide is recommended, which is administered as a constant intravenous infusion. It is initiated at least 12 h prior to surgery and continued for up to 48 h postoperatively [50]. Similar prophylactic measures may be required for the problems associated with pancreatic NETs, for example, a glucose infusion for insulinomas and potassium replacement therapy for VIPomas.

13.2.1.3 Liver Resection: Results

To date, no prospective trials have been conducted to determine the results of palliative liver resections for NELM. A number of retrospective studies have attempted to assess the results of liver resections for NETs; however, frequently these trials have included both curative and palliative procedures. Primarily due to the small number of patients involved in these studies, outcome measures for the two groups are often not reported separately. Table 13.4 shows studies which detail outcome measures, in terms of either endocrine symptoms or survival, specifically for cohorts of patients who have undergone palliative liver resections.

Palliative liver resections can partially or completely relieve systemic endocrine-related symptoms in more than 80 % of patients with NELM [54, 56, 60, 63, 64]. Although variability does exist in the definition of symptom relief between studies, overall the literature does suggest excellent palliation of hormone-related symptoms. Over a decade ago, Que et al. showed similar initial symptomatic response rates in patients undergoing liver resections for NELM regardless of whether these procedures were undertaken with curative or palliative intent [56]. The distinguishing feature was the earlier recurrence of symptoms in patients who had undergone palliative rather than curative resections (11.3 vs. 20.4 months). Palliative resections were undertaken if the primary tumour and 90 % or more of the hepatic disease were deemed resectable. Although few other studies specifically report the duration of symptom relief in those undergoing palliative resections, where reported the figures are similar to those obtained by Que et al. [54, 58].

The 5-year survival of patients with NELM treated with only medical therapy is 20–40 % [68, 69]. Sarmiento et al. report one of the largest single-institution studies of hepatic resections for NELM [62]. This series of 170 patients revealed 5- and 10-year survival rates of 61 and 35 %, respectively. However, curative resections were undertaken in 44 % of patients, and the survival figures provided do not distinguish between those procedures undertaken with curative and palliative intent. Considering palliative resections only, up to 48 % of patients survive for 5 years [67]. Table 13.4 highlights the inter-study variability in survival figures for palliative resections. This variability reflects differences between studies in terms of the types of tumours included and the criteria for palliative resections. For example, Hibi et al. report a 5-year survival rate of 0 % following palliative resections for NELM, but this group consists of a disproportionate number of patients with lung and pancreatic NETs, which have comparatively poor survival outcomes [64]. Overall, current evidence suggests that palliative resection for NELM does prolong survival.

There is a paucity of data regarding changes in quality of life following treatment of NELM.

A study by Knox et al. [70] that included patients undergoing hepatic resections for metastatic carcinoid tumours revealed a statistically significant improvement in quality of life indices from the third postoperative month. These effects were sustained for in excess of 4 years, and further assessment was limited by follow-up. When symptoms of carcinoid syndrome did recur, these were less severe than they had been initially and did not significantly affect quality of life.

13.2.1.4 Adjuncts to Surgery

Hepatic resection may be combined with a number of ablative techniques such as radiofrequency ablation (RFA) and cryoablation to provide effective cytoreduction. Osborne et al. reports the use of RFA in patients with bilobar or scattered disease. Of the 23 patients in the study who underwent palliative cytoreductive surgery, 11 had formal liver resections, six had a wedge resection with RFA and six received RFA alone. All patients experienced relief from associated endocrine symptoms, and the mean survival was 32 months [55]. Other studies have also described similar encouraging results from the use of RFA in the palliative setting [63, 67]. Cryoablation in combination with palliative resection is also an efficient method of cytoreduction in terms of symptom relief and survival [54, 66]. Although results suggest ablative techniques may be a beneficial adjunct to surgical resection in the palliative setting, all studies are limited by the relatively small number of patients involved.

In summary, NELM are one of the main indications for a palliative liver resection. Cytoreductive surgery to reduce tumour volume by in excess of 90 % is associated with improvements in associated symptoms and prolonged survival. Although each individual case should be considered in terms of the potential risks and benefits involved, the literature does provide clear justification for the role of palliative resection in NELM.

13.2.2 Epithelial Ovarian Cancer

More than 35 years ago, a landmark study by Griffiths first conclusively demonstrated an inverse relationship between the diameter of residual ovarian tumour tissue remaining following surgery and patient survival [71]. Current standard treatment for advanced epithelial ovarian cancer (stages III–IV, Table 13.5) consists of cytoreductive surgery to minimise residual tumour volume followed by platinum- and taxane-based chemotherapy.

Intraperitoneal chemotherapy improves survival compared to intravenous chemotherapy alone; however, to be effective, patients must first undergo maximal debulking surgery [72]. Optimal cytoreduction, which is usually defined as residual disease <1 cm, correlates with improved survival [72]. The median survival for

Table 13.4 Cohorts of patients who have undergone palliative liver resections for neuroendocrine tumours

Author	Number	Primary neuroendocrine tumour	Ablative techniques in addition to liver resection	Endocrine symptoms (%)	Proportion of endocrine symptoms relieved (%)	30-day mortality (%)	Survival, months
McEntee et al. [58]	20	GI tract, pancreas	None	80	50, complete relief	–	Mean, 11
Grama et al. [59]	5	Functional pancreatic tumours	None	100	NR	NR	Median, 36
Que et al. [53]	46	GI tract, pancreas	None	91	83, complete relief	4	Median, 23.6
Chamberlain et al. [60]	6	GI tract, pancreas, lung, unknown	None	NR	100	NR	Median, 66
Nave et al. [61]	21	GI tract, pancreas, lung	None	NR	NR	0	26 % alive at 5 years
Chung et al. [54]	29	GI tract, pancreas, lung, thyroid	Cryosurgery, RFA	100	90, complete relief	3	31 % 5 years survival
Sarmiento et al. [62]	95	GI tract, pancreas, unknown	None	NR	NR	NR	Median,16
Osborne et al. [55]	23	GI tract, pancreas, lung, unknown	RFA	100	NR	4	Mean, 32
Jensen et al. [63]	13	GI tract, pancreas, unknown	RFA	100	32, complete relief; 68, partial relief	NR	NR
Hibi et al. [64]	7	GI tract, pancreas, lung, unknown	RFA, ethanol injection	86	83, complete relief; 17, partial relief	0	0 % 5-year survival
Mayo et al. [65]	65	GI tract, pancreas, lung, unknown	Yes	NR	NR	NR	Median, 77.5
Saxena et al. [66]	26	GI tract, pancreas, lung, uterus, gall bladder, unknown	Cryosurgery	NR	NR	NR	Median, 27
Cusati et al. [67]	32	Non-functional pancreatic tumours	RFA	0	–	0	93.8, 48.1 and 32.1 % alive at 1, 5 and 10 years, respectively

NR not reported, *RFA* radiofrequency ablation; this table only includes data from studies and cohorts of patients who have undergone palliative liver resections

Table 13.5 International Federation of Gynaecology and Obstetrics (FIGO) staging of ovarian cancer

Stage of ovarian cancer	Description
I	Limited to one or both ovaries
II	Pelvic extension or implants
III	Peritoneal implants outside of the pelvis; or limited to the pelvis with extension to the small bowel or omentum
IV	Distant metastases

advanced ovarian cancer is 3.5 years, and most patients develop chemoresistance after 24–36 months.

Although the liver is rarely the only site of metastatic disease in advanced ovarian cancer, a liver resection can be a component of primary or interval cytoreductive surgery. For example, when primary cytoreduction in patients with stage IV disease included a liver resection for metastases arising from peritoneal seeding, the 5-year progression-free survival rate and overall 5-year survival were very similar to those in patients undergoing cytoreduction for stage IIIc disease. No patients experienced any complications related to hepatic resection, including hemihepatectomy [73]. Bristow et al. describe outcome data for 37 patients with stage IV disease and liver metastases [74]. Of these, optimal cytoreduction of both hepatic and extrahepatic disease was achieved in six patients who had a median survival of 50 months. This compares to a median survival of 27 months in patients who underwent cytoreduction to achieve optimal control of extrahepatic disease, but suboptimal control of hepatic disease.

Hepatectomy has also been advocated in the setting of recurrent disease. Yoon et al. report a study of 24 patients who underwent cytoreductive surgery including a liver resection, mostly for recurrent ovarian cancer in 21 patients [75]. The median duration between the primary treatment and hepatic resection was 5 years, and median survival following liver resection was 62 months (range 6–94 months). Ideal candidates for a liver resection for metachronous disease are those with a good performance status and favourable tumour biology [75].

Studies concerning the role of cytoreductive liver resection for ovarian tumours are limited by the small numbers of patients involved and the lack of suitable control groups. Palliative liver resections for epithelial ovarian tumours are advocated by some authors but are currently generally limited to a highly select group of patients [73, 74, 76]. A palliative liver resection may be considered in patients with a good performance status, a favourable prognosis and disease that is suitable for optimal cytoreduction (<1 cm).

13.2.3 Testicular Germ Cell Tumours

There are a number of situations in which resection of liver metastases from testicular germ cell tumours is indicated. Firstly, patients with metastases from non-seminomatous tumours treated with chemotherapy that persist on follow-up imaging, with normalisation of tumour markers, should be resected. Secondly, residual disease should be resected after salvage chemotherapy when tumour markers normalise or plateau. Thirdly, resection should be considered if progression is evident despite salvage chemotherapy [77]. Some authors have termed liver resections in these situations "cytoreductive"; however, they should only be undertaken if complete resection of the tumour is feasible [78]. Unlike the situation with ovarian cancer, there is no evidence to support liver resection in situations where macroscopic disease cannot be resected in full [77]. This point is illustrated in a study reported by Rivoire et al. that included 37 patients who underwent a liver resection for metastatic testicular germ cell tumours [79]. Complete resection was achieved in all but two patients who subsequently died at 20 and 34 months. These patients had a significantly poorer prognosis compared to the group as a whole, who had a 63 % 5-year survival rate.

13.2.4 Breast Cancer

Although breast cancer is common, isolated liver lesions occur in only 1–5 % of patients with metastatic disease. Studies reporting liver resections undertaken for breast cancer metastases generally include small numbers of patients, lack suitable control groups and are retrospective, making it difficult to draw firm conclusions. Some authors advocate consideration of a liver resection in selected patients with no extrahepatic disease in whom negative margins are thought possible [80, 81]. Evidence concerning liver resections undertaken with positive margins and in the presence of extrahepatic disease is far more contradictory and the procedures controversial.

The anticipated likelihood of undertaking R0 liver resection has been a selection criterion in many studies. Although a number of studies report improved survival in the presence of negative hepatic resection margins [82–84], a notable study by Elias et al. refutes this [85]. This study included 54 patients with metastatic breast cancer, 44 of whom underwent R0 liver resection, with R1/R2 resections in the remainder. Median survivals in patients with R0 and R1/R2 resections were 40 and 31 months, respectively. No statistically significant difference in survival was evident between the groups. However, it could be that the effects of surgical margins in the study were confounded by the use of intra-arterial chemotherapy [86].

Evidence relating to liver resection in the presence of extrahepatic disease is similarly contradictory. Some studies have reported good results for liver resections undertaken in the presence of extrahepatic disease, but these series included few patients and those with extrahepatic disease represented a small proportion of the total number included [83, 87]. Bone metastases from breast cancer have a more indolent course than metastases involving other sites. Isolated bone metastases should therefore not necessarily preclude consideration of a liver resection; however, again, the number of patients involved in studies has been small [80, 81].

13.2.5 Renal Cell Carcinoma

Up to 50 % of patients with renal cell carcinoma (RCC) develop metastases, and in 20 % there is involvement of the liver. The liver is rarely the sole site of metastatic spread, and involvement usually indicates the presence of widespread disease. Whilst debulking liver resections are not indicated for metastatic RCC, there is evidence to support resections despite the presence of extrahepatic disease, which is itself amenable to treatment. Two large studies report series of patients who underwent liver resections for metastatic RCC. In both studies, the presence of extrahepatic disease, which was amenable to treatment, did not significantly impact on overall survival. Overall 5-year survival rates of 26 and 43 % were reported for liver resections undertaken for RCC [88, 89]. Favourable outcomes in the presence of widespread disease reflect the relatively indolent nature of RCC. Prognostic factors predicting long-term survival after liver resection for RCC include a disease-free interval of >24 months prior to liver resection and tumour-negative hepatic resection margins [90].

13.2.6 Intrahepatic Cholangiocarcinoma

There are minimal data, including only a small number of patients, on the role of non-curative resection of intrahepatic cholangiocarcinomas (ICC). Palliative resection of ICC has been associated with a survival benefit [91]; however, this is not a consistent finding throughout all studies [92]. When reported, the survival gain associated with palliative resection, compared to nonsurgical treatment, is in the region of a month (10 vs. 9 months) [91]. Given the survival benefit associated with a palliative resection is minimal and the overall prognosis is poor, palliative approaches other than surgery are appropriate for the vast majority of patients with ICC that is not amenable to curative resection.

13.2.7 Symptom Relief

A number of debilitating symptoms may arise from the presence of liver tumours, including intractable pain caused by stretching of the liver capsule, persistent pyrexias, malaise and nausea resulting from tumour infarction and necrosis and acute complications such as bleeding and infection. A palliative liver resection may be considered in these circumstances when all other conservative treatments have failed. The risks associated with a liver resection, in the very small minority of patients with advanced disease who fail to adequately respond to conservative treatments, are substantially higher than in those undergoing curative surgery. The associated risks and benefits therefore need to be carefully considered; however, in a highly select group of patients, a palliative liver resection can be a very effective way of relieving troublesome, refractory symptoms.

Evidence specifically relating to the symptomatic benefits associated with palliative liver resections is sparse. One study reports six patients who underwent palliative liver resections for debilitating symptoms, mostly uncontrollable pain. All experienced adequate palliation so that they were able to return to activities of daily living independently following recovery from surgery [93]. A small number of reports describe the beneficial effects of palliative liver resection in patients with bleeding arising from hepatocellular carcinomas, occurring either via spontaneous rupture or through invasion of the gastrointestinal tract [94].

Ablative techniques, including electrolysis, RFA, cryoablation and microwave ablation, are appealing alternatives to palliative liver resections undertaken for symptomatic relief. Although they can be undertaken surgically, percutaneous approaches under local anaesthetic are preferable in this situation to reduce the morbidity associated with the procedure. A recent study detailed the results of percutaneous RFA alone, alcohol ablation alone and combined ablation techniques included 20 patients with advanced malignant disease. Complete and partial relief of visceral pain was reported by 45 and 30 % of patients, respectively. The remainder reported no change in their pain. Pain relief, either complete or partial, was reported by all patients in the cohort who had liver tumours treated [95].

Conclusion

The symptoms arising from cholestasis associated with cholangiocarcinomas can be debilitating and significantly affect quality of life. In select cases where endoscopic drainage has failed or patients are found to have unresectable disease at exploratory laparotomy, a surgical bypass can provide excellent palliation of symptoms.

Neuroendocrine tumours are the main indication for undertaking a palliative liver resection. In this circumstance, cytoreductive surgery can be associated with both enhanced survival and symptom relief. There is limited evidence for undertaking cytoreductive hepatic resections in other malignancies. A small proportion of patients with epithelial ovarian cancer may benefit from cytoreductive liver surgery. Renal tumours are associated with a comparatively favourable prognosis, and the presence of extrahepatic disease, which is amenable to treatment, is not necessarily an absolute contraindication to liver resection.

Palliative liver resection may be indicated for symptom relief in a small number of patients in a wide range of tumours of different pathological types where all available conservative treatments have failed.

References

1. Pichlmayr R, Weimann A, Klempnauer J, Oldhafer KJ, Maschek H, Tusch G, et al. Surgical treatment in proximal bile duct cancer. A single-center experience. Ann Surg. 1996;224(5):628–38.
2. Li HM, Dou KF, Sun K, Gao ZQ, Li KZ, Fu YC. Palliative surgery for hilar cholangiocarcinoma. Hepatobiliary Pancreat Dis Int. 2003;2(1):110–3.
3. Witzigmann H, Lang H, Lauer H. Guidelines for palliative surgery of cholangiocarcinoma. HPB. 2008;10(3):154–60.
4. Singhal D, van Gulik TM, Gouma DJ. Palliative management of hilar cholangiocarcinoma. Surg Oncol. 2005;14(2):59–74.
5. Dennison AR, Maddern GJ. Operative solutions in hepatobiliary and pancreatic surgery. Oxford: Oxford University Press; 2010.
6. Jarnagin WR, Burke E, Powers C, Fong Y, Blumgart LH. Intrahepatic biliary enteric bypass

provides effective palliation in selected patients with malignant obstruction at the hepatic duct confluence. Am J Surg. 1998;175(6):453–60.
7. Traynor O, Castaing D, Bismuth H. Left intrahepatic cholangio-enteric anastomosis (round ligament approach): an effective palliative treatment for hilar cancers. Br J Surg. 1987;74(10):952–4.
8. Baer HU, Rhyner M, Stain SC, Glauser PW, Dennison AR, Maddern GJ, et al. The effect of communication between the right and left liver on the outcome of surgical drainage for jaundice due to malignant obstruction at the hilus of the liver. HPB Surg. 1994;8(1):27–31.
9. Guthrie CM, Banting SW, Garden OJ, Carter DC. Segment III cholangiojejunostomy for palliation of malignant hilar obstruction. Br J Surg. 1994;81(11):1639–41.
10. Launois B, Catheline JM, Maddern GJ. Intrahepatic anastomoses for malignant and benign biliary obstruction. Arch Surg. 1995;130(2):137–42.
11. Suzuki S, Kurachi K, Yokoi Y, Tsuchiya Y, Okamoto K, Okumura T, et al. Intrahepatic cholangiojejunostomy for unresectable malignant biliary tumors with obstructive jaundice. J Hepatobiliary Pancreat Surg. 2001;8(2):124–9.
12. Chaudhary A, Dhar P, Tomey S, Sachdev A, Agarwal A. Segment III cholangiojejunostomy for carcinoma of the gallbladder. World J Surg. 1997;21(8):866–70.
13. Kapoor VK, Pradeep R, Haribhakti SP, Singh V, Sikora SS, Saxena R, et al. Intrahepatic segment III cholangiojejunostomy in advanced carcinoma of the gallbladder. Br J Surg. 1996;83(12):1709–11.
14. Blumgart LH, Hadjis NS, Benjamin IS, Beazley R. Surgical approaches to cholangiocarcinoma at confluence of hepatic ducts. Lancet. 1984;1(8368):66–70.
15. Blumgart LH, Baer HU. Hilar and intrahepatic biliary-enteric anastomosis. In: Blumgart LH, editor. Surgery of the liver and biliary tract. 2nd ed. Edinburgh: Churchill Livingstone; 1994. p. 1051–67.
16. Becker CD, Glattli A, Maibach R, Baer HU. Percutaneous palliation of malignant obstructive jaundice with the Wallstent endoprosthesis: follow-up and reintervention in patients with hilar and non-hilar obstruction. J Vasc Interv Radiol. 1993;4(5):597–604.
17. Moss AC, Morris E, Leyden J, MacMathuna P. Malignant distal biliary obstruction: a systematic review and meta-analysis of endoscopic and surgical bypass results. Cancer Treat Rev. 2007;33(2):213–21.
18. Smith AC, Dowsett JF, Russell RC, Hatfield AR, Cotton PB. Randomised trial of endoscopic stenting versus surgical bypass in malignant low bileduct obstruction. Lancet. 1994;344(8938):1655–60.
19. Andersen JR, Sorensen SM, Kruse A, Rokkjaer M, Matzen P. Randomised trial of endoscopic endoprosthesis versus operative bypass in malignant obstructive jaundice. Gut. 1989;30(8):1132–5.
20. Shepherd HA, Royle G, Ross AP, Diba A, Arthur M, Colin-Jones D. Endoscopic biliary endoprosthesis in the palliation of malignant obstruction of the distal common bile duct: a randomized trial. Br J Surg. 1988;75(12):1166–8.
21. Kuhlmann KF, van Poll D, de Castro SM, van Heek NT, Busch OR, van Gulik TM, et al. Initial and long-term outcome after palliative surgical drainage of 269 patients with malignant biliary obstruction. Eur J Surg Oncol. 2007;33(6):757–62.
22. Nieveen van Dijkum EJ, Romijn MG, Terwee CB, de Wit LT, van der Meulen JH, Lameris HS, et al. Laparoscopic staging and subsequent palliation in patients with peripancreatic carcinoma. Ann Surg. 2003;237(1):66–73.
23. Muller MW, Friess H, Koninger J, Martin D, Wente MN, Hinz U, et al. Factors influencing survival after bypass procedures in patients with advanced pancreatic adenocarcinomas. Am J Surg. 2008;195(2):221–8.
24. Engelken FJ, Bettschart V, Rahman MQ, Parks RW, Garden OJ. Prognostic factors in the palliation of pancreatic cancer. Eur J Surg Oncol. 2003;29(4):368–73.
25. Gouma DJ, van Geenen R, van Gulik T, de Wit LT, Obertop H. Surgical palliative treatment in biliopancreatic malignancy. Ann Oncol. 1999;10 Suppl 4:269–72.
26. Mann CD, Thomasset SC, Johnson NA, Garcea G, Neal CP, Dennison AR, et al. Combined biliary and gastric bypass procedures as effective palliation for unresectable malignant disease. ANZ J Surg. 2009;79(6):471–5.
27. Lillemoe KD, Cameron JL, Hardacre JM, Sohn TA, Sauter PK, Coleman J, et al. Is prophylactic gastrojejunostomy indicated for unresectable periampullary cancer? A prospective randomized trial. Ann Surg. 1999;230(3):322–8; discussion 8–30.
28. Tarnasky PR, England RE, Lail LM, Pappas TN, Cotton PB. Cystic duct patency in malignant obstructive jaundice. An ERCP-based study relevant to the role of laparoscopic cholecystojejunostomy. Ann Surg. 1995;221(3):265–71.
29. Tischendorf JJ, Hecker H, Kruger M, Manns MP, Meier PN. Characterization, outcome, and prognosis in 273 patients with primary sclerosing cholangitis: A single center study. Am J Gastroenterol. 2007;102(1):107–14.
30. MacCarty RL, LaRusso NF, Wiesner RH, Ludwig J. Primary sclerosing cholangitis: findings on cholangiography and pancreatography. Radiology. 1983;149(1):39–44.
31. May GR, Bender CE, LaRusso NF, Wiesner RH. Nonoperative dilatation of dominant strictures in primary sclerosing cholangitis. AJR Am J Roentgenol. 1985;145(5):1061–4.
32. van Milligen de Wit AW, van Bracht J, Rauws EA, Jones EA, Tytgat GN, Huibregtse K. Endoscopic stent therapy for dominant extrahepatic bile duct strictures in primary sclerosing cholangitis. Gastrointest Endosc. 1996;44(3):293–9.
33. Olsson RG, Asztely MS. Prognostic value of cholangiography in primary sclerosing cholangitis. Eur J Gastroenterol Hepatol. 1995;7(3):251–4.
34. Ponsioen CY, Lam K, van Milligen de Wit AE, Huibregtse K, Tytgat GN. Four years experience with

short term stenting in primary sclerosing cholangitis. Am J Gastroenterol. 1999;94(9):2403–7.
35. Stiehl A, Rudolph G, Kloters-Plachky P, Sauer P, Walker S. Development of dominant bile duct stenoses in patients with primary sclerosing cholangitis treated with ursodeoxycholic acid: outcome after endoscopic treatment. J Hepatol. 2002;36(2):151–6.
36. Tischendorf JJ, Kruger M, Trautwein C, Duckstein N, Schneider A, Manns MP, et al. Cholangioscopic characterization of dominant bile duct stenoses in patients with primary sclerosing cholangitis. Endoscopy. 2006;38(7):665–9.
37. Glasbrenner B, Ardan M, Boeck W, Preclik G, Moller P, Adler G. Prospective evaluation of brush cytology of biliary strictures during endoscopic retrograde cholangiopancreatography. Endoscopy. 1999;31(9):712–7.
38. Prytz H, Keiding S, Bjornsson E, Broome U, Almer S, Castedal M, et al. Dynamic FDG-PET is useful for detection of cholangiocarcinoma in patients with PSC listed for liver transplantation. Hepatology. 2006;44(6):1572–80.
39. Pawlik TM, Olbrecht VA, Pitt HA, Gleisner AL, Choti MA, Schulick RD, et al. Primary sclerosing cholangitis: role of extrahepatic biliary resection. J Am Coll Surg. 2008;206(5):822–30.
40. Cameron JL, Pitt HA, Zinner MJ, Herlong HF, Kaufman SL, Boitnott JK, et al. Resection of hepatic duct bifurcation and transhepatic stenting for sclerosing cholangitis. Ann Surg. 1988;207(5):614–22.
41. Ahrendt SA, Pitt HA, Kalloo AN, Venbrux AC, Klein AS, Herlong HF, et al. Primary sclerosing cholangitis: resect, dilate, or transplant? Ann Surg. 1998;227(3):412–23.
42. Aljiffry M, Renfrew PD, Walsh MJ, Laryea M, Molinari M. Analytical review of diagnosis and treatment strategies for dominant bile duct strictures in patients with primary sclerosing cholangitis. HPB. 2011;13(2):79–90.
43. Cameron JL, Gayler BW, Sanfey H, Milligan F, Kaufman S, Maddrey WC, et al. Sclerosing cholangitis. Anatomical distribution of obstructive lesions. Ann Surg. 1984;200(1):54–60.
44. Martin FM, Rossi RL, Nugent FW, Scholz FJ, Jenkins RL, Lewis WD, et al. Surgical aspects of sclerosing cholangitis. Results in 178 patients. Ann Surg. 1990;212(4):551–6.
45. Ismail T, Angrisani L, Powell JE, Hubscher S, Buckels J, Neuberger J, et al. Primary sclerosing cholangitis: surgical options, prognostic variables and outcome. Br J Surg. 1991;78(5):564–7.
46. Farges O, Malassagne B, Sebagh M, Bismuth H. Primary sclerosing cholangitis: liver transplantation or biliary surgery. Surgery. 1995;117(2):146–55.
47. Yao JC, Hassan M, Phan A, Dagohoy C, Leary C, Mares JE, et al. One hundred years after "carcinoid": epidemiology of and prognostic factors for neuroendocrine tumors in 35,825 cases in the United States. J Clin Oncol. 2008;26(18):3063–72.
48. Lee SY, Cheow PC, Teo JY, Ooi LL. Surgical treatment of neuroendocrine liver metastases. Int J Hepatol. 2012;2012:146590.
49. Rorstad O. Prognostic indicators for carcinoid neuroendocrine tumors of the gastrointestinal tract. J Surg Oncol. 2005;89(3):151–60.
50. Ramage JK, Ahmed A, Ardill J, Bax N, Breen DJ, Caplin ME, et al. Guidelines for the management of gastroenteropancreatic neuroendocrine (including carcinoid) tumours (NETs). Gut. 2012;61(1):6–32.
51. Sarmiento JM, Que FG. Hepatic surgery for metastases from neuroendocrine tumors. Surg Oncol Clin N Am. 2003;12(1):231–42.
52. Steinmuller T, Kianmanesh R, Falconi M, Scarpa A, Taal B, Kwekkeboom DJ, et al. Consensus guidelines for the management of patients with liver metastases from digestive (neuro)endocrine tumors: foregut, midgut, hindgut, and unknown primary. Neuroendocrinology. 2008;87(1):47–62.
53. Que FG, Sarmiento JM, Nagorney DM. Hepatic surgery for metastatic gastrointestinal neuroendocrine tumors. Cancer Control. 2002;9(1):67–79.
54. Chung MH, Pisegna J, Spirt M, Giuliano AE, Ye W, Ramming KP, et al. Hepatic cytoreduction followed by a novel long-acting somatostatin analog: a paradigm for intractable neuroendocrine tumors metastatic to the liver. Surgery. 2001;130(6):954–62.
55. Osborne DA, Zervos EE, Strosberg J, Boe BA, Malafa M, Rosemurgy AS, et al. Improved outcome with cytoreduction versus embolization for symptomatic hepatic metastases of carcinoid and neuroendocrine tumors. Ann Surg Oncol. 2006;13(4):572–81.
56. Que FG, Nagorney DM, Batts KP, Linz LJ, Kvols LK. Hepatic resection for metastatic neuroendocrine carcinomas. Am J Surg. 1995;169(1):36–42.
57. Hodul P, Malafa M, Choi J, Kvols L. The role of cytoreductive hepatic surgery as an adjunct to the management of metastatic neuroendocrine carcinomas. Cancer Control. 2006;13(1):61–71.
58. McEntee GP, Nagorney DM, Kvols LK, Moertel CG, Grant CS. Cytoreductive hepatic surgery for neuroendocrine tumors. Surgery. 1990;108(6):1091–6.
59. Grama D, Eriksson B, Martensson H, Cedermark B, Ahren B, Kristoffersson A, et al. Clinical characteristics, treatment and survival in patients with pancreatic tumors causing hormonal syndromes. World J Surg. 1992;16(4):632–9.
60. Chamberlain RS, Canes D, Brown KT, Saltz L, Jarnagin W, Fong Y, et al. Hepatic neuroendocrine metastases: does intervention alter outcomes? J Am Coll Surg. 2000;190(4):432–45.
61. Nave H, Mossinger E, Feist H, Lang H, Raab H. Surgery as primary treatment in patients with liver metastases from carcinoid tumors: a retrospective, unicentric study over 13 years. Surgery. 2001;129(2):170–5.
62. Sarmiento JM, Heywood G, Rubin J, Ilstrup DM, Nagorney DM, Que FG. Surgical treatment of neuroendocrine metastases to the liver: a plea for resection to increase survival. J Am Coll Surg. 2003; 197(1):29–37.
63. Jensen EH, Kvols L, McLoughlin JM, Lewis JM, Alvarado MD, Yeatman T, et al. Biomarkers predict outcomes following cytoreductive surgery for hepatic

metastases from functional carcinoid tumors. Ann Surg Oncol. 2007;14(2):780–5.
64. Hibi T, Sano T, Sakamoto Y, Takahashi Y, Uemura N, Ojima H, et al. Surgery for hepatic neuroendocrine tumors: a single institutional experience in Japan. Jpn J Clin Oncol. 2007;37(2):102–7.
65. Mayo SC, de Jong MC, Pulitano C, Clary BM, Reddy SK, Gamblin TC, et al. Surgical management of hepatic neuroendocrine tumor metastasis: results from an international multi-institutional analysis. Ann Surg Oncol. 2010;17(12):3129–36.
66. Saxena A, Chua TC, Sarkar A, Chu F, Liauw W, Zhao J, et al. Progression and survival results after radical hepatic metastasectomy of indolent advanced neuroendocrine neoplasms (NENs) supports an aggressive surgical approach. Surgery. 2011;149(2):209–20.
67. Cusati D, Zhang L, Harmsen WS, Hu A, Farnell MB, Nagorney DM, et al. Metastatic nonfunctioning pancreatic neuroendocrine carcinoma to liver: surgical treatment and outcomes. J Am Coll Surg. 2012;215(1):117–24.
68. Modlin IM, Lewis JJ, Ahlman H, Bilchik AJ, Kumar RR. Management of unresectable malignant endocrine tumors of the pancreas. Surg Gynecol Obstet. 1993;176(5):507–18.
69. Moertel CG, Lefkopoulo M, Lipsitz S, Hahn RG, Klaassen D. Streptozocin-doxorubicin, streptozocin-fluorouracil or chlorozotocin in the treatment of advanced islet-cell carcinoma. N Engl J Med. 1992;326(8):519–23.
70. Knox CD, Feurer ID, Wise PE, Lamps LW, Kelly Wright J, Chari RS, et al. Survival and functional quality of life after resection for hepatic carcinoid metastasis. J Gastrointest Surg. 2004;8(6):653–9.
71. Griffiths CT. Surgical resection of tumor bulk in the primary treatment of ovarian carcinoma. Natl Cancer Inst Monogr. 1975;42:101–4.
72. Armstrong DK, Bundy B, Wenzel L, Huang HQ, Baergen R, Lele S, et al. Intraperitoneal cisplatin and paclitaxel in ovarian cancer. N Engl J Med. 2006;354(1):34–43.
73. Lim MC, Kang S, Lee KS, Han SS, Park SJ, Seo SS, et al. The clinical significance of hepatic parenchymal metastasis in patients with primary epithelial ovarian cancer. Gynecol Oncol. 2009;112(1):28–34.
74. Bristow RE, Montz FJ, Lagasse LD, Leuchter RS, Karlan BY. Survival impact of surgical cytoreduction in stage IV epithelial ovarian cancer. Gynecol Oncol. 1999;72(3):278–87.
75. Yoon SS, Jarnagin WR, Fong Y, DeMatteo RP, Barakat RR, Blumgart LH, et al. Resection of recurrent ovarian or fallopian tube carcinoma involving the liver. Gynecol Oncol. 2003;91(2):383–8.
76. Naik R, Nordin A, Cross PA, Hemming D, de Barros Lopes A, Monaghan JM. Optimal cytoreductive surgery is an independent prognostic indicator in stage IV epithelial ovarian cancer with hepatic metastases. Gynecol Oncol. 2000;78(2):171–5.
77. Albers P, Albrecht W, Algaba F, Bokemeyer C, Cohn-Cedermark G, Fizazi K, et al. EAU guidelines on testicular cancer: 2011 update. Eur Urol. 2011;60(2):304–19.
78. Hahn TL, Jacobson L, Einhorn LH, Foster R, Goulet Jr RJ. Hepatic resection of metastatic testicular carcinoma: a further update. Ann Surg Oncol. 1999;6(7):640–4.
79. Rivoire M, Elias D, De Cian F, Kaemmerlen P, Theodore C, Droz JP. Multimodality treatment of patients with liver metastases from germ cell tumors: the role of surgery. Cancer. 2001;92(3):578–87.
80. Ruiterkamp J, Ernst MF. The role of surgery in metastatic breast cancer. Eur J Cancer. 2011;47 Suppl 3:S6–22.
81. Howlader M, Heaton N, Rela M. Resection of liver metastases from breast cancer: towards a management guideline. Int J Surg. 2011;9(4):285–91.
82. Adam R, Aloia T, Krissat J, Bralet MP, Paule B, Giacchetti S, et al. Is liver resection justified for patients with hepatic metastases from breast cancer? Ann Surg. 2006;244(6):897–907.
83. Hoffmann K, Franz C, Hinz U, Schirmacher P, Herfarth C, Eichbaum M, et al. Liver resection for multimodal treatment of breast cancer metastases: identification of prognostic factors. Ann Surg Oncol. 2010;17(6):1546–54.
84. Thelen A, Benckert C, Jonas S, Lopez-Hanninen E, Sehouli J, Neumann U, et al. Liver resection for metastases from breast cancer. J Surg Oncol. 2008;97(1):25–9.
85. Elias D, Maisonnette F, Druet-Cabanac M, Ouellet JF, Guinebretiere JM, Spielmann M, et al. An attempt to clarify indications for hepatectomy for liver metastases from breast cancer. Am J Surg. 2003;185(2):158–64.
86. Chua TC, Saxena A, Liauw W, Chu F, Morris DL. Hepatic resection for metastatic breast cancer: a systematic review. Eur J Cancer. 2011;47(15):2282–90.
87. Sakamoto Y, Yamamoto J, Yoshimoto M, Kasumi F, Kosuge T, Kokudo N, et al. Hepatic resection for metastatic breast cancer: prognostic analysis of 34 patients. World J Surg. 2005;29(4):524–7.
88. Aloia TA, Adam R, Azoulay D, Bismuth H, Castaing D. Outcome following hepatic resection of metastatic renal tumors: the Paul Brousse Hospital experience. HPB. 2006;8(2):100–5.
89. Ruys AT, Tanis PJ, Iris ND, van Duijvendijk P, Verhoef C, Porte RJ, et al. Surgical treatment of renal cell cancer liver metastases: a population-based study. Ann Surg Oncol. 2011;18(7):1932–8.
90. Thelen A, Jonas S, Benckert C, Lopez-Hanninen E, Rudolph B, Neumann U, et al. Liver resection for metastases from renal cell carcinoma. World J Surg. 2007;31(4):802–7.
91. Li FH, Chen XQ, Luo HY, Li YH, Wang F, Qiu MZ, et al. Prognosis of 84 intrahepatic cholangiocarcinoma patients. Chin J Cancer. 2009;28(5):528–32.
92. Kawarada Y, Yamagiwa K, Das BC. Analysis of the relationships between clinicopathologic factors and survival time in intrahepatic cholangiocarcinoma. Am J Surg. 2002;183(6):679–85.

93. Teo MC, Tan YM, Chung AY, Chow PK, Cheow PC, Soo KC, et al. Metastectomy for non-colorectal, non-neuroendocrine liver secondaries. ANZ J Surg. 2006;76(7):575–8.
94. Lin TL, Yap AQ, Wang JH, Chen CL, Iyer SG, Low JK, et al. Long term survival in patients with hepatocellular carcinoma directly invading the gastrointestinal tract: case reports and literature review. Surg Oncol. 2011;20(4):e207–14.
95. Nair RT, van Sonnenberg E, Shankar S, Morrison PR, Gill RR, Tuncali K, et al. Visceral and soft-tissue tumors: radiofrequency and alcohol ablation for pain relief-initial experience. Radiology. 2008;248(3):1067–76.

Small Bowel

14

Matthias W. Wichmann

Contents

M.W. Wichmann, MD, FRACS
Department of General Surgery, Mount Gambier General Hospital, Flinders University—Rural Medical School, 276 Wehl Street North, Mount Gambier, SA 5290, Australia
e-mail: matthias.wichmann@health.sa.gov.au

Malignant small bowel obstruction is frequently seen in patients suffering from peritoneal carcinomatosis. Primary cancers of the small bowel are rare but due to late diagnosis also can present with obstruction. In the case of peritoneal carcinomatosis, the primary cancer usually is not localized within the small bowel. Primary lesions in these patients most commonly are in the large bowel, stomach, ovaries or pancreas. Surgery is the treatment of choice for the cure as well as palliation of small bowel cancers. In a palliative situation, treatment most of all must follow the principle to "first do no harm", and decisions must be based on the patient's wishes, fitness for surgery, oncologic treatment options and prognosis. If the patient is considered fit for surgery, only a short conservative treatment attempt should be made followed by surgery. If possible, enteroenteric bypass should be preferred over stoma formation. Peritoneal carcinomatosis should be assessed using the Peritoneal Cancer Index prior to treatment planning. In patients unfit for surgery, stent insertion (endoscopic or radiological), venting gastrostomy and feeding jejunostomy should be considered depending on symptoms. Medical treatment of nausea and vomiting as well as analgesia must be provided in close cooperation with the palliative care team.

M. Wichmann, G. Maddern (eds.), *Palliative Surgery*,
DOI 10.1007/978-3-642-53709-7_14,

14.1 Introduction

When treatment objectives change from cure to palliation, the maxim "primum non nocere" – most of all do no harm – must be at the centre of all surgical and medical decisions.

Involvement of the small bowel within peritoneal carcinomatosis is a common finding with various malignancies. Primary malignancies of the small bowel continue to be a rare diagnosis but appear to be on the rise.

14.2 Primary Small Bowel Malignancies

Less than 3 % of gastrointestinal malignancies arise from the small bowel [1]. The annual incidence has been reported to vary between 9.9 and 19.7 per million people [2, 3]. The SEER data review of malignant small bowel tumours by Chow et al. [2] indicates that the four most common histological types of cancer within the small bowel are:

- Malignant carcinoid tumours and neuroendocrine tumours (annual incidence 3.8/1,000,000) [4, 5]
- Adenocarcinomas (annual incidence 3.7/1,000,000) [5–9]
- Sarcomas (annual incidence 1.3/1,000,000) [10]
- Lymphomas (annual incidence 1.1/1,000,000) [5]

Other primary lesions of the small bowel are gastrointestinal stromal tumours (GIST) and small cell carcinoma [5, 11].

Most patients (90 %) are older than 40 years of age at the time of diagnosis. Due to unusual symptoms, the rarity of the disease as well as difficult imaging of the small bowel, the diagnosis is frequently made with a significant delay [1, 2].

Surgery is the treatment of choice for the cure as well as palliation of small bowel cancers.

14.3 Peritoneal Carcinosis/Carcinomatosis

The peritoneal cavity and the small intestine are frequently involved with advanced intra- as well as extra-abdominal malignancies. Usually, the primary cancer is not localized within the small bowel.

Malignancies frequently associated with peritoneal carcinomatosis are colorectal cancer (up to 30 % of all patients), gastric cancer (up to 50 % of all patients), ovarian cancer (up to 80 % of patients with first diagnosis) and pancreatic cancer (up to 10 % of all patients). In approximately 5 % of patients with CUP syndrome (carcinoma of unknown primary), peritoneal involvement can be observed [12, 13]. Other cancers known to involve the small bowel are malignant melanoma and lung cancer [14–18].

The extent of peritoneal involvement can be assessed with the Peritoneal Cancer Index (PCI), which was first described by Sugarbaker et al. [19]. This index evaluates 12 areas within the abdomen, and the tumour involvement is graded from 0 (not visible) to 3 (larger than 5 cm). The maximum PCI score is 39, and a score below 13 has been reported to be associated with better survival [20]. A PCI of less than 20 indicates a potential for multimodal treatment (cytoreductive surgery + intraoperative chemotherapy followed by systemic chemotherapy) with curative intent [1]. This option must always be considered when assessing a patient with peritoneal carcinosis.

14.4 Small Bowel Obstruction: To Operate or Not to Operate?

Decision making on whether or not to operate on a patient presenting with small bowel obstruction can be difficult. The decision depends on the patient's wishes, the disease prognosis as well as the patient's performance status.

A study by Zielinski et al. [21] revealed that free intraperitoneal fluid, mesenteric oedema, lack of faeces in the small bowel and vomiting are independent predictors favouring surgical exploration in patients with small bowel obstruction. Within the context of palliative surgery, however, patient performance status and disease prognosis are of special relevance for the decision-making process.

14.5 Preoperative Considerations

14.5.1 Fitness for Surgery

Fitness for surgery should be assessed by a team approach including the surgeon and the anaesthetist. It is best to discuss surgical goals and intraoperative risks with the patient and his or her family while both the surgeon and the anaesthetist are present. This approach avoids misunderstanding and poor information of the patient regarding the expected procedure and the potential benefits/risks of the intervention. Optimization of patient physiology – within the limits of bowel obstruction – should be attempted immediately before surgery.

14.5.2 Oncologic Treatment Options

Absence of or existing oncologic treatment options are of relevance for the treatment decision. Recent years have seen significant improvement of palliative chemotherapy as well as radiation treatment regimens (see Chaps. 23 and 24). This is of significance since surgical trauma and/or complications may delay the start of palliative chemotherapy/radiotherapy in some patients, while other patients may benefit from tumour debulking prior to the start of palliative chemotherapy and/or radiotherapy. Close cooperation between the surgeon, the medical oncologist and the radiation oncologist are of great importance to achieve best treatment results in this setting.

The decision for or against surgery should not only be based on the question whether or not this intervention is technically possible and will be survived by the patient. This necessitates close cooperation between different fields of medicine, and it can best be achieved within the setting of a multidisciplinary care team. This approach also allows for additional contributions from palliative care and dieticians. Careful documentation of the treatment recommendation is of great importance since a number of the decisions made within this setting cannot be based on reliable evidence and are usually tailored for the individual patient.

14.5.3 Prognosis

Malignant small bowel obstruction carries a poor prognosis and usually survival is not expected to exceed 1 year [12]. With regard to this, it is important to note that patients who already survived for a long period of time with inoperable cancer have a better prognosis than those who have only recently been diagnosed with the same disease (the so-called conditional survival) (see Chap. 23). Consideration of the underlying disease process and knowledge about "conditional survival" are important for the decision making within the setting of palliative surgery for malignant small bowel obstruction as well as other conditions.

14.6 Patient Fit for Surgery

Provided that clinical factors indicate that the patient will survive surgery, only a short trial of nasogastric decompression should be made [13].

Escalation of treatment in the setting of malignant bowel obstruction has been reported to improve survival but at the same time puts a significant financial burden on the system, and patients do suffer from significant morbidity and mortality [22]. Within the multitude of disease processes that can lead to malignant small bowel obstruction, patients with primary colorectal cancer appear to have better survival and palliation when treated with surgical intervention for malignant small bowel obstruction [23].

The choice of surgical approach (laparotomy vs laparoscopy) depends on the surgeon's experience and the available infrastructure. A low threshold for conversion to open surgery is mandatory since bowel laceration and enterotomies cause significant morbidity and delay patient recovery. Furthermore, sufficient tumour material has to be collected for histological evaluation, and the cause of obstruction must be clearly identified and treated (where possible) during this procedure. An additional factor to consider is the length of surgery, which usually is longer with extensive laparoscopic surgery when compared to the open approach: this additional stress directly impacts upon the patient's recovery. A potential benefit of laparoscopy, however, is the reduced risk of permanent leakage of malignant ascites from the trocar sites when compared to a laparotomy wound.

14.7 Surgical Technique

As stated previously, primary lesions of the small bowel causing malignant bowel obstruction are rare; therefore, only limited evidence exists regarding optimal surgical and oncologic treatment. Usually the same principles applied to large bowel malignancies are used for the treatment of these conditions. Resection of the primary lesion and clearance of metastatic lymph nodes and other metastatic lesions are the main parts of surgical therapy.

If radical surgery is possible – even in the setting of metastatic disease – this should be attempted to prevent local complications (obstruction, bleeding, pain), establish a clear diagnosis and achieve tumour debulking for better effects of (palliative) chemotherapy.

The author favours a side-to-side anastomosis (hand-sutured or stapled) following tumour resection. The use of a covering stoma should be avoided in view of the significant problems associated with high output stomas in the small bowel (electrolyte imbalance, dehydration, malnutrition, renal failure, maceration of the skin around the stoma, problems for patients/family to manage a high output stoma).

Frequently, radical resection for cure is impossible due to advanced and metastatic disease. In the palliative setting, intestinal bypass or stoma formation needs to be considered. For the aforementioned reasons, an intestinal bypass should always be preferred over a stoma for the treatment of a non-resectable malignant small bowel obstruction. Single or multiple side-to-side enteroenterostomies are the surgical method of choice.

Depending on the patient's overall condition and the (assumed) underlying primary disease, tumour debulking (cytoreduction) must be discussed within a multidisciplinary approach. A diagnostic laparotomy/laparoscopy with collection of sufficient tumour material for histological evaluation without resection should therefore not be considered a failure, but part of a multimodal treatment approach.

Interventional treatment options in the palliative situation involve the endoscopic placement of stents. These devices can be used as an alternative to bypass surgery provided a minimal lumen is still available for placement of a guidewire through the tumour stenosis. Here it may be necessary to sometimes think "out of the box": a colonoscope can reach deeper into the small bowel than a gastroscope [24–27]. Evidence supports the use of gastrointestinal stents to re-establish gastrointestinal patency – this endoscopic intervention has been shown to be of benefit even for patients treated in non-metropolitan hospitals [28]. Improved nutrition and overall well-being may also allow for additional oncologic treatment with dual interventional therapy (stent + chemoperfusion) [29].

Another palliative treatment option that is of relevance for patient comfort is the endoscopic or radiological placement of a venting gastrostomy [30] (see Chap. 25). Sometimes a combination of endoscopy and radiology may be necessary to avoid bowel laceration during this intervention. The venting gastrostomy significantly improves nausea and vomiting and can allow for oral fluid intake for patient comfort despite inoperable bowel obstruction.

The potential need for a feeding jejunostomy should be considered early, and this feeding device can then be inserted during the initial surgery [31]. Specifically designed feeding tubes can be implanted, but a urinary catheter (with minimal inflation of the balloon to avoid bowel obstruction) can also be used. The feeding jejunostomy is attached to the abdominal wall with dissolvable stitches and can be tunnelled. The catheter may be removed after 6 weeks – if not replaced by a new catheter, the small stoma site closes without permanent fistula formation. Interventional radiology also offers the option of direct percutaneous jejunostomy (see Chap. 25).

14.8 Emergencies

Progression of malignant disease or complications of medical treatment may result in an emergency situation where decision making needs to be fast. These situations include faeculent vomit (Miserere), symptomatic blood loss and bowel perforation (due to extensive dilatation or as a result of chemotherapy) [14].

Anticipation of these complications, discussion of treatment options if these problems should occur with the patient/family and exact documentation of the decisions made with regard to the treatment goals are very important parts of palliative (surgical) care. When no treatment directive exists for the emergency situation, the assessment steps and considerations outlined for "elective palliative surgery" should be adhered to whenever possible.

14.9 Patient Not Fit for Surgery

If the patient is considered unfit for surgery and would not survive surgery independent of where it is being performed, palliative nonsurgical treatment measures have to be initiated. Some of the described endoscopic and radiological palliative treatment options (feeding jejunostomy, venting gastrostomy) can still be discussed for patients who are considered unfit for surgery. In addition to these measures, a low residue diet and medical interventions to treat nausea, vomiting and adequate pain control must be provided (see Chaps. 3, 7, 16, 23, and 24).

14.10 Conclusion/Summary

Treatment decisions in palliative situations are challenging. Decisions have to be made within a short period of time, and the treatment expectation of the surgeon on one side and the patient/family on the other side may vary more than in the usual general surgical population. A clear definition of treatment goals and the possible outcome need to be agreed upon early during the patient's admission for malignant small bowel obstruction and/or peritoneal carcinomatosis. Early assessment of the patient's fitness for surgery is important to help identify treatment options. Other factors influencing the decision for or against surgery are oncologic treatment options and prognosis. A patient fit for surgery should only have a short trial of conservative management followed by surgery. Surgery should result in a definitive diagnosis, radical resection of the obstructing lesion or bypass formation. If possible, a stoma should be avoided. Stent placement, venting gastrostomy and feeding jejunostomy are additional endoscopic/radiological interventions that help to improve quality of life in patients suffering from malignant small bowel obstruction. Patients not fit for surgery may still be fit for endoscopic intervention – in addition they will require medical management of nausea, vomiting and pain.

References

1. Boursi B, Arber N. Small bowel malignancies: why are they so rare? Harefuah. 2004;143(10):727–32.
2. Chow JS, Chen CC, Ahsan H, Neugut AI. A population-based study of the incidence of malignant small bowel tumours: SEER, 1973-1990. Int J Epidemiol. 1996;25(4):722–8.
3. Lu Y, Fröbom R, Lagergren J. Incidence patters of small bowel cancer in a population-based study in Sweden: increase in duodenal adenocarcinoma. Cancer Epidemiol. 2012;36(3):e158–63.
4. Gulec SA, Mountcastle TS, Frey D, Cundiff JD. Cytoreductive surgery in patients with advanced-stage carcinoid tumors. Am Surg. 2002;68(8): 667–71.
5. Brücher BLDM, Roder JD, Fink U, Stein HJ, Busch R, Siewert JR. Prognostic factors in resected primary small bowel tumors. Dig Surg. 1998;15(1):42–51.
6. Nicholl MB, Ahuja V, Conway WC, Vu VD, Sim MS, Singh G. Small bowel adenocarcinoma: understaged and undertreated? Ann Surg Oncol. 2010;17(10): 2728–32.
7. Ting-Jung W, Yeh CN, Chao TC, Yi-Yin J, Chen MF. Prognostic factors of primary small bowel adenocarcinoma: univariate and multivariate analysis. World J Surg. 2006;30(3):391–8.
8. Agrawal S, McCarron EC, Gibbs JF, Nava HR, Wilding GE, Raipur A. Surgical management and outcome in primary adenocarcinoma of the small bowel. Ann Surg Oncol. 2007;14(8):2263–9.
9. Moon YW, Rha SY, Shin SJ, Chang H, Shim HS, Roh JK. Adenocarcinoma of the small bowel at a single

Korean institute: management and prognosticators. J Cancer Res Clin Oncol. 2010;136(3):387–94.
10. Howe JR, Karnell LH, Scott-conner C. Small bowel sarcoma: analysis of survival from the National Cancer Data Base. Ann Surg Oncol. 2001;8(6): 496–508.
11. Brümming P, Andersson J, Meis-Kindblom JM, Klingenstierna H, Engström K, Stierner U, et al. Neoadjuvant, adjuvant and palliative treatment of gastrointestinal stromal tumours (GIST) with imatinib: a centre-based study of 17 patients. Br J Cancer. 2003; 89(3):460–4.
12. Piso P, Arnold D. Multimodal treatment approaches for peritoneal carcinosis in colorectal cancer. Dt Ärztebl International. 2011;108(47):802–8.
13. Miller G, Boman J, Shrier I, Gordon PH. Small-bowel obstruction secondary to malignant disease: an 11-year audit. Can J Surg. 2001;43(5):353–8.
14. Schellhaas E, Loddenkemper C, Schmittel A, Buhr HJ, Pohlen U. Bowel perforation in non-small cell lung cancer after bevacizumab therapy. Invest New Drugs. 2009;27(2):184–7.
15. Murphy EM, Sexton R, Moran BJ. Early results of surgery in 123 patients with pseudomyxoma peritonei from a perforated appendiceal neoplasm. Dis Colon Rectum. 2007;50(1):37–42.
16. Garofalo A, Valle M. Laparoscopy in the management of peritoneal carcinomatosis. Cancer J. 2009;15(3):190–5.
17. Roviello F, Caruso S, Marrelli D, Pedrazzani C, Neri A, De Stefano A, et al. Treatment of peritoneal carcinomatosis with cytoreductive surgery and hyperthermic intraperitoneal chemotherapy: state of the art and future developments. Surg Oncol. 2011;20(1):e38–54.
18. Benizri EI, Bernard JL, Rahili A, Benchimol D, Bereder JM. Small bowel involvement is a prognostic factor in colorectal carcinomatosis treated with complete cytoreductive surgery plus hyperthermic intraperitoneal chemotherapy. World J Surg Oncol. 2012; 10(1):56.
19. Sugarbaker PH, Jablonski KA. Prognostic features of 51 colorectal and 130 appendiceal cancer patients with peritoneal carcinomatosis treated by cytoreductive surgery and intraperitoneal chemotherapy. Ann Surg. 1995;221:124–32.
20. Shehata M, Chu F, Saunders V, Kam PC, Links M, Morris DL. Peritoneal carcinomatosis from colorectal cancer and small bowel cancer treated with peritonectomy. ANZ J Surg. 2006;76(6):467–71.
21. Zielinski MD, Eiken PW, Bannon MP, Heller SF, Lohse CM, Huebner M, et al. Small bowel obstruction – who needs an operation? A multivariate prediction model. World J Surg. 2010;34(5):910–9.
22. Englert ZP, White M, Fitzgerald TL, Vadlamudi A, Zervoudakis G, Zervos E. Surgical Management of malignant bowel obstruction: at what price palliation. Am Surg. 2012;78(6):647–52.
23. Blair SL, Chu DZJ, Schwarz RE. Outcome of palliative operations for malignant bowel obstruction in patients with peritoneal carcinomatosis from nongynecological cancer. Ann Surg Oncol. 2001;8(8): 632–7.
24. Jeurnink SM, Repici A, Luigiano C, Pagano N, Kuipers EJ, Siersema PD. Use of a colonoscope for distal duodenal stent placement in patients with malignant obstruction. Surg Endosc. 2009;23(3): 562–7.
25. Gutzeit A, Binkert CA, Schoch E, Sautter T, Jost R, Zollikofer CL. Malignant gastroduodenal obstruction: treatment with self-expanding uncovered wallstent. Cardiovasc Interven Radiol. 2009;32(1):97–105.
26. Larssen L, Medhus AW, Hjermstad MJ, Körner H, Glomsaker T, Søberg T, et al. Patient-reported outcomes in palliative gastrointestinal stenting: a Norwegian multicenter study. Surg Endosc. 2011; 25(10):3162–9.
27. Johnsson E, Thune A, Liedman B. Palliation of malignant gastroduodenal obstruction with open surgical bypass or endoscopic stenting: clinical outcome and health economic evaluation. World J Surg. 2004; 28(8):812–7.
28. Baerlocher MO, Asch MR, Vellahottam A, Puri G, Andrews K, Myers A. Safety and efficacy of gastrointestinal stents in cancer patients at a community hospital. Can J Surg. 2008;51(2):130–4.
29. Wang Z, Chen K, Gong J, Zheng Y, Wang T. Combined arterial infusion and stent implantation compared with metal stent alone in treatment of malignant gastroduodenal obstruction. Cardiovasc Interven Radiol. 2009;32(5):1011–8.
30. Brooksbank MA, Game PA, Ashby MA. Palliative venting gastrostomy in malignant intestinal obstruction. Palliat Med. 2002;16(6):520–6.
31. Sparrow P, David E, Pugash R. Direct percutaneous jejunostomy – an underutilized interventional technique? Cardiovasc Intervent Radiol. 2008;31(2): 336–41.

Large Bowel and Rectum

15

Albert Tuca

Contents

A. Tuca, MD, PhD
Support and Palliative Care Unit,
Medical Oncology, Hospital Clinic Barcelona,
Villarroel 170, Barcelona 08036, Spain
e-mail: atuca@clinic.ub.es

At diagnosis, between 20 and 30 % of patients with colorectal cancer (CRC) present with metastatic spread. The main complications of advanced CRC, potentially suitable for palliative surgery, are bleeding and/or obstruction of the digestive tract. Surgery can re-establish digestive transit of malignant bowel obstruction (MBO) in some cases. However, its indication should be assessed carefully on an individual basis, especially in patients with advanced cancer due to the high rate of surgical mortality and morbidity. Factors limiting surgical success in MBO are advanced age, malnutrition, the presence of multiple occlusive levels, extra-abdominal metastatic disease, refractory ascites, poor performance status, previous abdominal radiotherapy, and the lack of specific treatment options for advanced cancer (chemotherapy). Self-expanding colonic stents are effective and safe alternatives in patients with a single level of occlusion, who are considered unfit for surgery or require a "bridge to surgery". Palliative medical treatment of inoperable MBO is multimodal and based on the combined use of glucocorticoids, antiemetics, antisecretors, and potent analgesic opioids. Palliative surgery, laser ablation, and radiotherapy are effective palliative treatments for colorectal bleeding. This chapter reviews and summarizes epidemiology, diagnosis, and therapeutic alternatives in these complications in advanced cancer patients.

M. Wichmann, G. Maddern (eds.), *Palliative Surgery*,
DOI 10.1007/978-3-642-53709-7_15, © Springer-Verlag Berlin Heidelberg 2014

15.1 Introduction

Colorectal cancer (CRC) is one of the most common malignancies in developed countries. At diagnosis, between 20 and 30 % of patients with CRC have synchronous distant metastases. Radical surgery is suitable for localized tumours or a small group of patients with hepatic metastases who are suitable for resection of the primary and metastatic lesions.

In advanced disease, the aim of palliative treatment may be improvement of survival, but most important is symptom control. The most frequent symptoms in CRC are bleeding and bowel obstruction. Palliative surgery plays an important role for control of these symptoms. Indications must be assessed carefully, due to the high rates of surgical mortality and morbidity. Primary objectives of surgery must be improved quality of life and consideration of the individual patient's treatment choices.

15.2 Basic Epidemiology of Colorectal Cancer and Complications of Advanced Disease

Considering both sexes, the overall incidence of CRC in developed countries is 28 cases per 100,000 habitants, and the 5-year survival ranges between 74 and 6 % depending on the stage of disease (stages I and IV, respectively). In Europe more than 450,000 patients are diagnosed with colorectal cancer each year. It is the fourth most frequent cancer, after lung, breast, and prostate tumours, and represents the second leading cause of cancer death, after lung tumours. Taking patient gender into account, CRC is the second most frequent cancer after breast tumours in women, and the third most frequent after lung and prostate tumours in men [1].

At diagnosis, between 20 and 30 % of patients with CRC present with metastatic disease. The main complications at diagnosis or during evolution of CRC are bleeding and/or obstruction of the digestive tract. Chronic anaemia secondary to occult blood loss is one of the most common symptoms in CRC (80–90 %), while severe bleeding occurs in less than one fifth of the patients.

About 65 % of patients with stage IV CRC present with severe local symptoms requiring invasive treatment. Surgical resection of tumour may be suitable for 30 % of patients. Surgical or endoscopic interventions, without primary tumour resection (stent, stoma, or bypass), may be indicated in 35 % of patients. About 35 % of patients only receive best supportive care, with non-invasive measures, because they do not present with severe local symptoms or they present in extremis. Considering overall data of invasive measures in metastatic CRC, there are no statistically significant differences between median survival of patients treated with resection surgery (11–22 months) and of patients treated with intervention without tumour resection (7–22 months). The median survival of patients receiving best supportive care only does not exceed 2–3 months [2].

Malignant bowel obstruction (MBO) is a frequent complication in patients with advanced cancer, especially of digestive or gynaecological origin. The incidence of MBO is estimated to range between 3 and 15 % of all cancer patients and reaches 20–50 % in ovarian cancer patients and 10–29 % in patients with colon cancer.

Primary cancers of abdominal origin that most frequently produce MBO are malignancies of colon (25–40 %), ovary (16–29 %), stomach (6–19 %), pancreas (6–13 %), bladder (3–10 %), and endometrium (3–11 %). Primary cancers of extra-abdominal origin most frequently leading to MBO due to peritoneal infiltration are breast (2–3 %) and malignant melanoma (3 %). Mean age of patients presenting with MBO is 61 years (58–65 years) and 64 % (59–69 %) are women. MBO is the initial presentation of malignant disease in 22 % (13–32 %) of patients in surgical series. One quarter of advanced and terminal cancer patients with this complication had previous episodes of intestinal obstruction (mean 1.37 sub-occlusive episodes per patient, SD ± 0.7).

Spontaneous resolution of the occlusive picture, with conservative management only, occurs in about 36 % (31–42 %) of patients with MBO. In these cases, the recurrence rate of obstruction is greater than 60 % [3–10].

15.3 Malignant Bowel Obstruction: Definition and General Considerations

Bowel obstruction is any mechanical or functional obstruction of the intestine that prevents physiological transit and digestion. This is a generic definition and includes very different benign or malignant clinical situations. An international consensus group recently proposed an operative, specific definition of MBO with the aim of unifying the diagnostic criteria of this complication. According to this definition, the diagnostic criteria of MBO are (a) clinical evidence of bowel obstruction, (b) obstruction distal to the Treitz ligament, (c) the presence of a primary intra-abdominal or extra-abdominal cancer with peritoneal involvement, and (d) the absence of reasonable possibilities for a cure [11].

The clinical management of MBO requires a specific and individualized approach based on disease prognosis and the objectives of care. Palliative surgery, as the only treatment option available which restores digestive transit in a consolidated MBO, must always be considered, but it should not be routinely performed. The decision-making process is difficult, especially in advanced phases of cancer, and depends on the level of obstruction, the presence of single or multiple occlusive levels, the extent of the cancer, the associated comorbidities, and the performance status of the patient. When surgical or endoscopic treatment is not possible, a devastating clinical picture develops, which leads to intense symptoms, rapid deterioration of the patient's general status, and a short life expectancy. At this time, palliative medical treatment aimed at reducing symptoms and providing the highest level of comfort possible becomes the priority of care.

15.4 Physiopathology of MBO

MBO may appear at any time during the evolution of the disease, but is more frequent in cases of advanced cancer. Obstruction may originate in the small (61 %) or large bowel (33 %) or in both simultaneously (20 %) [6, 12]. Obstruction may be complete or partial and may appear as a sub-occlusive crisis or may involve one or multiple intestinal levels. In advanced and inoperable patients, multiple occlusive levels are present in 80 % of cases, and peritoneal carcinomatosis has been previously diagnosed in more than 65 % of these patients [6]. Abdominal tumour growth may lead to MBO by extrinsic intestinal compression, endoluminal obstruction, intramural infiltration, or extensive mesenteric infiltration. Intraluminal tumours may occlude the bowel lumen or provoke intussusception. Intramural infiltration through the mucosa may obstruct the lumen or impair peristaltic movements. Mesenteric and omental tumour involvement may angulate the bowel and provoke extramural bowel occlusion. Infiltration of the enteric or celiac plexus can cause severe impairment in peristalsis and subsequent obstruction due to dysmotiliy. Factors that can contribute to the development of MBO but are not directly dependent on abdominal tumour growth include paraneoplastic neuropathies, chronic constipation, intestinal dysfunction induced by opioids, inflammatory bowel disease, renal insufficiency, dehydration, mesenteric thrombosis, surgical adhesions, and radiogenic fibrosis.

Fluid retention and intestinal gases proximal to the occlusive level produce a marked increase in endoluminal intestinal pressure. This abdominal distension favours the release of 5-HT3 by the intestinal enterochromaffin cells which, in turn, activates the enteric interneuronal system through its different mediators (P substance, nitric oxide, acetylcholine, somatostatin, and vasoactive intestinal peptide). This stimulates the secretomotor neurons that are especially mediated by the vasoactive intestinal peptide, which leads to splanchnic vasodilatation and hypersecretion of the cells of the intestinal crypts. As results of these pathophysiological changes, intense intestinal oedema develops, digestive fluids are being retained, and endoluminal pressures increase. All of these are mechanisms that perpetuate the pathophysiological process of MBO (Fig. 15.1) [6, 13–15].

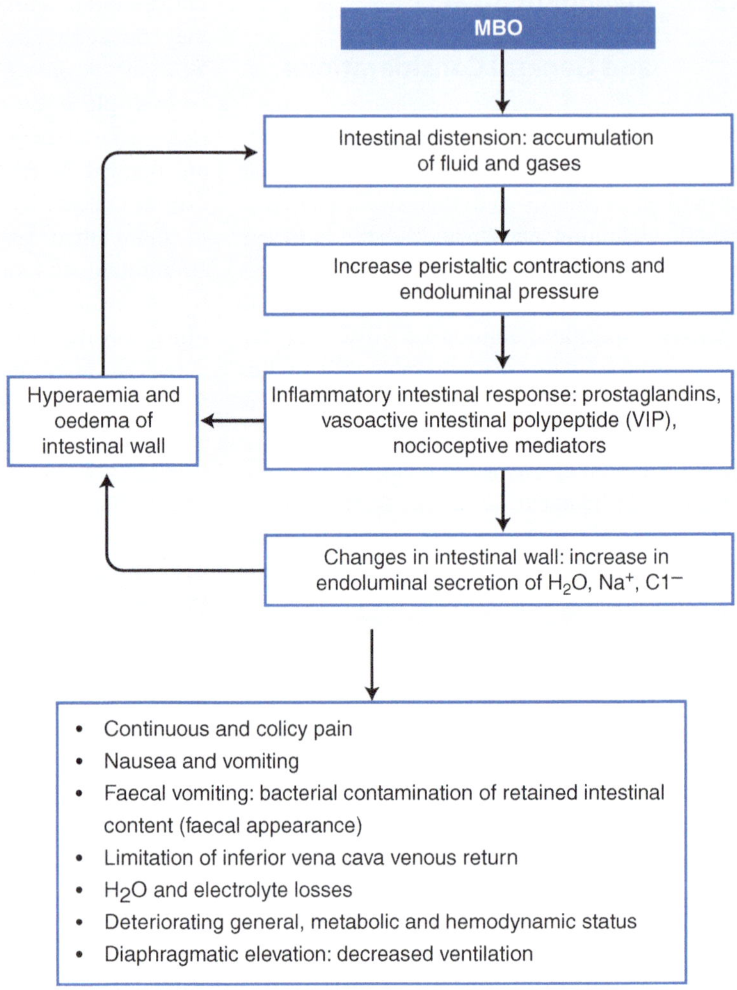

Fig. 15.1 Pathophysiology of MBO

15.5 Clinical Manifestations of MBO

The onset of MBO may be subacute with the presence of colic pain, abdominal distension, nausea, and vomiting, which spontaneously cease (subocclusive crisis). The symptoms observed in consolidated MBO are nausea 100 %, vomiting 87–100 %, colic pain 72–80 %, pain due to distension 56–90 %, and absence of bowel motions or passing of gases during the previous 72 h in 85–93 % [3, 6, 8, 9]. In upper gastrointestinal MBO, nausea is intense and presents early, vomiting occurs frequently with an aqueous, mucous or biliary appearance and has little odour. Vomiting in lower obstruction usually occurs later, is dark, and has a strong odour. Bacterial liquefaction of the retained intestinal content in the zone proximal to the obstruction confers the characteristic appearance and smell of fecaloid vomit. Cases with partial obstruction may present liquid stools due to bacterial liquefaction of the digestive content and intestinal hypersecretion. The colic pain is due to giant peristaltic waves and spasms in the bowel with increased endoluminal pressure and no possibility of effective transit. Intestinal distension and tumour infiltration of the abdominal structures are responsible for the continuous pain [2, 6, 16]. During physical examination, abdominal distension is noted and is more marked in lower obstructions.

At the onset, borborygmus, fighting peristalsis, may be heard on auscultation. On consolidation of MBO, the peristalsis may decrease or even cease to present isolated metallic sounds thereafter due to hydroaerial tension on auscultation. In patients with advanced cancer, MBO is also associated with anaemia (70 %), hypoalbuminaemia (68 %), alterations in hepatic enzymes (62 %), dehydration and prerenal renal dysfunction (44 %), cachexia (22 %), ascites (41 %), palpable abdominal tumour masses (21 %), and marked cognitive deterioration (23 %) [6].

15.6 Radiological Diagnosis of MBO

Plain radiography of the abdomen in the erect position is the imaging method of choice for the detection of suspected MBO and is also used to assess the patient's evolution after treatment. The radiological signs of MBO are distension of the intestinal loops, fluid retention, and gases with the presence of air-fluid levels in the zone proximal to the occlusion as well as a reduction in gas and stools in the segments distal to the obstruction. In upper gastrointestinal occlusions, distension of the loops and air-fluid levels may be absent.

Radiological techniques using contrast may be necessary to evaluate the surgical approach. Barium contrast provides excellent radiological definition, but is not absorbed and may become impacted, thereby compromising other tests or endoscopic manoeuvres. In many cases, these imaging tests are limited by the presence of nausea and vomiting, which may prevent the ingestion of radiographic contrast or increase the risk of aspiration pneumonia. Gastrografin provides similar radiologic definition, and its hyperosmotic character may, in some cases, contribute to the resolution of obstructions in the small bowel. In fact, a recent meta-analysis confirms a reduction in the need for surgical intervention and hospital stay in patients with occlusion after the administration of Gastrografin in small bowel obstruction [17]. Computerized tomography (CT) can be helpful with identification of the extent of neoplastic disease and usually helps to find the level of obstruction. The diagnostic sensitivity of CT in determining the obstruction level is 93 %, with a specificity of 100 % and a predictive value of 83–94 %, which is significantly higher than that provided by abdominal ultrasound or plain X-rays [18, 19]. The precision for correct diagnosis of peritoneal carcinomatosis via CT is poor, with a predictive value of less than 20 % if the peritoneal lesions are less than 0.5 cm in size or if they are located in the pelvis, mesenterium, or small bowel [20, 21]. The sensitivity of magnetic resonance imaging (MRI) in diagnosing of the extension of the neoplasm and the level of the obstruction is 93–95 %, with a specificity of 63–100 % and a predictive value of 81–96 %. One study on the diagnostic possibilities of MRI compared with CT in MBO showed the significant superiority of MRI in terms of sensitivity, specificity, and predictive value [22, 23].

In summary:

- Plain abdominal radiography is sufficient in most cases to confirm the diagnosis of MBO.
- One should consider the use of contrast radiography, CT, or MRI, when the patient's performance status was good prior to the onset of MBO, the extent of malignant disease is unknown, a single level of occlusion is suspected, and the cancer is potentially resectable.
- Contrast radiography determines, with a reasonable degree of accuracy, the site or sites of obstruction and the degree of obstruction. It may be helpful to rule out a bowel occlusion due to motility disorder (opioid-induced intestinal dysfunction, pseudo-obstruction).
- CT or MRI should be reserved for cases where precise radiological information is needed to facilitate adequate decision-making regarding surgery (i.e. tumour characteristics at the site of obstruction, lymph node status, intra- and extra-abdominal metastatic spread).

15.7 Treatment of MBO

15.7.1 General Considerations

The decision-making process in advanced oncologic patients requires an individualized evaluation based on the extension of the neoplasm, the overall prognosis, the availability of specific cancer treatment options, the associated comorbidities, the performance status, and the specific treatment options available to the duly informed patient. Treatment options include surgery, endoscopic palliation (stent), digestive aspiration, and symptomatic palliative pharmacologic therapy.

15.7.2 Palliative Surgery in MBO

The aim of surgery is to re-establish digestive function and should always be considered in patients in the initial stages of the disease, with a good performance status and a single level of occlusion. The surgical treatment of MBO comprises tumour resection, intestinal bypass, and stoma formation proximal to the level of stenosis. Studies involving a series of surgical cases of MBO have shown a 30-day mortality of 25 % (9–40 %), postsurgical morbidity of 50 % (9–90 %), a rate of re-obstruction of 48 % (39–57 %), and a median survival of seven months (2–12 months) [6, 7, 10, 12, 24–29]. Age, advanced disease, malnutrition, and poor performance status are considered factors for poor prognosis even in cases where surgery may technically be possible [6, 12, 16]. A study on patients with colon cancer undergoing surgery for MBO reported an increase in surgical mortality associated with age, with an OR of 1.85 for each 10-year interval of age above 65 years. Using the American Society of Anaesthesia (ASA) scale to measure deterioration of general status, surgical mortality increased in patients with a score ≥2, compared to those with a score <2 (odds ratio 3.3) [30]. Furthermore, surgical mortality is threefold greater in patients with poor nutritional status and hypoalbuminaemia. In ovarian cancer, the presence of ascites greater than 3,000 mL and palpable tumour masses are significant contributors to a poor surgical outcome [6, 10, 31]. Pelvic and abdominal radiotherapy prior to MBO is associated with a high rate of surgical complications and an increase in operative mortality in patients with gynaecological cancer, a fact that has not been fully confirmed in cancer of other etiologies [10, 32]. These findings on ascites and previous pelvic radiotherapy may be of relevance for other primary cancer sites although there is a lack of published evidence in this field.

Medical treatment prior to surgery for MBO is based on no oral intake, parenteral hydration, nasogastric aspiration, and antiemetic and analgesic drugs. The aims of these measures are to control the symptoms, re-establish the physiological balance of electrolytes, favour spontaneous resolution, and gain the time necessary to establish a diagnostic process to facilitate individualized surgical decisions. With these measures, adequate control of the symptoms can be achieved in 80 % of cases if low-residue diet and nasogastric aspiration are maintained. It is reasonable to assume that nasogastric aspiration at the onset of the obstruction may favour spontaneous resolution since it drastically reduces endoluminal pressure. However, long-term nasogastric aspiration is uncomfortable for the patient and has significant side effects (esophagitis, gastroesophageal reflux, nasal erosions, and bronchoaspiration). In a series of surgical cases, spontaneous resolution has been reported in 30 % of patients within a mean time of less than 8 days after diagnosis. For this reason, and considering the hypothesis that nasogastric aspiration may improve the rate of spontaneous resolution, there is no reason to maintain nasogastric aspiration for longer than 8 days, especially when adequate symptom control can be achieved with intensified palliative care treatment.

In summary, the following factors do limit the indication of surgery in MBO: advanced age, current or previous malnutrition or cachexia, peritoneal carcinomatosis, multiple levels of obstruction, palpable abdominal masses, refractory ascites, symptomatic extra-abdominal metastatic disease, poor performance status, renal or hepatic insufficiency, previous abdominal or pelvic radiotherapy, and lack of specific oncologic treatment options [3, 6, 12].

15.7.3 Stents in MBO

The use of stents has increased during recent years for the treatment of proximal small bowel as well as large bowel obstructions. The stent is formed by a network of metal filaments braided and assembled in a tube-like structure, which is capable of a radial self-expansion after placement in the area of an obstruction. The pressure exerted by the stent itself once deployed allows anchoring to the intestinal wall and prevents migration.

In the large bowel, their role is particularly useful in obstruction distal to the splenic flexure. Stent placement should be performed endoscopically or guided by fluoroscopy in interventional radiology. The full expansion of the stent may require several days after placement.

Successful insertion of a stent in colon cancer ranges from 80 to 100 % of the cases and improves symptoms in more than 75 % of the patients. The mean duration of colonic stent patency is 106 days (66–88 days). The most common complications of this technique are immediate or delayed perforation (4.5 %), migration (11 %), and obstruction (12 %) [33, 34]. Some studies show that the wall-covered stent provides a better long-term palliation because its cover prevents tumour growth into the lumen of the stent; the migration risk, however, appears to be greater. Recurrence of obstruction due to tumour growth through the mesh or endoluminal at the ends of the stent may require the placement of a second stent after reopening the lumen mechanically, with a laser (Nd:YAG laser) or with photodynamic therapy.

In summary, self-expanding metal stents can be considered a good option in patients with a single point of obstruction in whom palliative surgery has been ruled out or in those who do not want to undergo surgery. Endoscopic stents can also be used as a "bridge to surgery" where patients are being considered for cancer resection but require urgent resolution of bowel obstruction prior to definite or palliative surgery.

15.7.4 Percutaneous Endoscopic Gastrostomy for Aspiration in MBO

As mentioned previously, long-term aspiration using a nasogastric tube is uncomfortable and may produce severe secondary effects. The insertion of a percutaneous endoscopic gastrostomy (Venting-PEG) may be a highly effective and safe alternative for patients in whom surgery is ruled out and who require long-term nasogastric tube insertion. In MBO secondary to advanced ovarian cancer, the success of percutaneous endoscopic PEG placement is 94 % (94–98 %), which achieves adequate symptom control in 84 % of the patients for a mean duration of 70 days, even in patients presenting with peritoneal carcinomatosis, ascites, or gastric infiltration [35, 36]. These data on ovarian cancer can be applied to MBO due to peritoneal carcinomatosis of other primary origins.

15.7.5 Palliative Medical Management in Inoperable MBO

In 1985, Baines et al demonstrated that pharmacologic treatment, specifically palliative treatment for inoperable MBO, may provide adequate symptomatic control with measures aimed at maintaining the maximum comfort possible [5]. Palliative treatment for MBO has the following objectives: control of nausea, vomiting, and pain, allowing minimum food intake, avoiding or withdrawing permanent nasogastric tubes, and favouring outpatient treatment. This treatment is based on the use of antiemetic, potent analgesic, glucocorticoid, and antisecretor drugs in combination with the most comfortable route of administration to allow its application within the homecare setting [2, 5, 6].

More than 80 % of patients with MBO present with continuous pain and severe colic [5, 6, 8, 9]. The administration of analgesics for the treatment of MBO should be adjusted to the analgesic scale of the World Health Organization (WHO), which has demonstrated an efficacy rate greater than 80 % in cancer patients [37–40]. According to the European Society of Palliative Care and the WHO, it is now accepted that the majority of available strong opioids are effective for the treatment of cancer pain (morphine, methadone, oxycodone, fentanyl, hydromorphone, etc.) [41]. Some authors have reported that oxycodone may be more effective than other opioids for visceral pain treatment given its action on the kappa-opioid receptors, although this has yet to be confirmed in controlled clinical studies [42]. A meta-analysis of five controlled clinical trials by Tassinari et al in 2009 confirmed that fentanyl is a potent opioid that produces less constipation as a secondary effect [43]. A recent descriptive analysis of MBO in advanced cancer shows that more than 60 % of the patients were treated with potent opioids prior to the occlusive episode and more than 80 % required these drugs for analgesia during the episode. In this study, no statistically significant differences were observed in the rate of spontaneous resolution under symptomatic treatment among patients treated with a potent opioid prior to or during the episode of MBO versus those who did not receive this type of drug [6]. The opioid dose should be titrated individually for adequate pain relief. The subcutaneous, intravenous, sublingual, or transdermal route for opioid administration should be used frequently because nausea and vomiting do not allow for oral administration.

Antiemetic treatment uses drugs from three pharmacological groups: anticholinergic, dopamine antagonists, and serotonin antagonists (5-HT3). The dopamine antagonists are divided into benzamides (metoclopramide), butyrophenones (haloperidol), and phenothiazines (chlorpromazine). Metoclopramide blocks the dopamine receptors (D2) at the central and peripheral level. Its action facilitates the release of acetylcholine and at high doses (120 mg/day) antagonizes the 5-HT3 receptors. The mixed, central, and peripheral actions result in an antiemetic and prokinetic digestive effect of metoclopramide. The usual metoclopramide doses range from 40 to 120 mg/day. Haloperidol and phenothiazines (chlorpromazine and levomepromazine) are neuroleptic drugs that block the dopamine receptors at the central level only. They have a potent antiemetic, but no prokinetic effect. Among these drugs, haloperidol is considered the best choice because it produces less somnolence and anticholinergic effects. Haloperidol doses range from 5 to 15 mg/day, which can be administered in divided doses subcutaneously or intravenously, or by continuous subcutaneous or intravenous infusion. Scopolamine and hyoscine butylbromide are anticholinergic drugs. The antiemetic effects result from blocking acetylcholine at the central and peripheral levels in association with a clear antisecretor effect. Hyoscine butylbromide doses range from 40 to 120 mg/day. The serotonin (5-HT3) receptor antagonists, such as ondansetron or granisetron, can be useful for emesis control in the treatment of MBO. A recent noncontrolled phase II study demonstrated an index greater than 80 % for the antiemetic control of MBO using granisetron (5-HT3 receptor antagonist), even in cases that have not responded to typical antiemetic treatment [8]. The ondansetron dose ranges from 12 to 24 mg/day, and the granisetron dose ranges from 1 to 3 mg/day. These drugs are usually well tolerated. Headache, dizziness, and constipation are the most commonly reported side effects associated with their use.

Glucocorticoids possess an antiemetic action, the mechanism of which is not well known, and an anti-inflammatory action that reduces peritumoural oedema. Therefore, most researchers recommend glucocorticoids in the palliative treatment of MBO. A meta-analysis of three controlled clinical trials published in 1999 demonstrates that the use of glucocorticoids, particularly dexamethasone at a dose ranging from 6 to 16 mg, collaborates with the antiemetic action and favours the spontaneous resolution of MBO in advanced gynaecological and digestive cancer. In this meta-analysis, the rate of spontaneous resolution was 62–68 % in patients treated with glucocorticoids compared to 33–57 % in those receiving placebo [32, 44, 45].

The objective of antisecretor drugs is to reduce intestinal hypersecretion and, secondarily, to improve nausea, vomiting, and pain. Anticholinergic drugs (scopolamine, hyoscine, and butylbromide) have traditionally been the antisecretor of choice. Octreotide, a somatostatin analogue, provides a more specific and prolonged antisecretor effect. The pharmacologic activity of octreotide is mediated by the inhibition of the secretion of vasoactive intestinal peptides. This pharmacologic activity reduces electrolyte retention in the intestinal lumen, as well as gastric secretions, intestinal motility, biliary flow, splanchnic hypervascularization, and intestinal parietal oedema. Furthermore, it increases the absorption of water and the production of intestinal mucous [46, 47]. Different studies on the effectiveness of octreotide at doses from 200 to 600 μg/day have shown a clear reduction in intestinal secretions, decreased need for nasogastric tubes, and a high grade of antiemetic and analgesic response with no relevant adverse effects [3, 6, 9, 48–52]. Two controlled clinical studies have compared the antiemetic, analgesic, and antisecretory efficacy of octreotide (300 μg/day) versus hyoscine butylbromide (60 mg/day) in the treatment of MBO. In both studies, the efficacy of octreotide was statistically greater in all the parameters of response (reduction in digestive hypersecretion and control of nausea and vomiting) [48–50]. A phase II study demonstrated that a long-acting formulation of octreotide (LAR Depot) in combination with corticosteroids is useful and safe for the treatment of MBO due to peritoneal carcinomatosis [53]. A recent review of the literature concludes that despite the limited number of controlled clinical trials, octreotide is the antisecretory agent of choice for the treatment of MBO based on the results from 15 consistent studies and the experience acquired from 20 years of its use [54]. Histamine-2 antagonists and proton pump inhibitors are useful for reducing gastric secretions. A recent meta-analysis confirmed that ranitidine is more effective than proton pump inhibitors as an antisecretory agent. Based on these data, the authors hypothesized that ranitidine would be useful as an adjuvant drug in antisecretory therapy for the treatment of MBO and suggested the development of specific research to confirm these findings [55, 56].

15.7.5.1 Parenteral Nutrition in Inoperable MBO

The aim of total parenteral nutrition (TPN) is the recovery of nutritional status in patients who are candidates for surgery. The palliative indication for TPN in advanced oncologic patients with inoperable MBO is more controversial. TPN is an invasive technique that requires specific training for use and frequent monitoring of electrolytes and hydration. It also predisposes patients to infection (central venous access), thrombosis, diarrhoea, liver dysfunction, and hyperglycaemia. The scarce studies that have evaluated the efficacy of long-term TPN for inoperable MBO have reported a mean survival rate of 4–6 months, a rate of complications associated with the procedure greater than 13 %, and maintained stability of nutritional parameters of only 2–3 months prior to death. These studies concluded that only 30 % of the patients surviving for more than 3 months benefit from the application of TPN [57, 58]. Routine use of TPN in MBO, therefore, is not recommended in inoperable patients. The decision for long-term TPN should be made with caution and should be reserved for patients with a good performance status prior to MBO, slow growing tumours, the possibility of response to chemotherapy, expected survival of more than 3 months, and without severe extra-abdominal complications due to the neoplasm.

15.7.5.2 Polymodal Medical Management of Inoperable MBO

The palliative treatment of MBO is multimodal and based on the combined use of different drugs for symptom control. According to most researchers and the recently published guidelines of clinical practice from the National Comprehensive Cancer Network [59], the initial treatment for inoperable MBO is the combined use of analgesia with opioids, antiemetics, antisecretors, glucocorticoids, and intravenous hydration. It is reasonable to consider the continuous infusion of fentanyl using an intravenous, subcutaneous, or transdermal route as the method of choice due to its fewer effects on intestinal motility and better tolerance in dehydrated patients. In complete MBO, the antiemetic of choice is haloperidol since the prokinetic effect of metoclopramide may increase pain and nausea [3]. Antagonists of the 5-HT3 receptors (ondansetron or granisetron) may be an alternative for patients who have had an inadequate response to previous antiemetic treatments [8]. The initial use of glucocorticoids is recommended due to their antiemetic effect and reduction of intestinal oedema, which may facilitate the spontaneous resolution of the occlusive picture [32, 44, 45]. Most researchers recommend the early use of octreotide or an antisecretor drug due to its clear superiority over other anticholinergic drugs [3, 48–54]. Nasogastric aspiration should only be considered for the treatment of inoperable MBO in the absence of a symptomatic response to multimodal palliative treatment. The rate of control for nausea, vomiting, and pain using different variations of the described multimodal palliative treatment strategy in inoperable MBO is greater than 80 %, with spontaneous resolution in more than 30 % of cases [3, 5, 6, 8, 12, 50]. The estimated median survival of patients with inoperable MBO is 1 month with a 6-month survival of less than 8 % [6].

15.7.5.3 Factors Affecting the Spontaneous Resolution of Inoperable MBO

The spontaneous resolution of the occlusive picture occurs in 30–40 % of patients with inoperable MBO [6–10]. Little is known about the factors that may influence the spontaneous resolution of this complication. Surgical studies describe patients undergoing surgery, but do not report the evolution of inoperable patients.

A prospective cohort study was conducted by the Catalan Institute of Cancer in 2007, which included 100 patients diagnosed with inoperable MBO who were selected out of 885 patients visited by the palliative care hospital support team (MBO prevalence = 11.3 %). Twenty-five percent of these patients had previous episodes of MBO with spontaneous resolution (overall mean of 1.37 episodes per patient; SD±0.7; range 1–4). An extensive record of the clinical characteristics of these patients was documented. Over 80 % of patients had multiple levels of obstruction, and more than 60 % had peritoneal carcinomatosis with radiological or cytological confirmation. Spontaneous resolution of inoperable MBO with symptomatic treatment was observed in 42 % of patients. Resolution occurred within the first seven days after diagnosis in 92 % of patients. During follow-up, the rate of intestinal re-obstruction was 74 %. The mean overall survival rate was 23 days (95 % CI=16.8–29.4). Clinical data for all patients were stratified according to their specific evolution (spontaneous resolution versus no resolution) in order to identify the factors influencing the spontaneous resolution of MBO. The mean survival was 12 days (95 % CI=9.0–14.1) for patients with no spontaneous resolution of MBO, and 57 days for patients with complete resolution ($P < 0.001$). In the group of patients who did not present with MBO resolution, some showed tolerance to minimal food intake, mainly liquids, without recovery of normal digestive transit and with the need to maintain antiemetic and antisecretory treatment. The mean survival rate of these patients (persistent sub-obstruction) was 23 days (95 % CI=3.9–36), which is lower than the full resolution cases and higher than those patients who did not tolerate the intake of liquids at any time ($P<0.001$). Multivariate analysis showed that the most relevant factors influencing the spontaneous resolution of MBO are cognitive failure, cachexia, dyspnoea at rest, palpable abdominal tumours, hepatic failure, upper intestinal obstruction, and dehydration [6].

It is important to know the risk of non-resolution of MBO in order to carefully establish therapeutic measures, define realistic expectations, and accurately report them to the patient and family.

It is relevant to determine whether there are pharmacological and non-pharmacological measures for prevention of re-obstruction in patients who previously had spontaneous resolution of MBO. Some researchers suggest that a low-residue diet, avoidance of osmotic laxatives, or use of long-term antisecretory drugs (e.g. long-acting octreotide) may decrease the likelihood of further obstructive episodes. However, this question remains unanswered. A pilot study conducted in 2005 including 15 ovarian cancer patients diagnosed with inoperable MBO documented peritoneal carcinomatosis. These patients were treated with immediate-release octreotide followed by long-acting octreotide administered on a monthly basis. Sixty percent of patients received at least one dose of long-acting octreotide. Three of the patients (20 %) had full recovery of digestive transit. These patients continued the antisecretory therapy with long-acting octreotide over a mean time of 9 months (3–15 months)

[60]. Due to the size of the study and confounding variables (chemotherapy, lack of report of some re-obstructions), this study does not allow to conclude that the long-acting octreotide is useful in preventing new episodes of MBO. At present, the measures for preventing intestinal re-obstruction remain under debate and have to be the focus of future research.

15.7.6 Bleeding

Significant bleeding from the large bowel occurs in 20 % of all CRC patients [2] and can be observed in more than 35 % of patients with rectal cancers. It is well recognized that laser ablation is a good treatment option for bleeding colon cancer. The neodymium:yttrium-argon-garnet. (Nd:YAG) is the most commonly used device for this indication. The intensity modulation of the laser energy can be adjusted to only obtain haemostasis or to vaporize the tumour. Laser treatment may be used in rectal cancer for bleeding or tenesmus. The laser therapy can achieve control of rectal bleeding in more than 80 % of patients. The cancer spread in a long segment of colon or involving all quadrants of intestinal perimeter reduces laser ablation efficacy. The main complication of laser therapy is perforation (less than 3 %).

Radiotherapy is also a good option to reduce pain, tenesmus, and bleeding in some cases of advanced rectal cancer. Also radiotherapy does not improve survival in advanced rectal cancers; it can provide adequate control of pain and bleeding in 75 % of patients.

Palliative surgery can be considered as a treatment option in large bowel bleeding. The criteria for surgical intervention and the risk factors contributing to mortality and morbidity are similar to those discussed for intestinal obstruction [61].

15.8 Summary and Key Points

- At diagnosis, between 20 and 30 % of patients with CRC present with metastatic spread. The main complications of advanced CRC, potentially suitable for palliative surgery, are bleeding and/or obstruction of the digestive tract. About 65 % of patients with stage IV CRC present with severe local symptoms requiring invasive treatment (tumour resection, bypass, stoma, stent).
- MBO is a frequent complication in patients with advanced CRC. The diagnosis of MBO is fundamentally based on anamnesis, physical examination, and plain X-rays of the abdomen. Use of contrast, CT, and MRI increases the diagnostic precision related to tumour extension and the level of obstruction. This is often necessary for decision-making and evaluation of the indication for surgery or endoscopic palliation.
- Surgery can re-establish digestive transit. However, its indication should be assessed carefully on an individual basis, especially in patients with advanced cancer due to the high rate of surgical mortality and morbidity. Factors limiting surgical success in MBO are advanced age, malnutrition, the presence of multiple occlusive levels, extra-abdominal metastatic disease, refractory ascites, poor performance status, previous abdominal radiotherapy, and the lack of specific treatment options for advanced cancer (chemotherapy).
- Self-expanding colonic stents are highly effective and safe alternatives in patients with a single level of occlusion, who are considered unfit for surgery or require a "bridge to surgery".
- Percutaneous gastrostomy (venting-PEG) allows for more comfortable and safe long-term digestive decompression than nasogastric tube insertion in patients with inoperable MBO and symptoms that are inadequately controlled by symptomatic medical management.
- Palliative medical treatment of inoperable MBO is multimodal and based on the combined use of glucocorticoids, antiemetics, antisecretors, and potent analgesic opioids. Due to their antiemetic action and reduction of mucosal oedema, glucocorticoids are indicated in the initial phases of this complication and may increase the rate of spontaneous resolution. Antiemetics of choice are neuroleptics (haloperidol). Prokinetic drugs can increase

pain and should be avoided in MBO. Antagonists of 5-HT3 receptors are effective for controlling emesis in the treatment of MBO, even in cases where the patient's response to other antiemetics is insufficient.

- Abdominal pain in MBO is highly prevalent, of great intensity, and often requires the use of potent opioid drugs. No controlled clinical trials have compared the different potent opioids in this indication. Fentanyl is the opioid that least affects intestinal motility, which has been confirmed by controlled clinical studies with different causes of MBO.
- Antisecretor drugs improve nausea, vomiting, and pain with an important reduction in intestinal hypersecretion proximal to the obstruction. Several controlled clinical studies have shown that octreotide, an analogue of somatostatin and a potent antisecretor drug, is clearly superior in this setting when compared with anticholinergic drugs. Continuous digestive aspiration via a nasogastric tube or percutaneous gastrostomy is only useful if multimodal palliative pharmacological treatment does not provide adequate symptom control.
- Symptom control is very high with multimodal medical treatment strategies and spontaneous resolution occurs in more than one third of patients.
- Life expectancy of patients suffering from advanced malignancies presenting with inoperable MBO is short, with a mean survival rate no longer than 4 weeks.
- The most relevant factors influencing non-resolution of MBO include cognitive failure, cachexia, dyspnoea at rest, palpable abdominal tumours, hepatic failure, upper intestinal obstruction, and dehydration.

References

1. Globocan 2008. Estimated cancer Incidence, Mortality, Prevalence and Disability-adjusted life years (DALYs) Worldwide in 2008. International Agency for Research on Cancer. World Health Organisation. http://globocan.iarc.fr/. Accessed Feb 2013.
2. Evans MD, Escofet X, Karandikar SS, Stamatakis JD. Outcomes of resection and non-resection strategies in management of patients with advanced colorectal cancer. World J Surg Oncol. 2009;7:28.
3. Ripamonti C, Easson AM, Gerdes H. Management of malignant bowel obstruction. Eur J Cancer. 2008;44(8):1105–15.
4. Dvoretsky PM, Richards KA, Angel C, Rabinowitz L, Beecham JB, Bonfiglio TA. Survival time, causes of death, and tumor. Treatment related morbidity in 100 women with ovarian cancer. Hum Pathol. 1988; 19(11):1273–9.
5. Baines M, Oliver DJ, Carter RL. Medical management of intestinal obstruction in patients with advanced malignant disease – a clinical and pathological study. Lancet. 1985;2(8462):990–3.
6. Tuca A, Guell E, Martinez-Losada E, Codorniu N. Malignant bowel obstruction in advanced cancer patients: epidemiology, management, and factors influencing spontaneous resolution. Cancer Manag Res. 2012;4:159–69.
7. Miller G, Boman J, Shrier I, Gordon PH. Small bowel obstruction secondary to malignant disease: an 11-year audit. Can J Surg. 2000;43(5):353–8.
8. Tuca A, Roca R, Sala C, et al. Efficacy of granisetron in the antiemetic control of nonsurgical intestinal obstruction in advanced cancer: a phase II clinical trial. J Pain Symptom Manage. 2009;37(2):259–70.
9. Arvieux C, Laval G, Stefani L, Villard ML, Mestrallet JP, Cardin N. Protocol for the treatment of malignant inoperable bowel obstruction: a prospective study of 80 cases at Grenoble University Hospital Center. J Pain Symptom Manage. 2006;31(6):502–12.
10. Blair SL, Chu DZ, Schwarz E. Outcome of palliative operations for malignant bowel obstruction in patients with peritoneal carcinomatosis from non-gynecological cancer. Ann Surg Oncol. 2001;8(8):632–7.
11. Anthony T, Baron T, Mercadante S, et al. Report of the clinical protocol committee: development of randomized trials for malignant bowel obstruction. J Pain Symptom Manage. 2007;34 Suppl 1:S49–59.
12. Ripamonti C, Twycross R, Baines M et al; for Working Group of the European Association for Palliative Care. Clinical-practice recommendations for management of bowel obstruction in patients with end-stage cancer. Support Care Cancer. 2001;9(4):223–33.
13. Bennett MI, Livingstone HJ, Costello P, Allen KR, Degg TJ. Symptom scores, serotonin and 5-hydroxyindole acetic acid levels in cancer patients with and without bowel obstruction. Palliat Med. 2007;21(2):157–9.
14. Jimenez-Garcıa A, Balongo-Garcıa R, Alconero FF, et al. Intestinal wall damage in simple ileus in rabbits: immune modulator role of somatostatin. Hepatogastroenterology. 2004;51(58):1030–6.
15. Goyal RK, Hirano I. Enteric nervous system. N Engl J Med. 1996;334(17):1106–15.
16. Helye L, Easson AM. Surgical approaches to malignant bowel obstruction. J Support Oncol. 2008;6(3): 105–13.

17. Branco BC, Barmparas G, Schnüriger B, Inaba K, Chan LS, Demetriades D. Systematic review and meta-analysis of the diagnostic and therapeutic role of water-soluble contrast agent in adhesive small bowel obstruction. Br J Surg. 2010;97(4):470–8.
18. Suri S, Gupta S, Sudhakar PJ, Venkataramu NK, Sood B, Wig JD. Comparative evaluation of plain films, ultrasound and CT in the diagnosis of intestinal obstruction. Acta Radiol. 1999;40(4):422–8.
19. Thompson WM, Kilani RK, Smith BB, et al. Accuracy of abdominal radiography in acute small bowel obstruction: does reviewer experience matter? AJR Am J Roentgenol. 2007;188(3):W233–8.
20. de Bree E, Koops W, Kröger R, van Ruth S, Witkamp AJ, Zoetmulder MA. Peritoneal carcinomatosis from colorectal or appendiceal origin: correlation of preoperative CT with intraoperative findings and evaluation of interobserver agreement. J Surg Oncol. 2004;86(2):64–73.
21. Jacquest P, Jelinek JS, Steves MA, Sugarbaker PH. Evaluation of computed tomography in patients with peritoneal carcinomatosis. Cancer. 1993;72(5):1631–6.
22. Low R, Chen S, Barone R. Distinguishing benign from malignant bowel obstruction in patients with malignancy: findings at MR imaging. Radiology. 2003;228(1):157–65.
23. Beall D, Fortman B, Lawler B, Regan F. Imaging bowel obstruction: a comparison between fast magnetic resonance imaging and helical computed tomography. Clin Radiol. 2002;57(8):719–24.
24. Chan A, Woodruf RK. Intestinal obstruction in patients with wide-spread intra-abdominal malignancy. J Pain Symptom Manage. 1992;7(6):339–42.
25. Lau PV, Lorenz PG. Results of surgery for malignant bowel obstruction in advanced, unresectable, recurrent colorectal cancer. Dis Colon Rectum. 1993; 36(1):61–4.
26. Jong P, Sturgeon J, Jamieson CG. Benefit of palliative surgery for bowel obstruction in advanced ovarian cancer. Can J Surg. 1995;38(5):454–7.
27. Yazdi GP, Miedema BW, Humphrey LJ. High mortality after abdominal operation in patients with large volume malignant ascites. J Surg Oncol. 1996;62(2):93–6.
28. Woolfson RG, Jennings K, Whalen GF. Management of bowel obstruction in patients with abdominal cancer. Arch Surg. 1997;132(10):1093–7.
29. Sun X, Li X. Management of bowel obstruction in advanced ovarian cancer: an analysis of 57 cases. Zhonghua Zhong Liu Za Zhi. 1995;17(1):39–42.
30. Tekkis P, Kinsman R, Thompsom M, Stamatakis J. The Association of Coloproctology of Great Britain and Ireland study of large bowel obstruction caused by colorectal cancer. Ann Surg. 2004;240(1):76–81.
31. Bryan D, Radbod R, Berek J. An analysis of surgical versus a chemotherapeutic intervention for the management of intestinal obstruction in advanced ovarian cancer. Int J Gynecol Cancer. 2006;16(1):125–34.
32. Feuer DJ, Broadley KE, Shepherd JH, Barton DP. Systematic review of surgery in malignant bowel obstruction in advanced gynecological and gastrointestinal cancer. Gynecol Oncol. 1999;75(3):313–22.
33. Watt AM, Faragher IG, Griffin TT, Rieger NA, Maddern GJ. Self-expanding metallic stents for relieving malignant colorectal obstruction: a systematic review. Ann Surg. 2007;246(1):24–30.
34. Khot UP, Lang AW, Murali K, Parker MC. Systematic review of the efficacy and safety of colorectal stents. Br J Surg. 2002;89(9):1096.
35. Campagnutta E, Cannizzaro R, Gallo A, et al. Palliative treatment of upper intestinal obstruction by gynecological malignancy: the usefulness of percutaneous endoscopic gastrostomy. Gynecol Oncol. 1996; 62(1):103–5.
36. Pothuri B, Montemrano M, Gerardi M, et al. Percutaneous endoscopic gastrostomy tube placement in malignant bowel obstruction due to ovarian carcinoma. Gynecol Oncol. 2005;96:330–4.
37. World Health Organization. Cancer Pain Relief – with a guide to opioid availability. 2nd ed. WHO Geneva 1996. Available in internet: http://whqlibdoc.who.int/publications/9241544821.pdf. Accessed May 2012.
38. Ventafridda V, Tamburini M, Caraceni A, De Conno F, Naldi F. A validation study of the WHO method for cancer pain relief. Cancer. 1987;59(4):850–6.
39. Zech DF, Grond S, Lynch J, Hertel D, Lehmann KA. Validation of World Health Organization Guidelines for cancer pain relief: a 10-year prospective study. Pain. 1995;63(1):65–76.
40. Mercadante S. Pain treatment and outcomes for patients with advanced cancer who receive follow-up care at home. Cancer. 1999;85(8):1849–58.
41. Caraceni A, Hanks G, Kaasa S, Bennett MI, Brunelli C, Cherny N, Dale O, De Conno F, Fallon M, Hanna M, Haugen DF, Juhl G, King S, Klepstad P, Laugsand EA, Maltoni M, Mercadante S, Nabal M, Pigni A, Radbruch L, Reid C, Sjogren P, Stone PC, Tassinari D, Zeppetella G, European Palliative Care Research Collaborative (EPCRC); European Association for Palliative Care (EAPC). Use of opioid analgesics in the treatment of cancer pain: evidence-based recommendations from the EAPC. Lancet Oncol. 2012;13(2):e58–68.
42. Riley J, Eisenberg E, Müller-Schwefe G, Drewes AM, Arednt-Nielsen L. Oxycodone: a review of its use in the management of pain. Curr Med Res Opin. 2008;24(1):175–92.
43. Tassinari D, Sartori S, Tamburini E, et al. Transdermal fentanyl as a front-line approach to moderate-severe pain: a meta-analysis of randomized clinical trials. J Palliat Care. 2009;25(3):172–80.
44. Laval G, Girardier J, Lassauumiere JM, Leduc B, Haond C, Schaerer R. The use of steroids in the management of inoperable intestinal obstruction in terminal cancer patients: do they remove the obstruction? Palliat Med. 2000;14(1):3–10.
45. Hardy JR, Ling PJ, Mansi J, et al. Pitfalls in placebo controlled trials in palliative care: dexamethasone for the palliation of malignant bowel obstruction. Palliat Med. 1998;12(16):437–43.
46. Neville R, Fielding P, Cambria RP, Modlin I. Vascular responsiveness in obstructed gut. Dis Colon Rectum. 1991;34(3):229–35.

47. Nellgard P, Bojo L, Cassuto J. Importance of vasoactive intestinal peptide and somatostatin for fluid losses in small bowel obstruction. Scand J Gastroenterol. 1995;30(5):464–9.
48. Ripamonti C, Mercadante S, Groff L, Zecca E, De Conno F, Cassucio A. Role of octreotide, scopolamine butylbromide and hydration in symptom control of patients with inoperable bowel obstruction having a nasogastric tube – a prospective, randomized clinical trial. J Pain Symptom Manage. 2000;19(1):23–34.
49. Mercadante S, Ripamonti C, Casuccio A, Zecca E, Groff L. Comparison of octreotide and hyoscine butylbromide in controlling gastrointestinal symptoms due to malignant inoperable bowel obstruction. Support Care Cancer. 2000;8(3):188–91.
50. Mercadante S, Casuccio A, Mangione S. Medical treatment for inoperable malignant bowel obstruction: a qualitative systematic review. J Pain Symptom Manage. 2007;33(2):217–23.
51. Watari H, Hosaka M, Wakui Y, et al. A prospective study on the efficacy of octreotide in the management of malignant bowel obstruction in gynecologic cancer. Int J Gynecol Cancer. 2012;22(4):692–6.
52. Hisanaga T, Shinjo T, Morita T, et al. Multicenter prospective study on efficacy and safety of octreotide for inoperable malignant bowel obstruction. Jpn J Clin Oncol. 2010;40(8):739–45.
53. Laval G, Rousselot H, Toussaint-Martel S, et al. SALTO: a randomized, multicenter study assessing octreotide LAR in inoperable bowel obstruction. Bull Cancer. 2012;99(2):1–9.
54. Mercadante S, Porzio G. Octreotide for malignant bowel obstruction: twenty years after. Crit Rev Oncol Hematol. 2012;83(3):388–92.
55. Clark K, Lam L, Currow D. Reducing gastric secretions-a role for histamine 2 antagonists or proton pump inhibitors in malignant bowel obstruction? Support Care Cancer. 2009;17(12):1463–8.
56. Clark K, Lam LT, Gibson S, Currow D. The effect of ranitidine versus proton pump inhibitors on gastric secretions: a meta-analysis of randomised control trials. Anaesthesia. 2009;64(6):652–7.
57. Fan BG. Parenteral nutrition prolongs the survival of patients associated with malignant gastrointestinal obstruction. JPEN J Parenter Enteral Nutr. 2007;31(6):508–10.
58. Bozzetti F, Cozzaglio L, Biganzoli E, et al. Quality of life and length of survival in advanced cancer patients on home parenteral nutrition. Clin Nutr. 2002;21(4):281–8.
59. http://www.nccn.org [homepage on the Internet]. Palliative Care. Practice Guidelines in Oncology of National Comprehensive Cancer Network. Accessed 19 Feb 2011. http://www.nccn.org/professionals/physician_gls/f_guidelines.asp#palliative. Accessed Dec 2012.
60. Matulonis UA, Seiden MV, Roche M, et al. Long-acting octreotide for the treatment and symptomatic relief of bowel obstruction in advanced ovarian cancer. J Pain Symptom Manage. 2005;30(6):563–9.
61. Ronnekleiv-Kelly SM, Kennedy GD. Management of stage IV rectal cancer: palliative options. World J Gastroenterol. 2011;17(7):835–47.

Brain and Vertebral Column 16

Nigel Jones

Contents

N. Jones, DPhil, FRACS, FFPMANZCA
Department of Surgery,
University of Adelaide,
270 Wakefield Street, Adelaide,
SA 5000, Australia
e-mail: nigeljones@internode.on.net

Palliative neurosurgery has benefited from recent technological advances allowing safer and less invasive procedures aimed at relieving symptoms from advanced disease. Conditions treated include malignant glioma, cerebral and spinal metastases, hydrocephalus, malignant meningitis and cancer-related pain.

16.1 Introduction

Dunn [1] defines palliative surgery as: "A surgical procedure used with the primary intention of improving quality of life or relieving symptoms caused by advanced disease. Its effectiveness is judged by the presence and durability of patient acknowledged symptom resolution."

Not only has the last decade seen a greater transition of general palliative care practices to the neurosurgical setting, but various technological advances have widened the scope of neurosurgical procedures suitable for palliation. From the definition provided previously, it can be seen that palliative surgical procedures must relieve symptoms and improve quality of life. While significant discomfort or even some degree of increased disability is often acceptable for curative surgery, palliative procedures are not aimed at offering a cure, and the treatment must not be worse than the underlying condition. Modern neurosurgery is much less invasive than even two decades ago, and it is much easier to tip the balance in favour of intervention for symptom reduction, even when prolongation of life may not be possible.

M. Wichmann, G. Maddern (eds.), *Palliative Surgery*,
DOI 10.1007/978-3-642-53709-7_16,

Frameless stereotaxy, high-resolution preoperative and intraoperative imaging, endoscopy and minimally invasive spinal surgical techniques have all widened the scope of palliative neurosurgery. Embracing the multidisciplinary nature of palliative care is stereotactic radiation therapy, or radiosurgery, utilised by neurosurgeons and radiation oncologists in both the brain and the spine. Destructive procedures for pain relief have largely been replaced by more technologically advanced methods of pain management.

16.2 Cranial

16.2.1 Glioma

Glioblastoma is the most common primary brain tumour in adults with an incidence of approximately five per 100,000 [2]. These tumours have always had a poor prognosis but that has improved somewhat in recent years, related more to improvements in adjuvant treatment than surgery [3]. While there is still debate about the influence of surgery on survival [4, 5], it can be very useful for palliation of symptoms including headache and neurological deficit.

Gliomas frequently contain cysts that can contribute as much as, or more than, the solid tumour to raised intracranial pressure and neurological deficit (Fig. 16.1). Radiation and chemotherapy have little effect on these cysts and surgical drainage is a simple and relatively safe procedure that can significantly improve symptoms. The use of frameless stereotaxy coupled with computerised tomography (CT) or magnetic resonance imaging (MRI) allows relatively safe and minimally invasive drainage of tumour cysts, decreasing intracranial pressure and improving neurological function. It can be done through a small incision and burr hole and under local anaesthesia if necessary.

More aggressive tumour resection is also possible due to better anatomical localisation. Prior to surgery, MRI can be utilised to show fibre tracts, and functional MRI can localise eloquent areas. These images can then be fused with the guidance image and utilised intraoperatively. The use of intraoperative neuronavigation is now standard and can improve extent of resection without prolonging operative time [6].

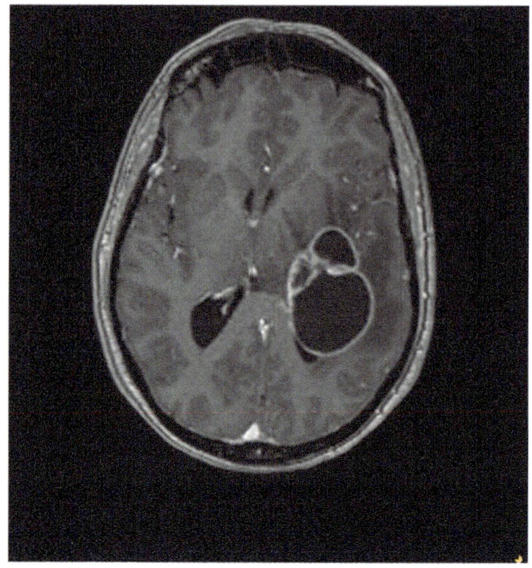

Fig. 16.1 T1-weighted, gadolinium-enhanced MRI showing a left deep-seated cystic glioblastoma

In some centres, intraoperative CT and even MRI [7, 8] can be used to further improve the extent of tumour removal and the addition of new techniques such as 5-ALA fluorescence-guided resection shows considerable promise [9]. While there still exists significant controversy regarding the survival advantages of this, in a palliative context it does allow symptomatic improvement from cytoreduction and resolution of peritumoural oedema with decreased risk of new neurological deficit.

Occasionally gliomas can be complicated by haemorrhage causing acute deterioration. Surgical evacuation of the haematoma, if done expeditiously, can be associated with good short-term outcomes but is often avoided in view of the poor overall prognosis in this condition. As the response to adjuvant treatment improves, these attitudes are changing.

Surgery may also be indicated for palliation of epilepsy, especially in patients with low-grade gliomas that otherwise may not have required surgical intervention. This can be very effective and lead to significant improvement in quality of life [10, 11].

16.2.2 Metastases

Metastatic tumours are the most common intracranial neoplasm in adults. Autopsy studies suggest that 20–25 % of cancer patients have brain metastases [12]. Eight to ten percent of adults with cancer will develop symptomatic brain metastases [13, 14]. As treatment of the primary malignancy improves, these figures are likely to increase further. Melanoma is the most likely primary tumour to spread to the brain, but numerically most cerebral metastases are from lung or breast primaries [15]. Prior to the 1970s, surgery was rarely considered appropriate for metastatic tumours in view of the high morbidity and poor survival. Improvements in surgical technique and, in particular, imaging have changed this, and now surgery has a well-defined role. As well as providing palliation of increased intracranial pressure and neurological deficit, it can provide tissue for histology in cases where no primary site is identified and in those patients where abscess or primary malignancy are in the differential.

Surgery is usually considered in patients with solitary metastases; however, many older series are not directly comparable with current clinical practice. Older series utilising CT will underestimate the incidence of multiple metastases compared with newer studies using MRI. There is some evidence supporting the treatment of up to three metastases [16], and for palliation of raised intracranial pressure or neurological deficit, a large metastasis may be removed even if the MRI reveals other smaller asymptomatic lesions. Metastases are usually very well defined and can be macroscopically removed with modern neurosurgical techniques. This immediately reduces intracranial pressure and surrounding oedema with improvement in symptoms. This can be quite dramatic, particularly with cerebellar metastases.

Another consideration is the improvement in technique with minimally invasive approaches made possible by the routine use of neuronavigation. The decreased surgical morbidity has made resection of symptomatic metastases more acceptable. Craniotomies can be made directly over the lesion and often through a small linear scalp incision rather than a large scalp flap. The hospital stay is usually very short and the morbidity minimal.

Radiosurgery, using either a linear accelerator or the Gamma knife, is often used for the treatment of symptomatic metastases. The advantages include the ability to treat multiple lesions and the non-invasive nature of radiosurgery. The disadvantages are the limited availability, and the fact that symptoms of raised intracranial pressure may be aggravated rather than relieved in the early stages [17]. Delayed radiation necrosis is another consideration [18]. Surgery will usually provide better palliation for accessible tumours in non-eloquent areas, but radiosurgery can be very useful for treating deep-seated tumours or those in eloquent areas.

Metastases may bleed causing acute deterioration. Melanoma and chorioncarcinoma are particularly prone to haemorrhage [19, 20], and craniotomy will usually be indicated in this situation, even in the presence of multiple lesions, especially if a tissue diagnosis has not yet been confirmed.

16.2.3 Meningioma

Many meningiomas are curable with simple excision, but a large number involve structures such as the dural venous sinuses or arise in relatively inaccessible areas such as the anterior foramen magnum, making complete excision impossible without unacceptable deficit. In such cases, surgical debulking may provide adequate palliation of symptoms, and the slow growth of many of these tumours often allows the residual to be treated by observation alone. When the histology is atypical suggesting a more aggressive nature, radiation therapy may be added. Surgical palliation of meningiomas may also be indicated for local control when these tumours threaten to erode through the skin.

Meningiomas are prone to haemorrhage which can be intratumoural, intracerebral or subdural, and in these instances surgery is usually indicated even if the underlying tumour cannot be completely removed [21].

16.2.4 Hydrocephalus

Hydrocephalus may occur in patients with primary or secondary malignancy due to obstruction of the cerebrospinal fluid (CSF) pathways. Ventriculoperitoneal shunting can provide dramatic palliation of symptoms of raised intracranial pressure with minimal morbidity [22]. In some cases, where there are malignant cells in the CSF, there can be a risk of peritoneal seeding as well as increased risks of shunt blockage. In this situation, endoscopic third ventriculostomy is a minimally invasive procedure that can give similar palliation without these risks. The results in tumour patients have been reported to be similar to those in patients with hydrocephalus due to non-neoplastic causes [23].

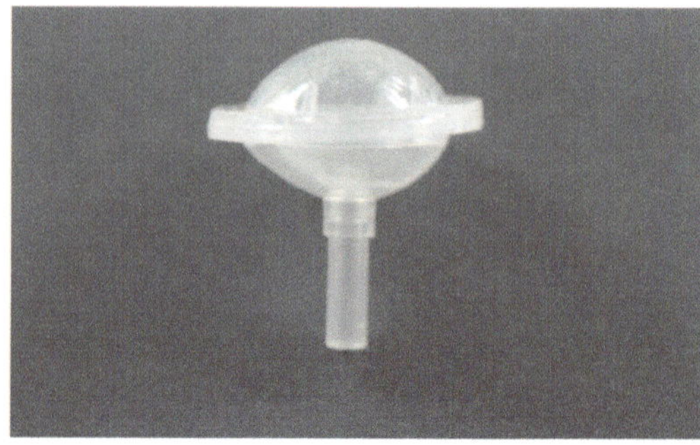

Fig. 16.2 An Ommaya reservoir (Accu-Flo CSF Reservoir, Codman, Johnson and Johnson)

16.2.5 Malignant Meningitis

Clinical diagnosis of malignant meningitis has become more frequent with the use of MRI [24], and it is found in up to 25 % of small cell lung cancer patients at post-mortem [25]. Malignant meningitis can cause a wide variety of neurological symptoms and signs and usually heralds a rapid decline. Some patients with malignant meningitis benefit from intrathecal chemotherapy but repeated lumbar punctures are often difficult and uncomfortable. There is also the risk of subdural or extradural injection [26]. In this situation, an Ommaya reservoir (Accu-Flo CSF Reservoir, Codman, Johnson and Johnson) can be inserted (Fig. 16.2). This is a simple procedure in which a ventricular catheter is passed, usually into the right frontal horn, and connected to a small chamber implanted permanently beneath the scalp. The incision is usually made anterior to the chamber so that the overlying scalp is numb. This makes repeated CSF access simple and much more comfortable than multiple lumbar punctures.

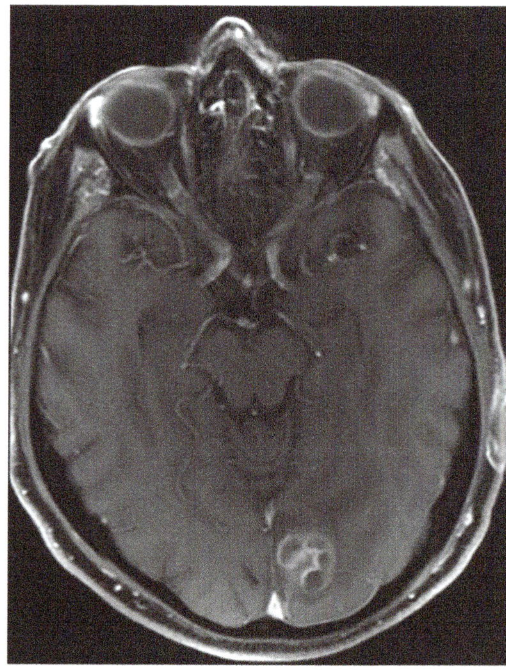

Fig. 16.3 T1-weighted, gadolinium-enhanced MRI showing a left occipital enhancing mass in an 84-year-old male with no predisposing factors for infection. It was thought to be glioblastoma but histologically proven to be nocardia

16.2.6 Infection

Patients with malignancy are more prone to infection, and this should always be considered in patients with undiagnosed cerebral or spinal lesions, especially in patients immunocompromised from steroids or chemotherapy. Apparent metastases or glioblastomas may be cerebral abscesses from nocardia or tuberculosis (Fig. 16.3). Magnetic resonance spectroscopy can be helpful in making the distinction, but often surgery is required to confirm the diagnosis even when treatment will be medical.

16.3 Spinal

16.3.1 Metastatic

Epidural spinal cord or cauda equina compression from metastatic disease can have a significant negative effect on quality of life. Treatment by posterior laminectomy often fails, partly because the compression is often ventral. In many cases, such surgery offers little benefit over radiotherapy alone. More aggressive treatment aimed at removing ventral tumour tends to be much more invasive and requires internal fixation to maintain stability. The benefits include better neurological outcomes and improvement in spinal pain [27]. This needs to be balanced with the increased morbidity and risks of the surgery. Modern minimally invasive surgery (MIS) techniques provide a compromise better suited to palliation of pain and neurological deficit. Using a combination of neuronavigation and MIS techniques, tumours can often be decompressed through the pedicle, and fixation can then be inserted percutaneously [28]. In some cases, percutaneous fixation can be used to treat pain without neurological deficit.

Vertebroplasty can also be useful in treating pain from spinal metastases. Using percutaneous techniques, polymethyl methacrylate (PMMA) cement is injected through the pedicle into the affected vertebral body [29, 30]. Care must be taken to avoid injecting cement into the canal, and this technique is contraindicated if the posterior cortex is not intact. Intramedullary spinal cord metastases are uncommon and surgery would rarely be indicated. With the advent of spinal stereotactic radiosurgery, it is possible to treat these and offer some palliation [31].

16.3.2 Primary

Although benign intra-dural tumours such as ependymoma and haemangioblastoma are usually surgically removable, occasionally the surgical risks are too great, and palliative options need to be considered. Even if debulking of the tumour itself is minimal or not possible, a simple duroplasty can sometimes buy considerable time with these slow-growing tumours (Fig. 16.4). Stereotactic radiosurgery is now an additional option and can be particularly useful in patients with multiple tumours such as those with type 2 neurofibromatosis.

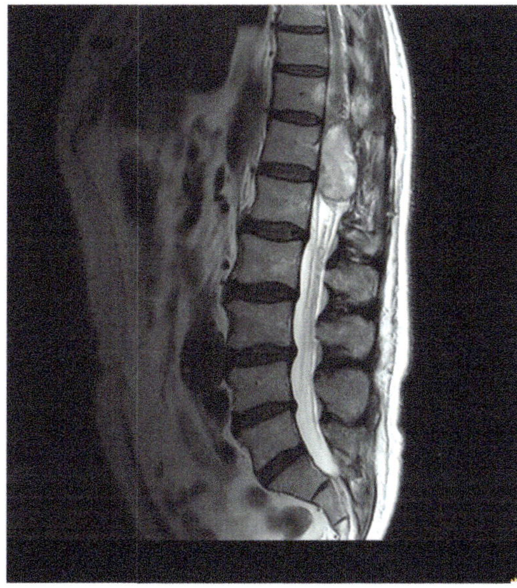

Fig. 16.4 T2-weighted MRI showing a highly vascular tumour at the conus that was causing significant neurological deficit but was not safely resectable. A duroplasty was performed with complete neurological recovery and abolition of back and leg pain. Five years later, his pain increased without neurological deficit and he was treated with stereotactic radiotherapy

16.3.3 Infection

Epidural spinal abscess should be considered in the differential of malignant spinal cord compression in the immunocompromised patient with malignancy.

16.4 Pain

Fleming [32] wrote in 1927 on the benefits of cordotomy and rhizotomy for cancer pain, but modern pain management techniques have largely supplanted these. In very selected cases, cordotomy or DREZ lesions can still be indicated [33], but neurosurgical input is more commonly limited to the insertion of epidural or intrathecal drug delivery systems [34]. A simple, tunnelled epidural catheter with an access port can provide excellent analgesia with acceptable infection risks in the short term. Implanted intrathecal programmable pumps are considerably more expensive, but in patients with a life expectancy of more than 3 months can be more cost-effective [35].

Spinal cord stimulation is used for chronic non-malignant pain but has not been shown to be beneficial or cost-effective in the palliative setting [36]. DBS (deep brain stimulation) is increasingly used in the treatment of chronic low back pain and neuropathic pain but has yet to have an impact on cancer pain, partly due to the costs involved.

References

1. Dunn GP. Surgical palliative care: recent trends and developments. Surg Clin North Am. 2011;91(2):277–92, vii.
2. Wrensch M, Minn Y, Chew T, Bondy M, Berger MS. Epidemiology of primary brain tumors: current concepts and review of the literature. Neuro Oncol. 2002;4(4):278–99.
3. Stupp R, Mason WP, van den Bent MJ, Weller M, Fisher B, Taphoorn MJ, Belanger K, Brandes AA, Marosi C, Bogdahn U, Curschmann J, Janzer RC, Ludwin SK, Gorlia T, Allgeier A, Lacombe D, Cairncross JG, Eisenhauer E, Mirimanoff RO, European Organisation for Research and Treatment of Cancer Brain Tumor and Radiotherapy Groups, National Cancer Institute of Canada Clinical Trials Group. Radiotherapy plus concomitant and adjuvant temozolomide for glioblastoma. N Engl J Med. 2005;352(10):987–96.
4. Vogelbaum MA. Does extent of resection of a glioblastoma matter? Clin Neurosurg. 2012;59:79–81.
5. Sanai N, Polley MY, McDermott MW, Parsa AT, Berger MS. An extent of resection threshold for newly diagnosed glioblastomas. J Neurosurg. 2011;115(1):3–8.
6. Wirtz CR, Albert FK, Schwaderer M, Heuer C, Staubert A, Tronnier VM, Knauth M, Kunze S. The benefit of neuronavigation for neurosurgery analyzed by its impact on glioblastoma surgery. Neurol Res. 2000;22(4):354–60.
7. Kubben PL, ter Meulen KJ, Schijns OE, ter Laak-Poort MP, van Overbeeke JJ, van Santbrink H. Intraoperative MRI-guided resection of glioblastoma multiforme: a systematic review. Lancet Oncol. 2011;12(11):1062–70.
8. Senft C, Franz K, Blasel S, Oszvald A, Rathert J, Seifert V, Gasser T. Influence of iMRI-guidance on the extent of resection and survival of patients with glioblastoma multiforme. Technol Cancer Res Treat. 2010;9(4):339–46.
9. Colditz MJ, Jeffree RL. Aminolevulinic acid (ALA)-protoporphyrin IX fluorescence guided tumour resection. Part 1: clinical, radiological and pathological studies. J Clin Neurosci. 2012;19(11):1471–4.
10. Bourgeois M, Sainte-Rose C, Lellouch-Tubiana A, Malucci C, Brunelle F, Maixner W, Cinalli G, Pierre-Kahn A, Renier D, Zerah M, Hirsch JF, Goutières F, Aicardi J. Surgery of epilepsy associated with focal lesions in childhood. J Neurosurg. 1999;90(5):833–42.
11. Packer RJ, Sutton LN, Patel KM, Duhaime AC, Schiff S, Weinstein SR, Gaillard WD, Conry JA, Schut L. Seizure control following tumor surgery for childhood cortical low-grade gliomas. J Neurosurg. 1994;80(6):998–1003.
12. Posner JB, Chernik NL. Intracranial metastases from systemic cancer. Adv Neurol. 1978;19:579–92.
13. Barnholtz-Sloan JS, Sloan AE, Davis FG, Vigneau FD, Lai P, Sawaya RE. Incidence proportions of brain metastases in patients diagnosed (1973 to 2001) in the Metropolitan Detroit Cancer Surveillance System. J Clin Oncol. 2004;22(14):2865–72.
14. Schouten LJ, Rutten J, Huveneers HA, Twijnstra A. Incidence of brain metastases in a cohort of patients with carcinoma of the breast, colon, kidney, and lung and melanoma. Cancer. 2002;94(10):2698–705.
15. Zimm S, Wampler GL, Stablein D, Hazra T, Young HF. Intracerebral metastases in solid-tumor patients: natural history and results of treatment. Cancer. 1981;48(2):384–94.
16. Bindal RK, Sawaya R, Leavens ME, Lee JJ. Surgical treatment of multiple brain metastases. J Neurosurg. 1993;79(2):210–6.
17. Breneman JC, Warnick RE, Albright Jr RE, Kukiatinant N, Shaw J, Armin D, Tew Jr J. Stereotactic radiosurgery for the treatment of brain metastases. Results of a single institution series. Cancer. 1997;79(3):551–7.
18. Shaw E, Scott C, Souhami L, Dinapoli R, Kline R, Loeffler J, Farnan N. Single dose radiosurgical treatment of recurrent previously irradiated primary brain tumors and brain metastases: final report of RTOG protocol 90-05. Int J Radiat Oncol Biol Phys. 2000;47(2):291–8.
19. Wakai S, Yamakawa K, Manaka S, Takakura K. Spontaneous intracranial hemorrhage caused by brain tumor: its incidence and clinical significance. Neurosurgery. 1982;10(4):437–44.
20. Kondziolka D, Bernstein M, Resch L, Tator CH, Fleming JF, Vanderlinden RG, Schutz H. Significance of hemorrhage into brain tumors: clinicopathological study. J Neurosurg. 1987;67(6):852–7.
21. Jones NR, Blumbergs PC. Intracranial haemorrhage from meningiomas: a report of five cases. Br J Neurosurg. 1989;3(6):691–8.

22. Gonda DD, Kim TE, Warnke PC, Kasper EM, Carter BS, Chen CC. Ventriculoperitoneal shunting versus endoscopic third ventriculostomy in the treatment of patients with hydrocephalus related to metastasis. Surg Neurol Int. 2012;3:97.
23. Chen CC, Kasper E, Warnke P. Palliative stereotactic-endoscopic third ventriculostomy for the treatment of obstructive hydrocephalus from cerebral metastasis. Surg Neurol Int. 2011;2:76.
24. Clarke JL, Perez HR, Jacks LM, Panageas KS, Deangelis LM. Leptomeningeal metastases in the MRI era. Neurology. 2010;74(18):1449–54.
25. Rosen ST, Aisner J, Makuch RW, Matthews MJ, Ihde DC, Whitacre M, Glatstein EJ, Wiernik PH, Lichter AS, Bunn Jr PA. Carcinomatous leptomeningitis in small cell lung cancer: a clinicopathologic review of the National Cancer Institute experience. Medicine (Baltimore). 1982;61(1):45–53.
26. Chamberlain MC. Neoplastic meningitis: diagnosis and treatment. In: Richard Winn H, editor. Youman's neurological surgery. 5th ed. Philadelphia: Saunders; 2004.
27. Quan GM, Vital JM, Aurouer N, Obeid I, Palussière J, Diallo A, Pointillart V. Surgery improves pain, function and quality of life in patients with spinal metastases: a prospective study on 118 patients. Eur Spine J. 2011;20(11):1970–8.
28. Zairi F, Arikat A, Allaoui M, Marinho P, Assaker R. Minimally invasive decompression and stabilization for the management of thoracolumbar spine metastasis. J Neurosurg Spine. 2012;17(1):19–23.
29. Burton AW, Rhines LD, Mendel E. Vertebroplasty and kyphoplasty: a comprehensive review. Neurosurg Focus. 2005;18(3):e1.
30. Eckel TS, Olan W. Vertebroplasty and vertebral augmentation techniques. Tech Vasc Interv Radiol. 2009;12(1):44–50.
31. Veeravagu A, Lieberson RE, Mener A, Chen YR, Soltys SG, Gibbs IC, Adler JR, Tian AG, Chang SD. CyberKnife stereotactic radiosurgery for the treatment of intramedullary spinal cord metastases. J Clin Neurosci. 2012;19(9):1273–7.
32. Fleming HW. Palliative neurosurgical methods. Cal West Med. 1927;27(3):386.
33. Gadgil N, Viswanathan A. DREZotomy in the treatment of cancer pain: a review. Stereotact Funct Neurosurg. 2012;90(6):356–60.
34. Wagemans FM, Zuurmond WA, De Lange J. Long-term spinal opioid therapy in terminally ill cancer pain patients. Oncologist. 1997;2:70–5.
35. Singh M, Cugati G, Singh P, Singh AK. Programmable morphine pump (an intrathecal drug delivery system) – a promising option for pain relief and palliation in cancer patients. Indian J Med Paediatr Oncol. 2012;33(1):58–9.
36. Lihua P, Su M, Zejun Z, Ke W, Bennett MI. Spinal cord stimulation for cancer-related pain in adults. Cochrane Database Syst Rev. 2013;(2):CD009389.

17 Head and Neck

Guy Rees

Contents

G. Rees, MBBS, FRCS, FRACS
Department of Otolaryngology and Head and Neck Surgery, The Royal Adelaide Hospital, 78 Harrow Road, Adelaide, SA 5000, Australia
e-mail: mail@entsurgeons.com.au, vivandguyrees@hotmail.com

The definition and range of care applicable to palliation of surgical patients is complex and involves multiple disciplines of the healthcare workforce. As surgeons, we must balance issues related *to* non-maleficence and beneficence whilst respecting the patient's autonomy. With regard to head and neck cancer, symptom control is complex and requires multidisciplinary care input to achieve the best ends for our patients. The importance of education and training in this area is emphasised. Ultimately, our patients should avoid suffering and maintain dignity, and as surgeons, we possess the skills to provide their care.

17.1 Introduction

What is palliative care? It is the support of physical, emotional and psychological suffering of patients with advanced illness regardless of age, diagnosis or life expectancy.

Palliative care (from Latin *palliare*, to cloak) is an area of healthcare that focuses on relieving and preventing the suffering of patients. *Palliative medicine* is appropriate for patients in all disease stages, including those undergoing treatment for

M. Wichmann, G. Maddern (eds.), *Palliative Surgery*,
DOI 10.1007/978-3-642-53709-7_17, © Springer-Verlag Berlin Heidelberg 2014

curable illnesses and those living with chronic diseases, as well as patients who are nearing the end of life. Palliative medicine utilises a multidisciplinary approach to patient care, relying on input from physicians, pharmacists, nurses, chaplains, social workers, psychologists and other allied health professionals in formulating a plan of care to relieve suffering in all areas of a patient's life. This multidisciplinary approach allows the palliative care team to address physical, emotional, spiritual and social concerns that arise with advanced illness.

With regard to head and neck cancer, symptom control is complex and requires multidisciplinary care input to achieve the best ends for our patients.

17.2 Characteristics of Palliative Care

Palliative care does the following:

- Provides relief from pain, shortness of breath, nausea and other distressing symptoms
- Affirms life and regards dying as a normal process
- Intends neither to hasten nor to postpone death
- Integrates the psychological and spiritual aspects of patient care
- Offers a support system to help patients live as actively as possible
- Offers a support system to help the family cope
- Uses a team approach to address the needs of patients and their families
- Will enhance quality of life
- Is applicable early in the course of illness, in conjunction with other therapies that are intended to prolong life, such as chemotherapy or radiation therapy

Whilst palliative care may seem to offer a broad range of services, the goals of palliative treatment are concrete: relief from suffering, treatment of pain and other distressing symptoms, psychological and spiritual care, a support system to help the individual live as actively as possible and a support system to sustain and rehabilitate the individual's family [1].

Patients at all stages of treatment need some kind of palliative care to comfort them. In some cases, medical specialty professional organisations recommend that patients and physicians respond to an illness only with palliative care and not with a therapy directed at the disease. The following items are indications named by the American Society of Clinical Oncology as characteristics of a patient who should receive palliative care but not any cancer-directed therapy [2]:

- Patient has low performance status, corresponding with limited ability to care for oneself.
- Patient received no benefit from prior evidence-based treatments.
- Patient is ineligible to participate in any appropriate clinical trial.
- The physician sees no strong evidence that treatment would be effective.

The aim is to prevent or alleviate suffering and to improve quality of life for patients with severe, complex illness.

17.3 Definitions of Surgical Palliative Care

Surgical palliative care is the treatment of suffering and the promotion of quality of life for seriously or terminally ill patients under surgical care [3].

Palliative surgery includes operations to relieve symptoms. The operations may be inclusive of treating disease with curative intent, but in all cases the management of symptoms should be an element of the intervention. Operations with curative intent in asymptomatic patients that result in residual disease or positive margins should be considered non-curative, non-palliative [4].

Surgical palliation for cancer is defined best as a procedure used with the primary intention of improving quality of life (QOL) or relieving symptoms caused by the advanced malignancy. The effectiveness of a palliative intervention should be judged by the presence and durability of patient-acknowledged symptom resolution [5].

Palliative surgery is an operation that is "largely intended for symptom relief *or* avoidance of symptoms or conditions anticipated secondary to progressive local disease, *and* is unlikely to alter the ultimate progression of disease in this patient or significantly impact patient survival" [6].

Palliative surgery is any invasive procedure in which the main intention is to mitigate physical symptoms in patients with non-curable disease without causing premature death [7].

Relief of suffering has always been the first priority of surgical care and this objective has never conflicted with the goal of cure [8, 9].

17.4 Principles of Surgical Palliative Care

The three cardinal surgical virtues in palliative caring are gentleness, skill and non-abandonment. These have been expanded on by Dunphy [10] discussing non- abandonment, Gaisford [11] on collegiality with colleagues and recognition of spiritual needs and Sugarbaker [12].

In 2005, the American Board of Surgery produced a statement of principles of Palliative Care [13]. This was an ethical compass for the conduct of care not only at end of life but in all encounters in which the relief of suffering and promoting quality of life are desired. It is an evolutionary step beyond the College's 1998 *Statement of Principles Guiding Care at End of Life*. The statement focused on an emphasis to provide palliative care alongside curative care and to understand when transition from one model to the other is appropriate. It was recognised that surgeons require training in procedural skills for palliation as well as cure [14].

When identifying surgical patients in need of palliative care, we should note that they have a serious or life-threatening condition, which is potentially responsive to a surgical intervention. At the same time, the patient's premorbid health conditions should not preclude surgical intervention as we recognise that these patients are at high risk for disease or treatment-related morbidity [15].

17.5 Principles of Palliative Surgery

Palliative surgery is frequently confused with or used interchangeably with non-curative surgery. A study performed by the Society of Surgical Oncology indicated that 95 % of respondents felt that palliative surgery was synonymous with gross residual tumour remaining on conclusion of an oncological procedure. When asked what should be included in a definition of palliative surgery, 43 % said it should be based on preoperative intent, 27 % on postoperative factors and 30 % on patient prognosis [16]. It is probably more accurate to say that the critical distinguishing principle separating palliative and non-curative surgery is that there is intent to provide asymptomatic patients with an oncological cure in non-curative surgery, whereas in palliative surgery, the intent is to relieve symptoms without consideration of any oncological benefit [17]. The primary aim in palliative surgery then is to durably alleviate symptoms, as acknowledged by the patient [15].

As surgical oncologists, 10–20 % of our practice is palliative surgery [18], a figure that is far greater if we move from malignancy as the underlying disease process to other chronic, life-limiting diseases. It is also important to understand that whilst there may be an association with end-of-life care, many palliative surgical procedures may be offered in patients with long-term survival. As surgeons, we are caring for the general needs of a patient, to alleviate their suffering as a whole, and so our management moves beyond surgical procedures to pain and nausea management, nutrition issues and psychological conditions associated with this patient group.

The costs related to palliative surgery are about 50 % of the resources in cancer surgery [19].

The moral and ethical questions about palliative surgery are those we face with any patient undergoing surgical care. The main challenge for us is to balance the moral duty to help with the ethical needs for non-maleficence and beneficence: primum non nocere. The patient's autonomy should not be overridden in the search to help, and giving advice to them is very difficult given the lack of evidence regarding outcomes of palliative surgery.

17.6 Cytoreductive/Aggressive Palliative Surgery

Surgery of this type is performed in the setting of advanced malignancy and may act to allow symptom control and in some cases to enhance disease control, possibly increasing the period of disease-free survival and rarely improving overall survival.

Patients who are offered this type of treatment must be carefully selected with regard to their age, comorbidities and performance status. In addition, the patient should be clear as to their aims and the quality and duration of survival whilst recovering from the morbidity of the procedure. In some cases, patients who are currently asymptomatic may be offered debulking surgery on the basis that future suffering and pain may be alleviated: this is a form of proactive palliative surgery.

17.7 Curative Resection of Primary Tumours with Short Anticipated Survival

In some instances, the morbidity of death from a primary tumour may outweigh the impact of distant metastatic disease. In these cases, whilst survival is not affected, the mode of death and the pathway to the end of life is alleviated: for example, total laryngectomy or glossectomy in a patient with pulmonary metastases. Patients in these situations may have a prolonged illness-free period, with better control of pain, and eventually succumb to the slow decline of chronic debility as the metastatic disease progresses. The critical issues here are to balance the quality-of-life impact of different modes of death, the duration of benefit and the morbidity of the procedure being performed.

17.8 End-of-Life Palliative Surgery

Sometimes palliative surgery occurs during the end-of-life period of care, but it may be offered well before this time is reached. In the end-of-life period, the escalating symptoms for the patient and the potentially short period of life left impact on the choice of procedures to be offered. In head and neck surgery, for example, the insertion of a naso-enteric feeding tube for fluid and nutrition may be offered, a tracheostomy may be performed to help deal with secretions or aspiration, or endovascular occlusion of feeding vessels causing bleeding into the airway may be performed. It is important to discuss these treatments with the patient and their family/support network as to the aims and outcomes of such interventions. Insertion of feeding tubes may prolong life through delivery of fluids and nutrition, but it is important to maximise other elements of symptom control at the same time, or the patient will just be delivered to a place of prolonged suffering.

17.9 Current Surgical Palliation

Obstruction of a viscus or airway by advanced malignancy often requires a surgical opinion and may be alleviated without the need for an open surgical procedure but by the placement of a stent. This draws into question whether this is actually a surgical procedure, as they can be inserted by nonsurgical colleagues, but the procedure to aid the patient is more important than the technician who supplies care. In addition, fixation of pathologic fractures may alleviate pain and aid speech and swallowing, if the mandible is affected, and endovascular stenting may improve blood flow and reduce the risk of major arterial bleed. Vessels may also be occluded endovascularly to stop bleeding [20].

17.10 Decision-Making in Palliative Surgery

It is a surgical skill to recognise when surgery will be too adventurous, ill advised or futile, given the condition of a patient. It is difficult to resist pressure to operate, whether this comes from the patient, relatives or medical colleagues, but it must be recognised that surgery cannot solve every problem [21].

Decision-making in palliative surgery requires superior surgical judgment owing to the narrow risk-benefit profile. Patient selection is critical and information is given to patients and family to allow best quality informed consent [16].

It had been assumed that palliative patients undergoing surgery have a higher operative morbidity and mortality rate, and thus they should not be considered for surgical intervention. This has been challenged in a study of stage and severity matched cases, who were being operated on with either curative or palliative intent, and had similar morbidity and mortality [6].

It is important to look beyond the immediate risk of the intervention to the patient towards to durability of benefit. It has been estimated that patients would need to survive for 60–90 days for the benefit of the surgical intervention to become apparent, as before this time, any benefits will be masked by the recovery time from the intervention itself [22].

The use of multidisciplinary clinics to give a forum to discuss palliative care allows the use of guidelines and evidence in many cases to be used. In some cases, the decision is made on the surgeon's experience and preferences. In these cases, the surgeons may be accurate in prediction of life expectancy, but less so in predicting benefit from the palliative intervention. There is a tendency to underestimate the success of the procedures, and hence it is possible that many patients will not be considered for interventions, and not be helped by these interventions [23].

17.11 Ethics of Palliative Surgery

Although surgery is an important part of palliative treatment, there has been relatively little focus on the moral aspects within palliative surgery [24].

In a study looking at moral dilemmas faced by surgeons when treating patients with palliative intent, it was notable that they used data including patient age, tumour biology, extent of disease and severity of symptoms when making treatment decisions. These individually tailored approaches have multiple areas of input, which also include surgical skills and preferences and not least, the patient's wishes. All factors must be balanced to make, what is a very complex decision in care planning [25]. The duty to help is a basic moral impetus in medicine, an essential obligation for all health professionals. This is especially so for those who are the weakest and face most suffering. This duty to help has been challenged in medicine as reports of overtreatment and the use of futile treatments are promulgated. There is a perception that surgeons have substantial professional autonomy and that most standard surgical therapies have never been subject to rigorous evaluation [26–28]. Thus, the duty of help can be interpreted too absolutely, without relevant balance, and especially so in palliative surgery with weak and vulnerable patients. It is part of our duty of care to ensure that we employ the best evidence for efficacy, effectiveness and efficiency in the options of care offered to these patients.

Duty of care to help is closely allied to another virtue: that of benevolence combined with compassion. Benevolence also requires consciousness of whether the actions actually help the patient in need, and one cannot offer drastic interventions on the basis of compassion and benevolence alone. It is important to be sensitive to the autonomy of the patient and not be excessively paternalistic wielding power with interventions.

Sometimes it is better to sit and watch rather than get up and do. This goes against patients and their relatives wanting everything possible to be done, in the support of hope of survival and continuance of life. Not doing anything is perceived as having given up on the patient [29]. The desire to do everything possible may enhance a misconceived duty to help, and it should be made clear to the patient the benefits or futility of intervention and also the health implications for the patient of having an intervention. Patients will come with a concept of the limitless ability of medicine in general and surgery in particular to cure them with little or no risk. If the efficacy, effectiveness and efficiency of palliative surgery are uncertain, it can be challenging to either offer or refuse intervention. At the same time, the patients should be supported emotionally, existentially and psychologically so that they retain hope and confidence in the treating team.

Informed consent is at the core of modern medicine and patient autonomy. This can be challenging in palliative surgery, as information about outcomes may be limited and the patients may be unable to comprehend the information given. Rapid changes in health status require forward thinking of care planning: what if? Questions must be raised and plans made by patients for the care they would like to be employed. Through this, options for care should be explored which may be surgical or nonsurgical and no sense of blame be carried by the patients with decisions taken. They should not feel pressured into "doing something for the family".

Priority is often given to patients with cancer requiring palliative surgery. As indicated previously, palliative surgery consumes approximately 50 % of the entire surgical oncology budget [19]. There may be an ethical imperative to decide where the health dollar should be spent: on delivering cure to patients or supporting during their inevitable decline to death. It is not clear that first world nations have grasped this nettle.

17.12 Priorities in Palliative Surgery: Future Considerations

We are faced with multiple competing elements driving our development of palliative surgical care. Primarily, we are responsible for high levels of fiscal responsibility in offering and delivering care. Increasing healthcare costs and health reforms aiming to curb those costs should be recognised. Secondly, we should strive to develop an evidence base to the care being offered with palliative surgery. This should be looking at the benefits and durability of symptom control, the cost of delivery of the care and the risk of such treatments to patients in terms of morbidity and mortality. The third issue reflects the empire growth effect in palliative care: we probably have only been treating the tip of an iceberg in palliative terms, but we should be wary of opening the Pandora's box too quickly and without planning and regulation of care delivery. It is best that this is regulated on a hospital basis through multidisciplinary clinics, with national bodies regulating the framework of care being offered through those clinics.

17.12.1 Education and Training

Life is a terminal disease, and it is sexually transmitted, according to John Cleese [30]. The development of improved education regarding palliative care should be encouraged in medical schools and form one of the core areas of education in surgical training. Patients with life-threatening conditions will articulate their needs and these should be our main goals of care. In order of importance, these would be as follows: pain and symptom control, avoidance of unnecessary and prolonged suffering, autonomy of care, to relive burden on their families and to strengthen relationships with loved ones [31]. We have a disconnect with these desires, and they increase as the severity of the disease increases, driving us towards more procedures and increased ICU care and resulting in lower satisfaction with care outcomes from patients and their families. To ease this, we should engage with patients and families to offer emotional support, involvement in decision-making and continued communication of key information of current and future expected changes and to offer treatment respectfully [32].

17.12.2 Multidisciplinary Care

The complexity of patient care escalates as they move from curative towards palliative intent in their treatment planning. The use of multidisciplinary clinics to bring together information with clinical and patient-derived input for discussion amongst skilled health professionals should allow better decision-making and a smoother coordination of care. The focus here is that the patient is at the centre of the clinic and all professionals involved are attempting to bring their best quality of care to that patient. A care plan is derived from the group and a recommendation of care or options of treatment is made. The implementation of that care plan occurs with the acceptance and involvement of the patient and their family. Feedback is given from the patient care interface back to the clinic to assess the impact of the care plan. This serves to improve quality of care and gives data to use in future patient care [33].

17.13 Head and Neck Palliative Surgery

Surgeons of this era are increasingly being asked to care for an older group of patients presenting with an increasing number of cancer-related diseases, on the background of comorbidity which comes with age. We should adapt to this by looking at illness rather than disease as our focus. We are taught to identify disease in organs and to treat those diseases, whereas illness, the individuals' experience of disease, occurs in people. As surgeons, we are specialists in the care of people afflicted with disease, rather than specialists in the surgical treatment of neoplastic disease [34].

In head and neck cancer (HNC), the disease processes are complex and the outlook uncertain, leading to the delivery of radical treatments whose intent is palliative. The spectrum of care delivery for palliation may range from primary treatment, through salvage therapy and to end-of-life terminal care.

The pattern of HNC is commonly one of initial treatment, with response, followed by relapse associated with significant symptomatology and impact on daily functioning with physical, emotional and psychological effects. It is important to realise that, in many areas of HNC, the management of advanced HNC has increased the disease-free interval, but overall cure rates have not changed. The mode of treatment failure and recurrence pattern has changed, and patients often live longer with quiescent subclinical disease.

Palliative care staff should be involved at an early stage in the treatment planning of patients where the treatment aim has changed from curative to supportive care with symptom control. Patients should feel that they have not been "abandoned" by their care team, but to realise that specialist input is being requested for a new phase in the management of their condition. Continuation of care by the team should be maintained through this period.

The location for delivery of palliative care should be centred upon the patient, their home and family support group, with the utilisation of community-based palliative support teams. Admission to hospital may be required for periods of stabilisation of symptoms and optimisation of care, with the aim to return the patient to their home, as and when clinically appropriate. If social and home support networks are lacking or if the disease process is too complex to manage, admission to institutional care may be the only sensible option.

The relationships developed between the patient and the surgical or oncology staffs are critical to the stability of care delivery at this time. Adaptability and response to change along with open access for communication are critical issues.

17.14 Relevance of Palliative Care in the Care of HNC

The incorporation of dedicated palliative care teams into the multidisciplinary care of HNC services is central to care in Australia and New Zealand. The major role of palliative care teams in this setting includes the management of symptoms, maintenance of quality of life and supervision of end-of-life care.

17.14.1 Quality of Life

QOL is a subjective phenomenon, encompassing physical, psychological, spiritual and social domains. Each of these may be individually or serially important and vary over the time course of the disease. All domains should be addressed at any time to deliver care, which covers the needs of the patient. Calman explored the concept of quality of life being a measure of the patient's expectation and the perceived experience of their current state of health [35]. This introduces the important variable of variability in the value patients attribute to certain measures of health. The aim therefore is to close the distance between expectation and reality as far as possible. Communication, education and response to needs are central elements of this process. In advanced disease, the clinician should not remove hope, but allow patients to make judgments of best use of time, allowing better use of life and planning for the eventuality of death.

17.14.2 Symptom Control

Patients with HNC have disease-specific and general physical problems, which may be multiple synchronously or metachronously. These problems may present at any stage of the disease (diagnosis, during treatment, during remission or during progression) and even during "cure" of disease. It is therefore important that palliative care professionals are available to be called upon throughout the entire time course of patient care.

Head and neck cancer may cause symptoms from the direct or indirect effect of the underlying cancer, the effects of cancer treatment and concomitant disease. Not all symptoms reported by patients relate to the cancer directly, and physical symptoms should be managed appropriate to their aetiology. The importance of detailed history taking and close attention to examination with appropriate relevant investigations will allow appropriate care delivery.

The pathway of care starts with initial assessment, treatment of the cause of the symptom, treatment of the symptom itself followed by reassessment. The treatment of the underlying cause of the symptom is most effective to produce significant and lasting symptom control, but sometimes this is not possible. The use of previous therapy, patient's health-related factors, their prognosis and wishes all impact on the delivery of care. It is important to realise that the range of palliative support options is wide and that a holistic approach to care delivery is employed, utilising skills of all members of the multidisciplinary care (MDC) HNC team, where appropriate.

17.15 Living with Head and Neck Cancer and Coping with Dying When Treatments Fail

It has been suggested that many cancer patients die an undignified death with poorly controlled symptoms [36]. In contrast, a "good death" is one which is pain free, peaceful and dignified in a place of the patient's choosing with relatives present and without futile interventions [37]. Although there may be a feeling that dying at home is a primary objective, acceleration of symptoms in the last couple of days may overwhelm patients and their families, who then opt for a skilled care environment [38]. The reasons put forward by patients and family members for the switch in care delivery site relate to effective pain relief and symptom management followed by preservation of dignity and hygiene as overriding concerns [39]. These factors appear to be particularly marked for head and neck cancer patients in comparison with the experience of other cancer patients [40].

When examining symptoms of patients at the end of life, pain is common (84 %) and generally managed well, mainly with opioids. Generally symptom control at this time is good, except for neuropsychological problems. Sixty-three percent died in hospital and only 22 % had a relative with them at the time of death. It is unusual to enact resuscitative measures at the time of death, or to use ICU care. The most common triggers for admission are airway bleeding, pain, dysphagia and breathing difficulties [38].

As mentioned previously, the aim of palliative care is to allow care delivery in the patient's own home surrounded by family and support. The complexity of care in the terminal period of life with HNC results in the admission of many patients. A recent study on the UK reported that 53 % of patients were hospitalised in their last month of life, due to bleeding (17 %), pain (9 %), breathing difficulties (9 %), swallowing difficulties (9 %), inability to cope (6 %) and fracture (3 %) [41]. Despite this, the terminal phase in HNC is often straightforward and, with appropriate levels of care and support, could occur in the home. The reality is that a UK study showed that 62 % died in a hospital, 19 % in a hospice, 16 % at home and 3 % in a nursing home [42]. The reasons for this are not entirely clear, but home death is more common in younger patients and in those with better symptom control.

Aside from palliative radiotherapy or chemotherapy, there are some areas where surgical palliation is the primary mode of care. The goal of palliative surgery is to improve the patient's quality of life by reducing symptoms without the additive effect of surgical complications [43].

Cancer of the head and neck often requires treatment to provide patients with adequate voice use and the ability to swallow. Endoluminal debulking of pharyngeal and laryngeal lesions can be useful palliation, avoiding the need for a tracheostomy and allowing them to use palliative chemotherapy or radiotherapy or to buy time for definitive palliative surgery. The use of laser allows clean, haemostatic tumour removal with predictable healing [44, 45]. In the Paleri study, the main indicators for duration of survival were tumour stage, site and performance score. One- and three-year survival rates were 15.8 and 1 % for oral cavity, 14.4 and 1.7 % for oropharynx, 27.8 and 1 % for larynx and 12 and 0 % for hypopharynx. There was noted to be a general tendency to offer treatment to a greater proportion of patients over time, albeit without any change in overall survival.

When examining the actual cause of death in head and neck palliative patients, more than half die of the effects of the cancer itself, with the others dying of pneumonia, respiratory failure, stroke and myocardial infarction [46].

In another study, again approximately half of all patients die of the effects of the head and neck tumour directly. Other cancer-related deaths were related to carotid artery invasion and bleeding, disseminated disease and second primary tumour. Non-cancer-related deaths included pneumonia and exacerbation of pulmonary disease, and these accounted for a quarter of all deaths [47].

Weight loss and malnutrition are major problems in patients with advanced head and neck cancer, with more than half having significant weight loss and cachexia [48], and approximately 20 % of all cancer-related deaths are caused by cachexia [49]. Cancer cachexia is different to starvation as it is associated with preferential loss of muscle over adipose tissue, increased proteolysis and lipolysis, increased metabolic activity of the liver and increased production of acute-phase proteins. This causes an inappropriate increase in resting energy expenditure even as dietary intake falls with anorexia [50]. The impact of weight loss directly reduces survival, with poorer responses to treatment and increased toxicity to treatment. This leads to increased risk of tumour recurrence [51, 52].

17.16 Summary

As surgical oncologists, we have a duty to care for the physical, emotional and psychological suffering of patients. In the case of surgical palliation, we may offer procedures used with the primary intention of improving quality of life (QOL) or relieving symptoms caused by the advanced malignancy. Our cardinal virtues as surgeons are gentleness, skill and non-abandonment. The main challenge for us is to balance the moral duty to help with the ethical needs for non-maleficence and beneficence.

In the case of head and neck cancer patients, issues related to function maintenance and control of pain are of particular importance with care for airway, nutritional intake and communication of specific interest. In the terminal stage of the disease process, head and neck cancer patients require symptom control and dignity: we are equipped to provide this care.

References

1. Walsh D, Gombeski W, Goldstein P, Hayes D, Armour M. Managing a palliative oncology program: the role of a business plan. J Pain Symptom Manage. 1994; 9(2):109.
2. American Society of Clinical Oncology. Five things physicians and patients should question. Choosing Wisely: an initiative of the ABIM Foundation. American Society of Clinical Oncology.
3. Cameron JL, editor. Current surgical therapy. 9th ed. Philadelphia: Mosby, Inc.; 2007. p. 1179.
4. Wagman LD. Palliative surgical oncology. Surg Oncol Clin North Am. 2004;13:XIIIeXIV.
5. Miner T. Palliative surgery for advanced cancer. Lessons learned in patient selection and outcome assessment. Am J Clin Oncol. 2005;28(4):411–4.
6. McCahill LE, Smith DD, Borneman T, Juarez G, Cullinane C, Chu DZJ. A prospective evaluation of palliative outcomes for surgery of advanced malignancies. Ann Surg Oncol. 2003;10:654–63.
7. Hofmann B, Håheim LL, Søreide JA. Ethics of palliative surgery in patients with cancer. Br J Surg. 2005;92:802–9.
8. Billroth T. Ueber esophagus resektion. Arch Klin Chir. 1872;13:65.
9. Halsted WS. The results of operations for the cure of cancer of the breast performed at the Johns Hopkins Hospital from June, 1899, to January, 1894. Johns Hopkins Hosp Rep. 1894–1895;4:297.

10. Dunphy JE. On caring for the patient with cancer. N Engl J of Med. 1976;295:313–9.
11. Gaisford JC. Palliative surgery. JAMA. 1972;221:83–4.
12. Sugarbaker PH, Barofsky I, et al. Quality of life assessment in extremity sarcoma trials. Surgery. 1982;91:17–23.
13. Statement of principles of palliative care. Task Force on Surgical Palliative care. Committee on Ethics. Bull Am Coll Surg. 2005;90(8):34–5.
14. Surgeons Palliative Care Workgroup. Report from the field. J Am Chem Soc. 2003;197(4):661–86.
15. Hanna J, Blazer DG, Mosca PJ. Overview of palliative surgery: principles and priorities. J Palliative Care Med. 2012;2:7.
16. McCahill LE, Krouse R, Chu D, Juarez G, Uman GC, et al. Indications and use of palliative surgery-results of Society of Surgical Oncology survey. Ann Surg Oncol. 2002;9:104–12.
17. Sallnow L, Feuer D. The role of surgery in the palliation of malignancy. Clin Oncol (R Coll Radiol). 2010; 22:713–8.
18. Dunn GP, Weissman DE. Surgical palliative care: a residents guide. Essex: American College of Surgeons/Cunniff-Dixon Foundation; 2009.
19. Giercksky K-E, Grønbech JE, Hammelbo T, Hirschberg H, Lundar T, Mjåland O. Use of palliative surgery in the treatment of cancer patients. Report 8. Oslo: The Norwegian Centre for Health Technology Assessment; 2003.
20. Sallnow L, Feuer D. The role of surgery in the palliation of malignancy. Clin Oncol. 2010;22:713–8.
21. National Confidential Enquiry into Perioperative Deaths. The report of the National Confidential Enquiry into Perioperative Deaths 1996/1997. London: NCEPOD; 1997.
22. Podnos YD, Juarez G, Pameijer C, Choi K, Ferrell B, Wagman LD. Impact of surgical palliation on quality of life in patients with advanced malignancy: results of the Decisions and Outcomes in Palliative Surgery (DOPS) trial. Ann Surg Oncol. 2007;14(2):922–8.
23. Smith DD, McCahill LE. Predicting life expectancy and symptom relief following surgery for advanced malignancy. Ann Surg Oncol. 2008;15(12):3335–41.
24. Foley KM, Gelbrand H. Improving palliative care for cancer. Washington, DC: National Academy Press; 2001.
25. McCahill LE, Krouse RS, Chu DZJ, Juarez G, Uman GC, Ferrell BG, et al. Decision making in palliative surgery. J Am Coll Surg. 2002;195:411–22.
26. Meakins JL. Innovation in surgery. Am J Surg. 2002; 183:399–405.
27. Woods WC. Design and interpretation of clinical trials. In: Morris PJ, Wood WC, editors. Oxford textbook of surgery. Oxford: Oxford University Press; 2000. p. 177–83.
28. Spodick DH. Numerators without denominators. There is no FDA for the surgeon. JAMA. 1975;232:35–6.
29. Jecker NS, Schneiderman LJ. When families request that "everything possible" be done. J Med Philos. 1995;20:145–63.
30. Cleese J. Life and how to survive it. London, GB: Publ Mandarin; 2004. ISBN 0749311088.
31. Singer PA, Martin DK, Kelner M. Quality end-of-life care: patient's perspectives. JAMA. 1999;281:163–8.
32. Teno JM, Mor V, Ward N, Roy J, Clarridge B, et al. Bereaved family member perceptions of quality of end-of-life care in U.S. regions with high and low usage of intensive care unit care. J Am Geriatr Soc. 2005;53:1905–11.
33. Rialon KL, Abernethy AP, Mosca PJ. Integration of palliative surgery into the palliative care delivery team. J Palliative Care Med. 2012;2:1–2.
34. Dunn GP. Principles and core competencies of surgical palliative care: an overview. Otolaryngol Clin North Am. 2009;42(1):1–13.
35. Calman KC. Quality of life in cancer patients—an hypothesis. J Med Ethics. 1984;10(3):124–7.
36. Ellershaw WC. Care of the dying patient: the last hours or days of life. BMJ. 2003;326:30–4.
37. Cohen LM, et al. A very good death: measuring quality of dying in end stage renal disease. J Palliat Med. 2001;4:167–72.
38. Fried T, et al. Older persons preference for site of terminal care. Ann Intern Med. 1999;131:109–12.
39. Steinhauser KE, et al. In search of a good death: observations of patients families and providers. Ann Intern Med. 2000;132:825–32.
40. van den Beuken MH, et al. Prevalence of pain with cancer: a systematic review of the past 40 years. Ann Oncol. 2007;18(9):1437–49.
41. Forbes K. Palliative care of patients with head and neck carcinoma. Clin Otol. 1997;22(2):117–22.
42. Talmi YP, et al. Pain experienced by patients with terminal head and neck carcinoma. Cancer. 1997;80(6):1117–23.
43. Forbes JF. Palliative surgery in cancer patients: principles and potential of palliative surgery in patients with advanced cancer. Recent Results Cancer Res. 1988;108:134–42.
44. Lim RY. Laser tumour debulking. W V Med J. 1989;85(12):530–2.
45. Paleri V, et al. Laser debulking in malignant upper airway obstruction. Head Neck. 2005;27(4):296–301.
46. Wutzl A, et al. Mortality and cause of death after multimodality treatment for advanced oral and oropharyngeal cancer. J Oral Maxillofac Surg. 2007;65(2):255–60.
47. Coatesworth AP. The cause of death in patients with head and neck squamous carcinoma. J Laryngol Otol. 2002;116:269–71.
48. Lees J. Incidence of weight loss in head and neck cancer patients commencing radiotherapy treatment at a regional oncology centre. Eur J Cancer Care. 1999;8: 133–6.
49. Inagki J, et al. Causes of death in cancer patients. Cancer. 1974;33:568–71.
50. Tisdale MJ. Cachexia in cancer patients. Nature. 2002;2:862–71.
51. Dewys WD. Weight loss and nutritional abnormalities in cancer patients: incidence, severity and significance. Clin Oncol. 1986;5:251.
52. Nguyen TV, et al. Weight loss predicts mortality after recurrent oral cavity and oropharyngeal carcinomas. Cancer. 2002;52:72–91.

Craniomaxillofacial Area

18

David J. David

Contents

D.J. David, MBBS, MD, FRCS, FRACS
Australian Cranio-Facial Unit, David David Medical Services, Women & Children's Hospital, Royal Adelaide Hospital, 226 Melbourne Street, North Adelaide, SA 5006, Australia
e-mail: ddavid@ddms.com.au

The meaning of palliation needs to be clearly defined. Once understood that it does not involve the intention to cure the underlying disease, the multidisciplinary task of relieving symptoms can be undertaken. Surgeons have a key role in this phase of the delivery of health care enlisting the wide range of procedures available to them to support their patients.

18.1 Introduction

In dealing with palliative surgery of the cranio-maxillofacial region, this chapter will focus only on those areas of the author's personal expertise and experience and that is essentially those structures bordering the maxillae, namely, the nasal cavity medially, the orbits and base of skull above, the oral cavity below and laterally and the covering integument and contained viscera.

18.2 Definition of Palliation

Fundamental to any consideration of this topic is a clear understanding of the meaning of the terms. A search of the recent literature on surgical palliation of the region under discussion revealed that all the publications dealt with malignant lesions [1]. These authors used the following definition: "any invasive procedure in which the main intention is to mitigate physical symptoms in patients with non-curable disease without causing premature death". They rightly

M. Wichmann, G. Maddern (eds.), *Palliative Surgery*,
DOI 10.1007/978-3-642-53709-7_18, © Springer-Verlag Berlin Heidelberg 2014

point out that the difficulty in defining palliative care is an epistemological and ethical one.

The current Oxford English Dictionary definition of the word palliative used as an adjective is "(of an action) intended to alleviate a problem without addressing the underlying cause". This latter definition suits my current task as it allows me to deal with a wider range of clinical problems and hence with some of the potential solutions.

This chapter will deal with some of the problems that are associated with benign conditions such as fibrous dysplasia and neurofibromatosis which fit under the latter definition.

18.3 Philosophical and Ethical Issues

The philosophical setting for modern western medical practice has been, like the rest of the culture developed from the ancient Greeks (Hippocrates), spread throughout the Roman Empire, was nurtured and preserved in the monasteries in the Middle Ages, value added by scientific Islam (Ibn Sina known mostly as Avicenna) and arrived at its present state via the Enlightenment.

Throughout this development the overall philosophical thrust that has informed medical ethical practice has been to put the patient first ahead of the physician's needs and those of the general body politic. This ethic is widely expressed in the various renditions of the Hippocratic Oath taken by new medical graduates.

Enduring as it has been, this patient-centred concept is under significant challenge in the post-modern world and its strange bedfellow "economic rationalism".

18.4 Clinical Setting

The clinical setting in which decisions are made about the institution of palliative care and its implementation is widely considered to be most appropriately a multidisciplinary one where the surgeon is one among equals rather than the team leader. Almost every paper reviewed that dealt with palliation of malignant disease drew attention to the necessity of a multifaceted team that in these circumstances extended itself beyond the hospital environment into the community via outreach nursing services and specialised palliative care centres [2, 3]. These two papers open a window to the extensive literature attempting to deal with this difficult problem.

So it is with management of the non-malignant but incurable conditions and the multidisciplinary approach for managing these conditions that has been set out and implemented for many years [4].

18.5 Six Principles of Health-Care Delivery

Such teams should be based on six principles of health-care delivery, namely:

1. Be multidisciplinary.
2. Be protocol driven.
3. Measure outcomes.
4. Manage the patient through the whole of development or through the whole disease process.
5. Have a research arm.
6. Be involved in teaching.

These principles are reflected throughout the literature on head and neck cancer as well as that on craniomaxillofacial surgery. Ledeboer et al. made the point that recently there has been more prospective work in the area, but very few randomised trials, and a review of the literature at the time indicated that little was known of the long-term influence of various treatment modalities for palliation [5].

With respect to malignant disease of the craniomaxillary region, few would now argue that the multidisciplinary approach is not necessary for management; in view of the almost static state of the survival rates and the increased emphasis on quality of life and relief of symptoms, the team approach is mandatory to establish protocols for the establishment of surgical palliation in each patient. Often patients will progress to the palliative stage without being considered suitable for potentially curable management [6]. Sorting out whether a patient is for palliation, salvage surgery or that vague indication of potential palliation based on knowledge of the natural history of the disease with a view to palliating a symptom likely to occur in the near future while the situation is propitious is most difficult without multidisciplinary input [7].

18.6 Types of Pathology

18.6.1 Malignant Tumours, Orbit, Maxilla, Oral Cavity/Mandible, and Skin

Each of these anatomical regions has its own set of problems when it comes to palliative treatment by surgery. The usual scenario is that of uncontrolled primary disease that recurs in an irradiated field.

The orbit may be the focus of palliative surgery when a previously exenterated and skin-grafted orbit exhibits local recurrence, or there is invasion from the adjacent paranasal sinuses. A less common but very vexing situation is that of the secondary sarcoma of the orbit occurring years after treatment of childhood malignancy such as rhabdomyosarcoma. The issues for palliation are fungation, ulceration, smell, altered appearance and pain.

The maxilla abutting as it does on the oral cavity, nasal cavity, orbit and infratemporal fossa can have advanced lesions that occur in a resected and skin-grafted primary surgical site; the extensive recurrence can be beneath the flap repair and the more or less sophisticated reconstruction; it may cause airway obstruction, may invade branches of cranial nerve V or indeed ulcerate through the facial integument.

The oral cavity and mandible are involved in the airway, speech, mastication, swallowing and social interaction. Problems to be palliated include the effects of fungating or ulcerating recurrent tumours, the effects of altered anatomy resulting from treatment as well as disease; this includes the radiation changes to the lining mucosa. Osteoradionecrosis mixed with recurrent cancer can be painful and malodorous. The presence of an exposed carotid artery in an adjacent irradiated field with overlying damaged skin poses a difficult potential situation with the possibility of carotid blow out which has high morbidity and mortality. This event is a frightening experience for all involved.

The skin may be affected with primary uncontrolled skin cancer, recurrent skin cancer and secondary deposits from distant sources and by underlying tumours fungating through the integument. A common clinical situation in the Australian setting is the elderly, unwell, male patient with advanced skin cancer of the balding scalp which is painful, difficult to clean and dress, bleeds and is unsightly.

18.6.2 Benign Tumours

18.6.2.1 Neurofibromatosis

Neurofibromatosis (neurofibromatosis type 1 is also known as von Recklinghausen disease) is a genetically inherited disorder in which the nerve tissue grows tumours (neurofibromas) that may be benign and may cause serious damage by compressing nerves and other tissues. The disorder affects all neural crest cells (Schwann cells, melanocytes and endoneurial fibroblasts). This can result in excessive tissue proliferation, in the case of the head and neck giving rise to gross facial distortion and loss of function around the orbits, facial soft tissue and oral cavity as well as throughout the body (Fig. 18.1). It is an incurable disease and the symptoms need palliation.

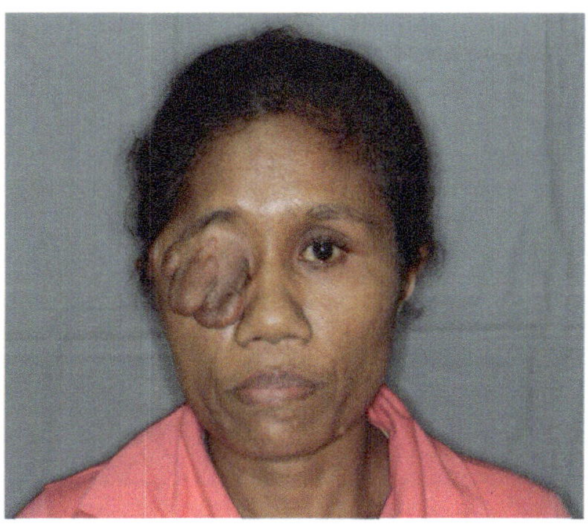

Fig. 18.1 Neurofibromatosis type 1, unsightly but incurable. An example of palliation in a benign condition

18.6.2.2 Fibrous Dysplasia

Fibrous dysplasia occurs when normal bone is replaced with fibrous bone tissue. This results in abnormal growth or swelling of bone. Fibrous dysplasia can occur in any part of the skeleton but the bones of the skull, thigh, shin, ribs, upper arm and pelvis are most commonly affected and there is no known cure. Fibrous dysplasia is not malignant.

Most lesions in the head and neck region are monostotic that is involving one or adjacent bones. When the lesions are identified early and are small enough to be excised in their entirety, the condition can be cured. However, when allowed to grow extensively throughout the craniofacial skeleton, the manifestations can be gross affecting the airway, eyes and calvarium (Fig. 18.2). It is at this stage that management is long term and surgical intervention palliative.

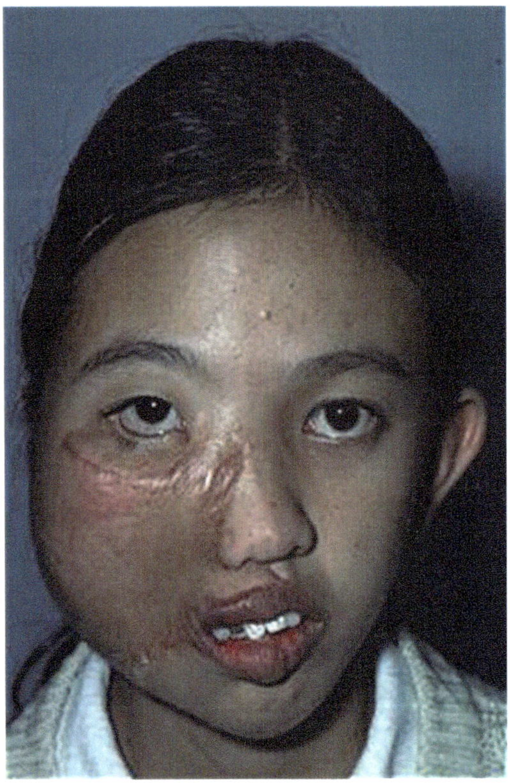

Fig. 18.2 Fibrous dysplasia, extending widely throughout the facial skeleton. The disease recurred relentlessly throughout this woman's life

18.6.3 Other Incurable Conditions Requiring Palliation in the Broad Sense

18.6.3.1 Post-trauma

The all too common panfacial fracture and the unfortunate increase in gunshot wounds of the head and face result, in spite of high-quality modern reconstructive techniques, in clinical situations requiring palliative surgery in the broad sense of the term. Permanent change of appearance, ever-increasing restriction of jaw movement, progressive premature loss of dentition and ongoing care of damaged eyes and orbits present continuing palliative challenges to surgeons and their teams (Fig. 18.3).

18.6.3.2 Congenital Deformities

There are now an increasing number of patients with severe deformities who because of advanced health-care systems can lead relatively full lives but are in need of continuing monitoring with a view of surgical and other palliative measures as the disease process continues to manifest itself with age. An example of such conditions is the craniosynostosis syndromes of Crouzon and Apert. Even after full protocol management severe symptoms such as eye exposure, airway obstruction and loss of dentition may occur with age requiring surgical intervention for palliation (Fig. 18.4).

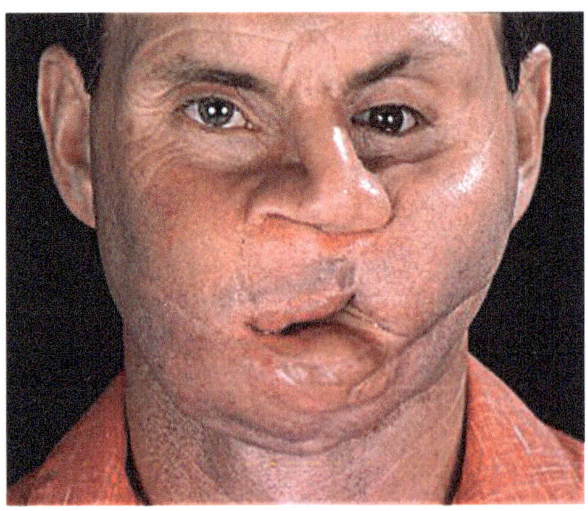

Fig. 18.3 Long-term follow-up of a devastating gunshot wound

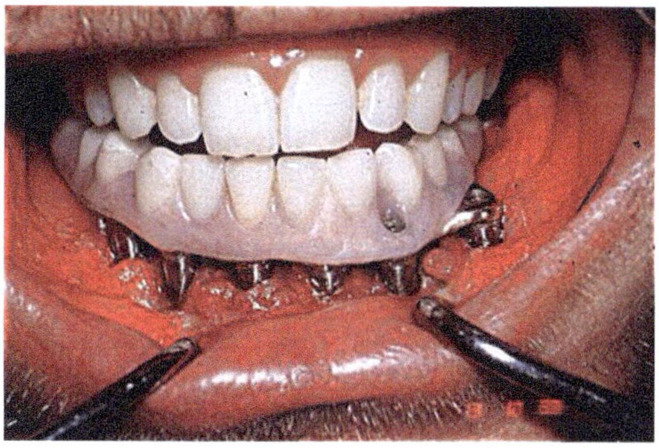

Fig. 18.4 Loss of dentition requiring osseo-integrated dental reconstruction as part of the palliative package

18.6.3.3 Some Degenerations

Other disease processes lend themselves to be considered in this context. Degenerations where bone and/or soft tissue withers and/or disappears over time such as Romberg's hemifacial atrophy or hypertrophy and aberrant growth of Proteus syndrome (elephant man syndrome) (Fig. 18.5a–c).

18.7 Planning

18.7.1 The Team, the Treatment Protocol and the Outcome Measures

The necessity of the team approach and systems-based practice is widely recognised in the literature if not so widely practiced in reality [5–9].

Those patients with cancer require a continuum of management as the disease progresses, and it is not always evident to the patient or treating specialists whether treatment is still being aimed at cure or for the relief of symptoms. If surgery is to be used for the dedicated purpose of relief of symptoms, this will need to be made clear. The decision processes necessary during the progress through incurable disease to death are best managed by a team so that the protocols can be adjusted, and all modalities of care necessary to palliate the patient are introduced in a timely and effective manner.

Some palliative measures may need to be introduced at a time when there is still a hope of cure and such therapies are in place, for example, airway protection, measures to reduce disfigurement and covering a potentially vulnerable vessel.

Measuring outcomes is intimately bound up with delivery of the service by a multidisciplinary team as surgeons and patients expectations may not match and the differences may not be communicated. The role of social worker, palliative nurses and others on the team is crucial in bridging this gap. Meaningful data on the outcomes of palliative surgery are understandably difficult to come by; however, it is clear that there is little time between decision to palliate and time of death placing an emphasis on surgeons not to make the surgical intervention more burdensome than the disease. Many of the problems encountered with meaningful outcome measures in this difficult area of practice are well described by Shuman and colleagues [10, 11]. These authors and others fully acknowledge that further research in the experience of managing patients with terminal head and neck malignancy is greatly needed.

There is little or no literature directed to the broader concept of palliation as applied to the nonfatal but incurable diseases mentioned previously.

18.8 Surgical Techniques for Palliation of Craniomaxillary Disease

At the point when attempts to cure give way to palliation, it is quality-of-life issues that become the patients and hence the treating team's primary concern. The following symptoms are the most common in those patients approaching death with their incurable disease.

Pain from head and neck cancer can be caused by direct stimulation of nerve endings, by ulceration and infection producing and open wound, by compression and invasion of sensory nerves (Fig. 18.6a, b) and by invasion of bone.

The referred pain from the tonsillar fossa tumour to the ear is an example of direct stimulation.

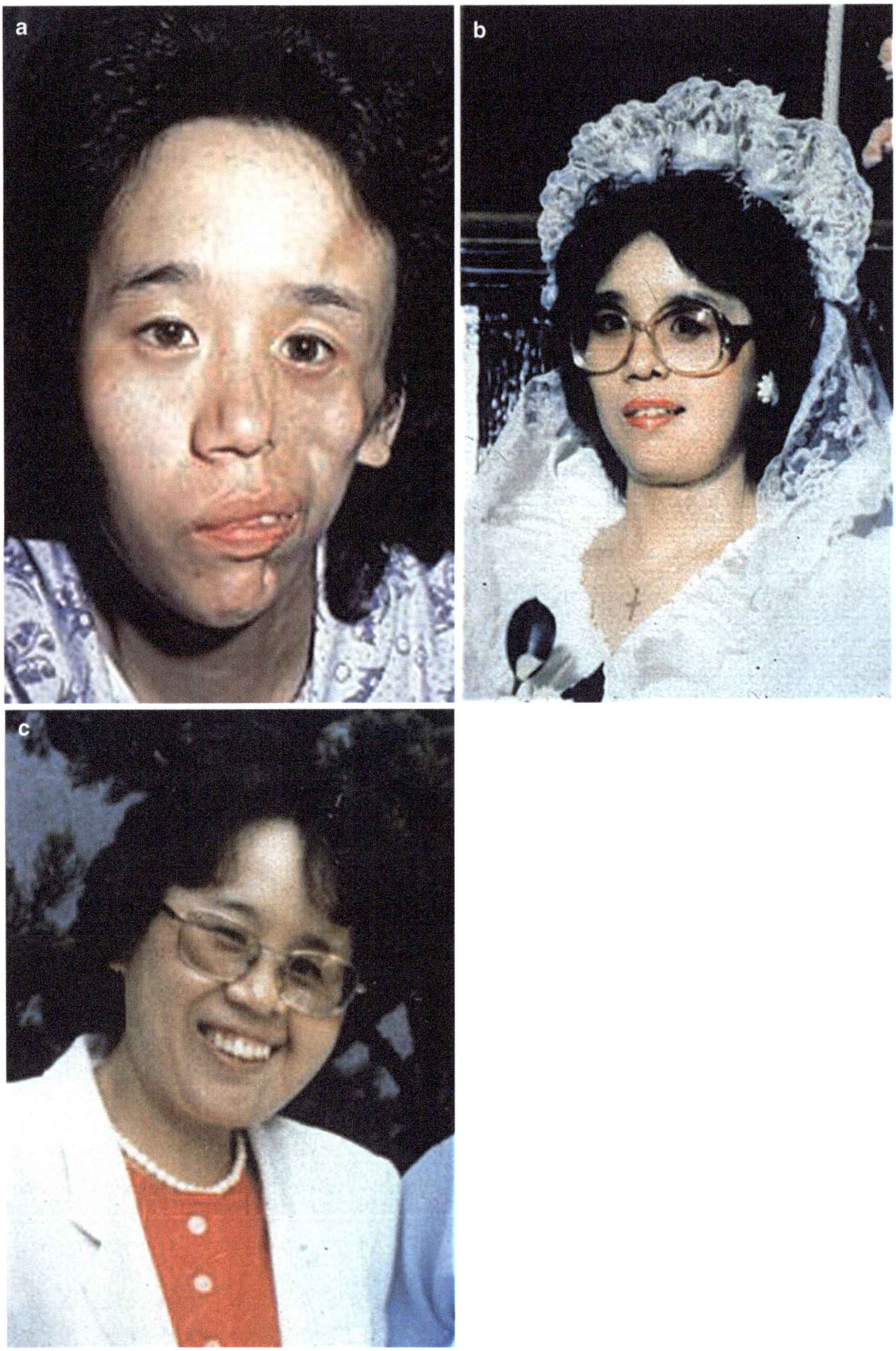

Fig. 18.5 (**a**–**c**) Romberg's hemifacial atrophy

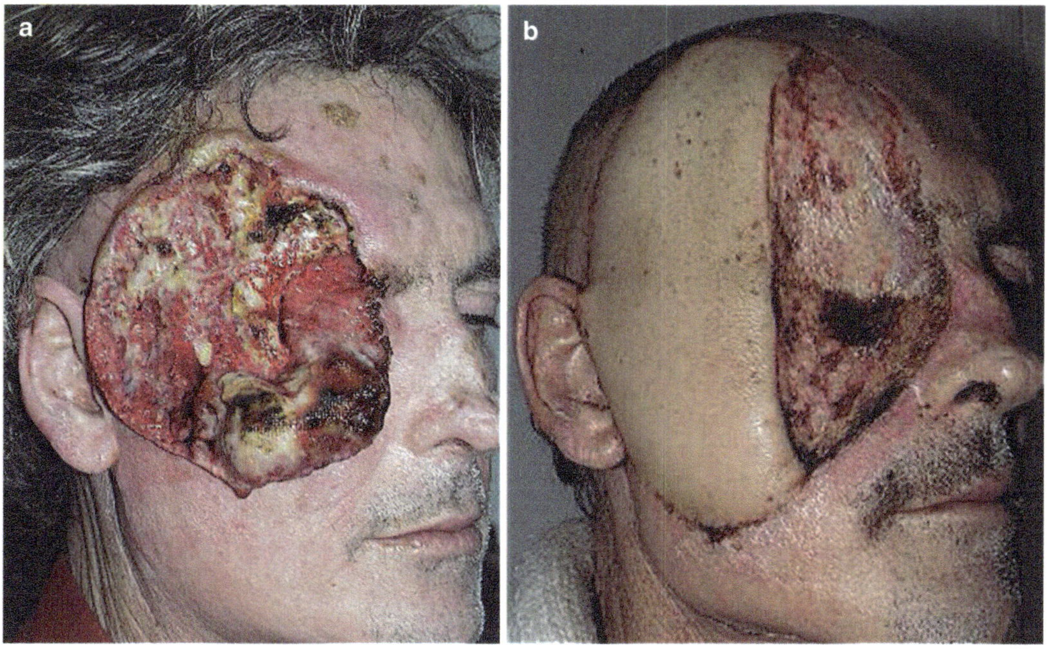

Fig. 18.6 (**a**, **b**) A massive painful fungating tumour (**a**) palliated by excision and flap coverage (**b**)

Ulceration and infection in the oral cavity produces pain that is exacerbated by irritant factors during eating and swallowing. Skin ulceration, for example, on the scalp, is often painful to debride, clean and dress.

Nerve invasion can result in tumour travelling through the cranial base foraminae to the Gasserian ganglion and beyond. Cranial nerves V and IX are most frequently involved in this manner.

Bone pain may be exacerbated by a pathological fracture, e.g., of the mandible, or associated with nerve pain as the tumour invades the skull.

The management of pain rarely falls in the realm of surgery and is most often managed by specific pain teams. The techniques of nerve blocks may be very helpful in this region. Irrespective of who is palliating these patients, it is the author's experience that the surgeon should maintain close contact with the patient who almost invariably considers this as a significant support.

It is worth revisiting the difficult situation of "salvage surgery" when the aim of the surgeon may be ambivalent, there being still some hope of cure, but emphasis is also on preventing pain caused by local recurrence. The poor outcomes in terms of complications and function place the emphasis on the surgeon to carefully consider the options [12]. A potentially short survival time together with a high complication rate from complex surgery is not a good combination.

However, if at the time of "salvage surgery" great care is given to reconstructive techniques such as using carefully constructed flap repair (pedicled or microvascular) which are sculpted to fit the defect and sensate where possible, the high proportion of such patients that proceed to palliative care will potentially have less of a local burden [13].

Painful ulcerating lesions of the scalp need careful dressing and debridement; once again the presence and guidance of the treating surgeon is much appreciated for the contact if nothing else. Excision and skin grafting can be of great help if done under local anaesthetic using regional blocks. Care must be taken to preserve a viable bed for the graft in what is often a much compromised region. Occasionally local rotation or transposition flaps can be used, employing similar regional anaesthetic techniques, when there is a risk of exposed bare bone or even

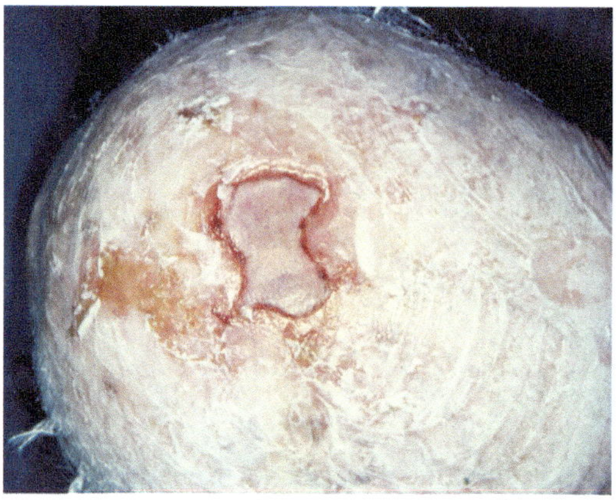

Fig. 18.7 A sun-affected scalp with advanced skin cancer, selective excision and grafting can keep the area clean and pain free

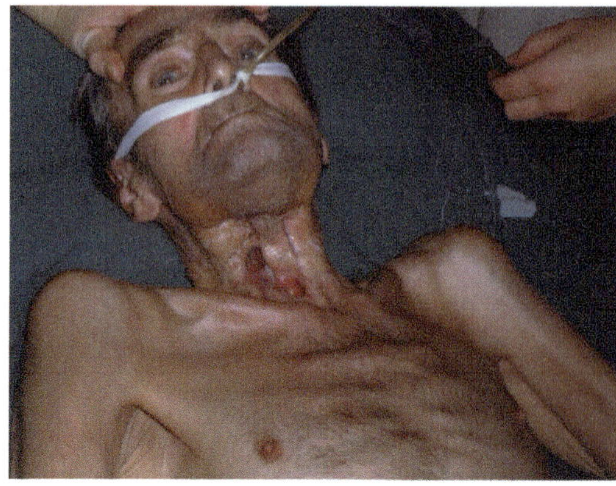

Fig. 18.8 Radiation, surgery, recurrent tumour, salivary fistula near the major vessels

exposed dura mater. The operator must exercise caution and judgement when working on sun-affected, tumour-infiltrated and often irradiated skin. Little flaps rarely work as large flaps usually have to be raised to cover relatively small defects (Fig. 18.7).

The problems of fungation, ulceration exposed vessels and potential catastrophic bleeding affect the unfortunate patient in a number of ways. We have noted the association of pain, but changed appearance, malodour and the bloody exudates can herald and hence fuel the fear if not terror of a burst carotid or other large artery. Depending on the patient's clinical situation, wound management alone may suffice best done with repeated wet dressings for gentle debridement [2].

The presence of an exposed carotid artery in an irradiated, ulcerated neck containing recurrent tumour is a surgical emergency requiring coverage of the vessel with a muscle or musculocutaneous flap (Fig. 18.8). If the sternomastoid muscle is still in situ and in good condition, it may suffice. The pectoralis major myocutaneous flap is useful in this circumstance as is the adjacent trapezius muscle flap. What is problematic is embarking on microsurgical transfer of issue as the recipient vessels are sure to be compromised and the complication rate from the intervention becomes its own problem as the incidence is high and the survival time for the patient is short. This problem/dilemma was well described by Shedd [14], and the results are no better in terms of survival today [6].

The role of microvascular free tissue transplant reconstruction in covering a non-healing area is difficult to describe, and the multidisciplinary team together with the patient has hard decisions to make. These can only be taken when there has been frank discussion as a basis for the acquisition of fully informed consent from the patient. The concept that dying from local disease is worse than dying from distant metastasis has not been substantiated by some studies and needs to be taken into account during this decision-making process [10, 11].

Free flap surgery is a major intervention, and the decision to do it is often taken in the grey area of holding out some hope of cure but with a strong element of symptom relief as already discussed. Such a scenario exists when there is radiation-induced osteoradionecrosis of the mandible producing pain infection, ulceration, fistula formation and dysphagia. A carefully planned and constructed composite flap of bone and skin from the hip, fibula or scapula generally has a good healing potential especially if the anastamoses can be performed outside the irradiated field (Fig. 18.9). The microvascular surgeon is therefore the most important member of the team.

By way of contrast, a similar situation in the upper jaw (maxilla), on many occasions, will

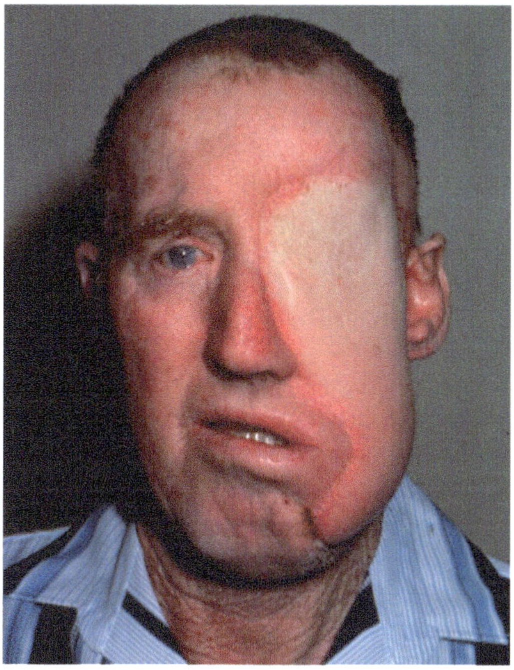

Fig. 18.9 A massive free flap to cover incompletely excised tumour in irradiated tissue with exposed vital structures

respond to excision of the affected area and dental prosthetic restoration. In the right circumstances this option allows inspection of the oral cavity and exposed walls of the sinus area, allows cleaning and with a functional prosthesis facilitates speech and mastication. Loss or limitation of these two faculties is a great burden for the terminal patient resulting in a much decreased quality of life. Filling the upper jaw cavity with a large insensitive flap is in many cases the lesser preferred option.

In the case of those benign but relentlessly persistent conditions mentioned previously, there is a necessity for repeated debulking, excising and reshaping excessive hard and soft tissue. The skin excesses of neurofibromatosis type 1 may affect an eyelid only or a whole face. The surgical possibilities are all those of plastic surgery of the face and include excisions, redraping, skin grafting and refashioning of specific structures such as eyelids and oral sphincters (Fig. 18.10a, b).

Fibrous dysplasia of the craniofacial skeleton may require repeated "paring" operations to

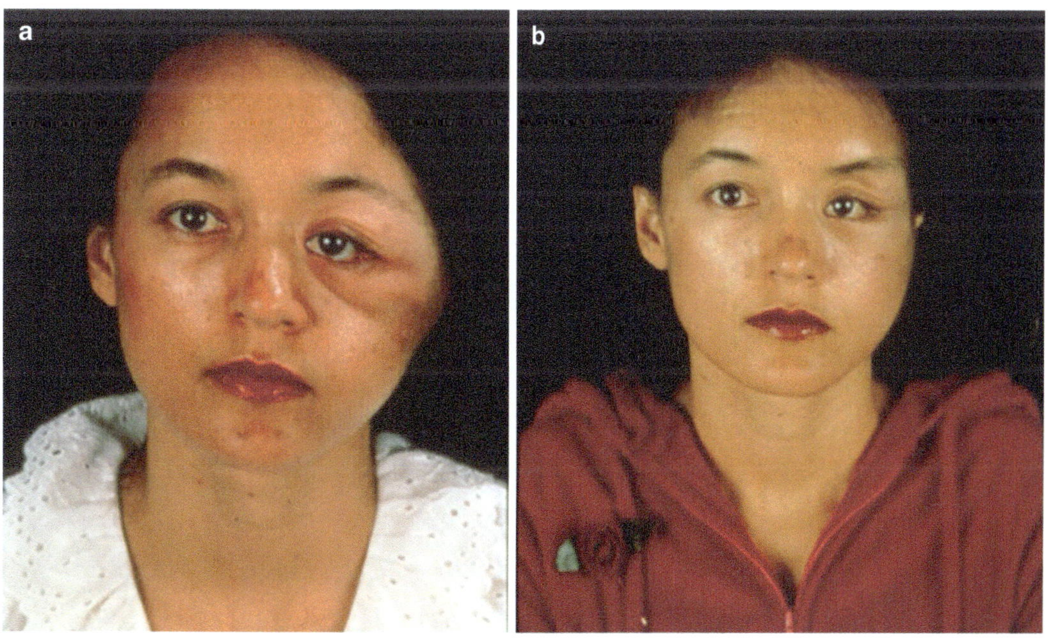

Fig. 18.10 (a) A case of extensive neurofibromatosis affecting the orbit, temporal bone and base of skull. (b) Extensive transcranial reconstruction has been undertaken but the disease is ongoing

reshape asymmetrical growth, debulking of expanded orbital walls producing proptosis and, rarely, complex transcranial resection around the orbital apex to decompress the optic nerve.

The surgeon's role in airway management is critical, and the management strategies are determined in the context of the multidisciplinary team. I do not intend to deal with those problems that emanate from laryngo-phyrangeal carcinoma where a tracheostomy has been part of the initial treatment. Patients with oral cancer and local recurrence in the head and neck may need tracheostomy as part of palliation. Timon and Reilly's study showed that almost a third of the patients in their series undergoing palliative care for head and neck malignancy required tracheostomy [2]. When the central compartment of the neck is widely infiltrated with tumour, a cricothyroidotomy may be considered [10].

The use of tracheostomy in palliative care offers a good option for airway management; however, the timing of the procedure in the progress of care requires extensive discussion involving patient and family. The indications include airway obstruction, chronic aspiration, the need for lung toilet and the need for long-term ventilation. Altered swallowing and loss of speech may make the patient decline the surgery.

As far as surgical technique is concerned, the open method using an inferiorly based tracheal flap sparing the upper two tracheal rings is the author's preferred method. The flap can be sutured to the skin or the investing layer of deep cervical fascia to create a smooth passage for changing the tube. Other techniques are widely used [15].

Forty-three percent of patients in Timon and Reilly's study required percutaneous gastrostomy to maintain nutrition. This form of surgical palliation is discussed in greater detail in another chapter.

In the chronic, incurable but non-malignant patients, there is a wide range of other surgical interventions that will serve to palliate symptoms and improve quality of life. They include tarsorrhaphy, partial or complete, temporary or permanent to protect the cornea and active and static slings to support the drooping face and nonfunctioning oral and ocular sphincters in patients with facial palsy.

Physical appearance plays a large role in quality of life for the terminally ill and for the chronically incurable with facial deformity. Fortunately there is now much greater acceptance of the fact that facial deformity raises levels of anxiety and causes depression [2, 7, 16]. Early recognition of this aspect of care in each individual patient enables the surgeon to understand the patient's needs more fully and when possible minimise deformity. In the continuum of care for the patient with malignancy, this should start early in the therapeutic process with carefully considered reconstructions where scars are placed in less obvious creases, where sections of the face are reconstructed as cosmetic units, and prosthetic reconstruction given due consideration. A simple example of the latter is the preference for prosthetic coverage of an exenterated orbit rather than a bulky and disfiguring flap repair (Fig. 18.11a, b).

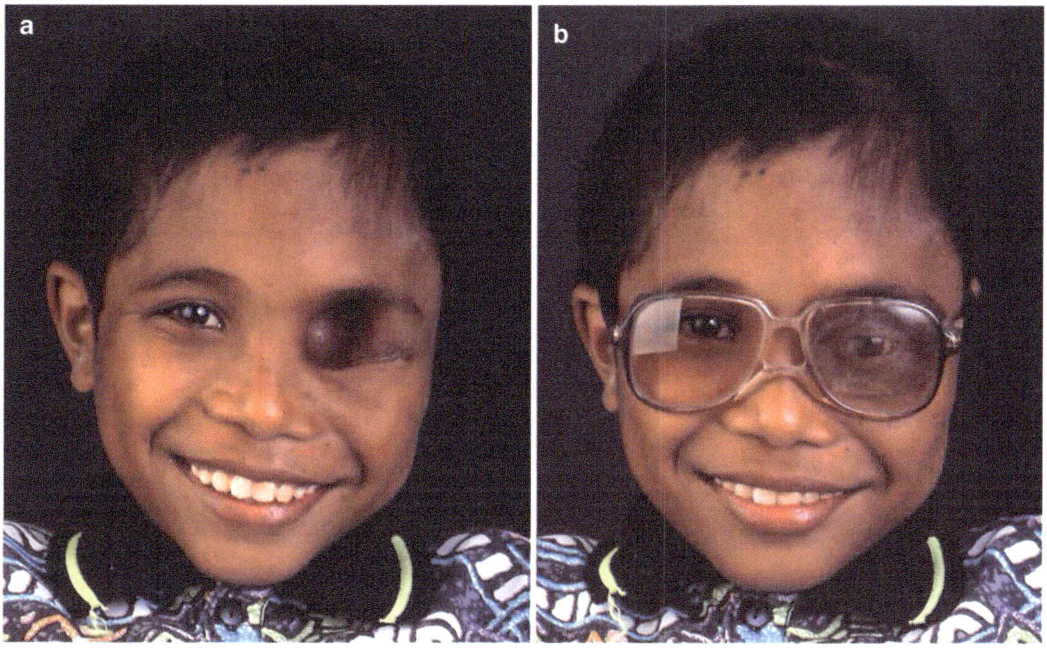

Fig. 18.11 (**a**, **b**) The prosthesis is not only more aesthetically pleasing but affords ease of inspection of the orbital cavity

Conclusion

By defining palliation in the broader sense, the surgeon's role can be extended from the treatment of final-stage cancer patients to those suffering incurable but benign diseases. The surgeon has much to offer all of these patients but always as a member of a multidisciplinary team dedicated to open and honest communication especially about when attempts to cure have ceased and relief of symptoms becomes the primary goal. Palliative care patients with head and neck cancer usually have a short survival time so the management needs to be intensive. Because of the variety of symptoms emanating from the facial region, the team should have surgical members with a variety of specialist skills. Palliation is about improving the quality and dignity of patient's lives. As a result there must be a commitment by surgeon and team to consistently make patient centric decisions.

Palliation of the effects of disease in the craniomaxillofacial region is particularly challenging because this small area of the body contains almost all of the faculties that make us truly human.

References

1. Hofmann B, Haleim LL, SAEreide JA. Ethics of palliative surgery in patients with cancer. Br J Surg. 2005;92:802–9.
2. Elackattu A, Jalisi S. Living with head and neck cancer and coping with dying when treatments fail. Otolaryngol Clin N Am. 2009;42:171–84.
3. Kurzweg T, Mockelmann N, Laban S, Knecht R. Current treatment options for recurrent/metastatic head and neck cancer: a post-ASCO 2011 update and review of last year's literature. Eur Arch Otorhinolaryngol. 2012;269:2157–67.
4. David DJ. A model for the development and delivery of craniofacial health care systems in developing countries. J Craniofac Surg. 2009;20 Suppl 2: 1661–3.
5. Ledeboer QCP, van der Velden L-A, de Boer MF, Feenstra L, Pruyn JFA. Physical and psychological correlates of head and neck cancer: an update of the literature and challenges for the future (1996-2003). Clin Otolaryngol. 2005;30:303–19.

6. Timon C, Reilly K. Head and neck mucosal squamous cell carcinoma: results of palliative management. J Laryngol Otol. 2006;120:389–92.
7. David DJ, Barritt JA. Psychological implications of surgery for head and neck cancer. Clin Plast Surg. 1982;9(3):327–36.
8. Dunn GP. Principles and core competencies of surgical palliative care: an overview. Otolaryngol Clin N Am. 2009;42:1–13.
9. Ledeboer QCP, van der Schroeff MP, Pruyn JFA, de Boer MF, Baatenburg de Jong RJ, van der Velden L. Survival of patients with palliative head and neck cancer. Head Neck. 2011;33(7):1021–6.
10. Shuman AG, Fins JJ, Prince ME. Improving end of life care for head and neck cancer patients. Expert Rev Anticancer Ther. 2012;12(3):335–42.
11. Shuman AG, Yang Y, Taylor JMG, Prince ME. End of life care among head and neck cancer patients. Otolaryngol Head Neck Surg. 2011;144(5):733–9.
12. Zafereo ME, Hanasono MM, Rosenthal DI, Stergis EM, Lewin JS, Roberts DB, Weber RS. The role of salvage surgery in patients with recurrent squamous cell carcinoma of the oropharynx. Cancer. 2009;115: 5723–33.
13. David D. Use of an innervated deltopectoral flap for intra oral reconstruction. PR&S. 1977;60:377.
14. Shedd DP, Shedd C. Problems of terminal head and neck cancer patients. Head Neck Surg. 1980;2: 476–82.
15. Chan T, Devaiah AK. Tracheostomy in palliative care. Otolaryngol Clin N Am. 2009;42:133–41.
16. Rumsey N, Clarke A, White P. Exploring the psychological concerns of outpatients with disfiguring conditions. J Wound Care. 2003;12(7):247–52.

Pleura, Chest Wall, Lung, and Mediastinum

19

Craig A. Jurisevic

Contents

C.A. Jurisevic, MBBS, MS, FRACS
Cardiothoracic Surgery Unit, Royal Adelaide Hospital, North Terrace, Adelaide, SA 5066, Australia
e-mail: jurisevic@ozemail.com.au

An objective approach to the surgical palliation of pleural, pulmonary, and mediastinal malignancy with a focus on minimally invasive, low-morbidity techniques

19.1 Introduction

When considering surgical palliation for conditions affecting the thorax, the treating surgeon must be guided by the overriding principle of palliation. That is, that the surgical intervention provides a reasonable chance of symptom relief without undue morbidity. Thus, minimally invasive procedures are preferable over those that require larger, more morbid approaches such as a thoracotomy or a median sternotomy. A point that is commonly overlooked when discussing surgical procedures on the chest is the high incidence of chronic pain after a thoracotomy. Chronic pain syndrome occurs in 20–70 % of patients who have undergone a thoracotomy [1]. Chronic pain following a thoracotomy is multifactorial but predominantly related to retraction neuropraxia at the time of rib spreading, resulting in chronic intercostal neuralgia. When the surgeon decides to proceed down the pathway of a thoracotomy, he/she should carefully consider the necessity for the procedure in the palliative setting, making an objective risk-benefit analysis. The surgeon must be steadfast in their decision not to operate when an assessment of the situation predicts a reduced quality of life with surgical intervention.

M. Wichmann, G. Maddern (eds.), *Palliative Surgery*,
DOI 10.1007/978-3-642-53709-7_19, © Springer-Verlag Berlin Heidelberg 2014

The main indications for thoracic surgical palliation in primary and secondary thoracic malignancies are:

- Cardiorespiratory compromise secondary to a malignant pleural effusion and/or pericardial effusion
- Pulmonary metastases from extra-thoracic primary malignancy
- Pain resulting from chest wall tumours
- Sepsis resulting from obstructive bronchogenic malignancy

Overwhelmingly, malignant pleural effusion is the main indication for surgical palliation in thoracic malignancy.

19.2 Malignant Pleural Effusion

Malignant pleural effusions arise as a result of malignant infiltration of the parietal and visceral pleurae, resulting in decreased reabsorption of pleural fluid and its subsequent accumulation within the pleural space. This results in extrinsic compression of the underlying lung parenchyma with secondary atelectasis, ventilation perfusion mismatch, and dyspnoea. In some instances the effusion may be under tension, resulting in decreased systemic venous return and a low cardiac output state. The pleura is a frequent site of metastatic disease from a host of primary tumours, including bronchogenic carcinoma, colorectal malignancies, uterine and ovarian carcinomas, breast carcinoma, and renal carcinoma, and a host of others. Primary pleural malignancies, predominantly malignant mesothelioma, frequently present with dyspnoea secondary to a malignant pleural effusion. It is generally accepted that pleurodesis not be attempted if the predicted survival of the patients is less than 3 months.

The prognosis for a patient with a malignant pleural effusion varies depending on the primary malignancy and the functional status of the patient and the median survival from time of diagnosis is in the order of 4 months [2]. A significant number of patients, however, die within 30 days of a procedure aimed at effecting a pleurodesis [3, 4], and accordingly, the treating surgeon must use all the information at hand to select the patients who will benefit from such treatment. Such patients generally have a symptomatic effusion, drainage of which results in a qualitative reduction in dyspnoea. Once a diagnosis of pleural malignancy has been made, one must identify any entrapment of the underlying lung by a malignant visceral pleural rind. This is a critically important point that is frequently overlooked and which will affect any attempted surgical palliation. Surgical treatment aims to remove the malignant pleural effusion, allows full expansion of the underlying lung, and prevents reaccumulation of the pleural fluid by affecting a pleurodesis. The extent of lung entrapment is inversely proportional to the amount of lung that can be effectively pleurodesed. This can usually be determined prior to surgery by tube thoracocentesis and draining the pleural space completely. If, on post-drainage plain chest x-ray, the lung re-expands completely, then one can be confident that complete pleural apposition can be achieved and any intervention to affect a pleurodesis will have a high likelihood of success. If, on the other hand, the lung fails to re-expand fully, indicating entrapment by a malignant pleural rind, then any attempt to achieve a pleurodesis will have a high failure rate.

Once the state of the visceral pleura (and, thus, lung expansion) has been established, one must select a minimally invasive option to achieve a permanent pleurodesis. In cases where it has been established that the lung has re-expanded fully after pleural drainage, the most effective surgical option is that of a *videoscopic talc pleurodesis*. This procedure requires general anaesthesia, double-lumen endotracheal intubation, and positioning of the patient in the lateral decubitus position. One or two sub-centimetre ports can be made in the 4th to 6th intercostal spaces between the mid- and anterior axillary lines. It is preferable to use a single intercostal space for all ports so as to minimise the number of intercostal nerves injured. The pleural fluid is aspirated, and under videoscopic visualisation, sterile talc is insufflated to effectively cover all areas of the visceral and parietal pleura. The standard dose is 5–10 g. A chest drain is then inserted (either through one of the ports or through a separate incision), the lung is re-expanded, and the remaining ports are closed. The patient is then extubated and the chest tube is left in situ (attached to an underwater sealed drainage bottle) for 48–72 h. Ideally the chest tube should be removed when less than 150 ml of pleural fluid is produced over a period of 24 h. This usually occurs at 48–72 h postoperatively. The success rate of a talc pleurodesis performed in this manner is in the order of 75–95 % [5, 6]. Talc is still the most effective sclerosant material available [7, 8] and is still the most widely used sclerosant outside of the experimental setting. Other substances such as anticancer drugs (bleomycin, cisplatin), antibiotics (tetracycline, erythromycin, doxycycline), and cytokines (interferon, transfer growth factor) are still undergoing investigation for widespread use as sclerosants [9].

Talc insufflation does have several common adverse effects including pyrexia, pleuritic pain, acute respiratory distress syndrome (ARDS), systemic inflammatory response, and pleural space infection. There is no evidence, however, that talc insufflation increases overall mortality

Less frequently used techniques in the situation where the lung re-expands fully after pleural drainage include videoscopic pleural abrasion, videoscopic parietal pleurectomy, and combinations of these two procedures.

In cases where the lung does not fully re-expand after pleural drainage, but where significant symptomatic relief is achieved by pleural drainage, standard surgical pleurodesis techniques will be unsuccessful. It is not uncommon for the upper lobes of the lung to re-expand fully whilst the lower lobe is trapped, and these patients present the most difficult therapeutic challenge. A standard videoscopic talc pleurodesis may result in pleurodesis of the upper lobe, but the lower lobe of the lung will remain trapped and there will be a persistent (obligatory) pleural effusion in the lower hemithorax. In such cases, particularly in those where significant symptomatic benefit is achieved by pleural drainage, a permanent indwelling tunnelled pleural catheter may be the most effective option. There are several such drainage systems available currently on the market including the PleurX (CareFusion Corp. San Diego, California) and Aspira (Bard Access Systems, Salt Lake City, Utah). These catheters are inserted under either local or general anaesthesia using a Seldinger technique with tunnelling of the catheter a certain distance under the skin and subcutaneous tissues in order to reduce the risk of pleural space infection. These systems allow for effective palliation of symptoms on an outpatient basis and allow the patients to drain their own effusion at intervals commensurate with their symptom deterioration [10].

In patients in whom a videoscopic talc pleurodesis is considered high risk from an anaesthetic viewpoint, or when the patient preference is for outpatient treatment, the permanent tunnelled pleural catheter may be the option of first choice [11].

Talc slurry, where talc is mixed with normal saline (5 g talc: 50–100 ml sterile normal saline) and instilled via an intercostal catheter, is a useful technique for achieving pleurodesis in the patient who is not fit for or declines surgical intervention. In this technique, performed at the bedside, the talc slurry is instilled via the intercostal catheter and the tube clamped. The patient is then positioned on each side in the supine position for approximately 20 min and then in the upright position, leaning left and right for a further 20 min. The procedure, by virtue of the acute pleuritis, can be quite painful and adequate analgesia should be provided to the patient.

Thoracoscopic talc pleurodesis has a significantly higher success rate than talc slurry (approximately 81 % for thoracoscopic pleurodesis versus 62 % for talc slurry) [5]. The effectiveness of talc slurry compared with permanent indwelling pleural catheter is comparable, and their cost-effectiveness as palliative treatments is currently under investigation [12].

Malignant pleural mesothelioma is the most common primary pleural malignancy. The choice of surgery in this condition is still controversial, as there is no effective cure, and data from randomised controlled trials are not available [11, 13–16]. There are currently various surgical options in patients with malignant pleural mesothelioma including pleurectomy/decortication (also known as total pleurectomy) and extra-pleural pneumonectomy (which involves en bloc resection of the parietal pleura, lung, ipsilateral diaphragm, and the pericardium) [17]. These two procedures will not yield complete resection of the tumour (RO resection) [18], and they have not been shown to improve survival when compared to systemic chemotherapy [16, 19]. As there is no level 1 evidence of survival benefit from pleurectomy, decortication, or extra-pleural pneumonectomy, the patient should be treated for symptoms relating to their malignant pleural effusion. For this reason it is recommended that videoscopic talc pleurodesis and insertion of a tunnelled indwelling pleural catheter are the most appropriate forms of palliation in patients with malignant pleural mesothelioma.

19.3 Malignant Pericardial Effusion

Malignant pericardial effusions can be effectively managed in the acute setting by percutaneous drainage via an ultrasound-guided catheter introduced using a Seldinger technique. For long-term management a pericardial window can be formed videoscopically on the left or right side. Using standard videoscopic techniques a 2×2 cm pericardial resection is performed in a pre-phrenic location on the right side and either pre- or post-phrenic on the left. The pericardial fluid will then drain into the pleural space making it available for absorption by the pleura. This technique does require essentially non-diseased pleura, and difficulty may arise when a patient has a malignant pleural and pericardial effusion. It is rare to have a malignant pericardial and bilateral malignant pleural effusion, and as such, a pericardial window can be performed in most patients with a malignant pericardial and unilateral pleural effusion.

19.4 Pulmonary Metastatectomy

Pulmonary metastases occur commonly in metastatic carcinoma of the colon or rectum, kidney, prostate, breast, thyroid, and oropharynx. The lungs are also common sites of metastases from various sarcomatous malignancies including osteosarcoma, soft tissue sarcoma, and Ewing's sarcoma.

The principles of patient selection for pulmonary metastatectomy have not altered significantly since the mid-1960s when Thomford et al. [20] outlined principles for patient selection. The criteria are as follows:

- The primary tumour process should be under control.
- The pulmonary metastases should be technically resectable.
- Any extra-thoracic metastatic disease should be excluded or, if limited, be resectable.
- Surgical morbidity and mortality should be minimal.

The choice of surgical procedure should be guided by the principle minimising surgical morbidity, and as such, a lung-sparing and minimally invasive approach is the preferred option. As the majority of pulmonary metastases are peripherally located within the lung parenchyma, wedge resections are the most common lung-sparing modality used. Anatomic resections such as a pulmonary segmentectomy or lobectomy are often also required if the tumour is located more centrally within the lobe or if there are multiple metastases within that lobe. Central metastases located near or involving hilar structures may necessitate a pneumonectomy, but great consideration should be given to perform such a radical resection in the palliative setting. Morbidity following pulmonary metastatectomy is determined predominantly by the patient's general medical status, the surgical approach used, and the extent of the surgical resection [21, 22].

There is significant variation in the indications for and results from pulmonary metastatectomy in the various malignancies that metastasize to the lungs [22]. Patients who have undergone a complete resection of pulmonary metastases have a 5-year survival of between 40 and 68 % [23]. In colorectal carcinoma unfavourable factors predicting poor prognosis include histologically confirmed thoracic lymph node metastases, a short disease-free interval, a raised serum carcinoembryonic antigen, and multiple lung metastases [23]. In the presence of synchronous liver metastases, survival rates of 42 % or more have been reported with sequential liver and lung metastatectomy [23]. Patients with pulmonary metastases from colorectal carcinoma have a significantly lower survival than those with only hepatic metastasis [24].

Renal cell carcinoma metastases treated by pulmonary metastatectomy can provide significant disease-free survival, particularly when mediastinal lymph node metastases are absent [25]. To date there are very few randomised controlled trials comparing surgical resection to nonsurgical options in patients with pulmonary metastatic disease. Patient selection should be considered in a multidisciplinary setting to achieve the best outcomes in these patients. Again, the overriding principle in these patients should be that of palliation where any intervention should not increase the patient's morbidity in view of their limited long-term survival prospects.

19.5 Stage IIIB and IV Non-small Cell Lung Carcinoma (NSCLC)

There are several situations in which a surgical intervention may be required in Stage IIIB and IV NSCLC. The most common situation is that in which malignant bronchial obstruction results in post-obstructive infection, often with cavitation, abscess formation, and persistent sepsis. Post-obstructive lung abscess results in symptoms related to sepsis and also precludes patients from ongoing chemotherapeutic treatment options. In this situation it may be necessary to perform a lobectomy or pneumonectomy, but such treatment must be undertaken after a thorough assessment of the patient's current medical status, predicted operative mortality and morbidity, and, of course, their prognosis.

Rarely, an anatomical resection (lobectomy or pneumonectomy) may be required to control haemorrhage from a bronchovascular fistula secondary to malignant erosion into pulmonary arterial or venous structures or from direct bronchial arterial erosion. In such situations, by virtue of the acuity of the presentation, one may be in a situation where resection is performed as a life-saving manoeuver in a patient with a very limited expected survival from the underlying malignant process.

19.6 Chest Wall Tumours

Chest wall involvement by direct extension from unresectable primary lung malignancies, sarcomatous tumours, breast carcinoma, and mesothelioma often results in significant pain. This pain is multifactorial and may involve any combination of pleuritic, intercostal neuralgic, and erosive bony pain. Furthermore, tumours that involve the chest wall often present as large ulcerated wounds with significant skin loss, exudation, and malodorous discharge. Pain management and wound care become major factors impacting on the patient's overall quality of life. Major chest wall tumour resection and myofascial and cutaneous reconstruction may be undertaken in such situations, but one must be aware that such procedures are unlikely to significantly reduce the pain aspect of the condition. In patients with significant pre-resection intercostal neuralgia, for example, resection of multiple ribs and neurovascular bundles may result in multilevel intercostal neuralgia with a consequent reduction in the patient's quality of life.

References

1. Wildgaard K, Ravn J, Kehlet H. Chronic post-thoracotomy pain: a critical review of pathogenic mechanisms and strategies for prevention. Eur J Cardiothorac Surg. 2009;36(1):170–80.
2. Heffner JE. Diagnosis and management of malignant pleural effusions. Respirology. 2008;13:5–20.
3. Bernard A, de Dompsure RB, Hagry O, et al. Early and late mortality after pleurodesis for malignant pleural effusion. Ann Thorac Surg. 2002;74:213–7.
4. Dresler CM, Olak J, Herndon II JE, et al. Phase III intergroup study of talc poudrage vs. talc slurry sclerosis for malignant pleural effusion. Chest. 2005;127:909–15.
5. Stefani A, Natali P, Casali C, Morandi U. Talc poudrage versus talc slurry in the treatment of malignant pleural effusion. A prospective comparative study. Eur J Cardiothorac Surg. 2006;30(6):827–32.
6. Lee P. Should thoracoscopic talc pleurodesis be the first choice management for malignant effusion? Yes. Chest. 2012;142(1):15–7.

7. Walker-Renard PB, Vaughan LM, Sahn SA. Chemical pleurodesis for malignant pleural effusions. Ann Intern Med. 1994;120:56–64.
8. Tan C, Sedrakyan A, Browne J, et al. The evidence on the effectiveness of management for malignant pleural effusion: a systematic review. Eur J Cardiothorac Surg. 2006;29:829–38.
9. Colt HG, Davoudi M. The ideal pleurodesis agent: still searching after all these years. Lancet Oncol. 2008;9:912–3.
10. Efthymiou CA, Masudi T, Thorpe JA, Papagiannopoulos K. Malignant pleural effusion in the presence of trapped lung. Five-year experience of PleurX tunneled catheters. Interact Cardiovasc Thorac Surg. 2009;9(6):961–4.
11. Fysh ET, Waterer GW, Kendall P, Bremner P, Dina S, Geelhoed E, et al. Indwelling pleural catheters reduce inpatient days over pleurodesis for malignant pleural effusion. Chest. 2012;142(2):394–400.
12. Davies H, Mishra E, Wrightson J, Stanton A. The second therapeutic intervention in Malignant Effusion Trial (TIME2): a randomized controlled trial to assess the efficacy and safety of patient controlled malignant pleural effusion by indwelling pleural catheter compared to chest tube and Talc Slurry. Am J Respir Crit Care Med. 2012;185:6860.
13. Tsao AS, Witsuba I, Roth JA, Kindler HL. Malignant pleural mesothelioma. J Clin Oncol. 2009;27:2081–90.
14. Kaufman AJ, Flores RM. Surgical treatment of malignant pleural mesothelioma. Curr Treat Options Oncol. 2011;12:201–16.
15. Kindler HL. Surgery for mesothelioma? The debate continues. Lancet Oncol. 2011;12:713–4.
16. Rice D. Surgical therapy of mesothelioma. Recent results. Cancer Res. 2011;189:97–125.
17. Maziak DE, Gagliardi A, Haynes AE, et al. Surgical management of malignant pleural mesothelioma: a systematic review and evidence summary. Lung Cancer. 2005;48:157–69.
18. Rice D, Rusch V, Passh H, et al. Recommendations for uniform definitions of surgical techniques for malignant pleural mesothelioma: a consensus report of the International Association for the Study of Lung Cancer International Staging Committee and the International Mesothelioma Interest Group. J Thorac Oncol. 2011;6:1304–12.
19. Tsao S, Witsuba I, Hasani A, Alvarez JM, Wyatt JM, et al. Outcome for patients with malignant pleural mesothelioma referred for tri-modality therapy in Western Australia. J Thorac Oncol. 2009;4: 1110–6.
20. Thomford N, Woolner L, Clagett O. The surgical treatment of metastatic tumors in the lungs. J Thorac Cardiovasc Surg. 1965;49:357–63.
21. Roth J, Pass H, Wesley M, White D, Putnam I. Comparison of median sternotomy and thoracotomy for resection of pulmonary metastases in patients with adult soft-tissue sarcomas. Ann Thorac Surg. 1986;42:134–8.
22. Vogt-Moykopf I, Krysa S, Bülzebruck H, Schirren J. Surgery for pulmonary metastases. The Heidelberg experience. Chest Surg Clin N Am. 1994;4:85–112.
23. Pfannschmidt J, Hoffmann H, Dienemann H. Reported outcome factors for pulmonary resection in metastatic colorectal cancer. J Thorac Oncol. 2010;5(6 Suppl 2):S172–8.
24. Neeff H, Hörth W, Makowiec F, Fischer E. Outcome after resection of hepatic and pulmonary metastases of colorectal cancer. J Gastrointest Surg. 2009;13: 1813–20.
25. Meimarakis G, Angele M, Schneider C, Weidenhagen R, Kalaitzis N, Molki A, et al. Bedeutung der systematischen Lymphknotendissektion im Rahmen der Resektion pulmonaler Metastasen solider extrapulmonaler Tumoren. Zentralbl Chir. 2010;135:556–63.

20 Breast

David C.A. Walsh

Contents

D.C.A. Walsh, MBBS, FRACS
Department of Surgery, The Queen Elizabeth Hospital, Woodville Road, Woodville, Adelaide
5081, SA, Australia
e-mail: leawalsh@ozemail.com.au

This chapter deals with the issue of locoregional recurrence in breast cancer. In the era of expanding option for systemic therapy, radical surgery and reconstruction may be an important consideration for patients previously considered untreatable. Similarly, the resection of primary breast cancer in the setting of disseminated disease may be appropriate. The role of surgery for breast cancer metastases remains controversial.

20.1 Introduction

The first attempts to perform controlled and standardised breast cancer surgery can be traced back to the hands of William Halsted [1]. By modern standards Halsted was dealing in aggressive locally advanced disease. His goal was essentially always palliative, with the faint hope of cure well in the background. Lack of effective systemic therapy and crude radiotherapy options meant that Halsted was forced to apply meticulous and practical surgical techniques for local control of breast cancer.

At the start of the twenty-first century, we are now dealing with a different spectrum of breast cancer presentations. Increasing public awareness and mass mammographic screening have led to the expectation that breast cancer will be encountered in an early stage, and the hope is for a permanent cure [2]. However, despite the earlier diagnosis of breast cancer and advances in both systemic therapies and radiation treatment,

M. Wichmann, G. Maddern (eds.), *Palliative Surgery*,
DOI 10.1007/978-3-642-53709-7_20, © Springer-Verlag Berlin Heidelberg 2014

locally advanced breast cancer is still an important entity. Uncontrolled locoregional (breast and axilla) breast cancer is now seen in the setting of relapsed, resistant disease or in the late presentation of breast cancer, despite the availability of screening measures. Women with metastatic breast cancer face remote disease as their dominant cause of death, but many will have concurrent locoregional relapse [3]. This is associated with major morbidity and suffering, even when breast cancer survival is unlikely [4].

The role of heroic surgery for upfront management of locally advanced breast cancer is currently limited. Most patients will benefit from systemic therapy and local irradiation, with local surgery waiting to deal with residual tumour. For those patients where the local tumour burden is considerable, the problem is challenging. The key to locoregional palliative surgical management is the establishment of durable tumour control. The key to this goal is tumour margin clearance.

20.2 Local Surgery

Traditionally, patients that will benefit from aggressive local surgical procedures have been limited in number and often difficult to identify [5]. Obstacles to patient identification have included the extent of metastatic disease and the likely overall survival after a time-consuming and morbid local surgical procedure.

Two factors have helped in this situation. Firstly, CT, MRI and PET imaging have allowed very accurate determination of the presence and extent of metastatic disease [6]. Patients with no or minimal tumour burden outside of the breast and axilla are clearly more appropriate candidates for aggressive surgery. In these cases survival can be anticipated to be longer; therefore, the value of local palliative surgery is increased, particularly if local symptoms are likely to be severe and prolonged. Secondly, the emergence of new systemic options apart from systemic chemotherapy, such as Her2 blockade, second- and third-line endocrine therapies and targeted therapies such as tyrosine kinase inhibitors, has increased survival for metastatic patients and provoked greater interest in surgical procedures for local disease control [7]. Clearly, any decision to proceed with local palliative surgery requires multidisciplinary specialist input, along with detailed patient and family counselling.

20.2.1 Breast Surgery

The most common palliative surgical procedure for breast cancer is simple mastectomy and axillary clearance. Often a standard mastectomy technique with carefully planned skin excision can remove a symptomatic, ulcerating cancer with primary closure of the skin and subcutaneous tissues [8]. Likewise a simple wedge of underlying chest wall muscle may also obtain resection of a locally advanced tumour. Palliative simple mastectomy can be combined with appropriate axillary dissection as dictated by the extent of local lymph node involvement. Appropriate local chest wall radiotherapy is an important adjunct therapy for these procedures [9].

Where possible a simple primary closure of the skin with healthy, viable flaps is the best palliative option. In many cases skin closure will not be possible and more complex techniques for soft issue coverage will be needed.

Historically, split-skin grafting has been widely employed when repairing skin defects post mastectomy. Skin grafting has problems with extent of graft take, coverage of large defects and healing when deployed over cartilage, bone or previously irradiated tissues. Cosmesis is usually poor. Vascularised omental grafts from the peritoneal cavity have been used extensively in the past to provide an improved soft tissue underlay for split-skin grafts on the chest wall [10]. They remain an option but are little used now in modern surgical practice. Negative-pressure wound therapy (VAC dressings) is now used to improve graft take in hostile wound beds and to simplify dressing care for patients. VAC dressings are the currently preferred dressing for split-skin grafting post mastectomy [11].

The modern practice of reconstructive breast surgery has made the use of local soft tissue flaps very routine. These are now the best option for skin and soft tissue closure after radical palliative mastectomy associated with extensive soft tissue excision.

Latissimus dorsi (LD) myocutaneous flaps are the simplest option for new skin and soft tissue. They can be mobilised and rotated into a post-mastectomy defect with relatively little surgical morbidity. An LD flap provides robust skin and muscle coverage, which allows postsurgical radiotherapy to be performed [12]. There is an issue with the potential for upper-limb dysfunction, and the skin paddle available for transfer can be limited for large defects.

In patients where large soft tissue defects are anticipated, or where the option of an LD flap has already been used, the next option to consider is a trans rectus abdominis (TRAM) myocutaneous flap. TRAM flaps can be rotated into position on the chest using a pedicle based on the superior epigastric vessels or can be a free flap employing a microvascular anastomoses [13]. In general the pedicled flaps are simpler to construct and have a lower failure rate than free TRAM flaps. Both types of TRAM flap are associated with considerable surgical morbidity, particularly at the abdominal wall harvest site.

As pedicled TRAM flaps depend on the integrity of the superior epigastric pedicle, they may be compromised during breast cancer therapy, such as local surgery and radiotherapy. In this situation double pedicle or super-charged TRAM flaps may be a useful option [14].

Free tissue transfer TRAM flaps represent the most complex of the local soft tissue coverage options. As such they have the largest rate of failure or flap loss [15]. This is particularly an issue in palliative surgery where the option of reverting to simple suture closure is not possible or when patients with a limited life expectancy can be subjected to major morbidity, impacting on their quality of life. In general, the need for robust soft tissue coverage, capable of withstanding post-operative radiotherapy, means that full muscle TRAM flaps are more appropriate in this setting. For this reason, muscle-sparing, perforator-type flaps (e.g. DIEP) are increasingly being used in breast reconstruction to reduce abdominal wall morbidity but are usually avoided in the setting of radical palliative breast surgery [16].

The key to success in free TRAM flap construction is selecting the site for microvascular anastomosis. Commonly internal mammary or subscapular pedicles are selected as anastomotic sites, but both can have been compromised by prior surgery or radiotherapy. Again, dual vascular anastomoses are an option to improve graft survival.

Although well described, attempts at chest wall resection and reconstruction are very rarely employed. If the patient's projected survival and extent of local disease warrant such an approach, the muscles, ribs, cartilages, sternum and pleura can all be resected en bloc and soft tissue coverage obtained. Such surgery is inappropriate if more than minimal disease exists at other sites and must have the reasonable expectation of obtaining clear local surgical margins. Incomplete resection is a failure of surgical selection. Likewise, any more than microscopic pleural involvement indicates that a patient is a poor candidate for such aggressive local surgery. The simplest soft tissue coverage is a prosthetic mesh placed into the chest wall defect. PFTE, which is nonpermeable, is favoured for this task. A robust soft tissue flap, either LD or TRAM, is then used to provide outer coverage. Large chest wall resections can compromise the mechanics of ventilation, and there has been some experience with rigid prosthetic supports to deal with this problem [17].

20.2.2 The Axilla

Local axillary involvement can be extremely symptomatic for patients. Prior surgery and local radiotherapy create considerable surgical challenges in this region.

In many cases axillary dissection to level III can be a very important palliative surgical procedure. Sometimes, a palliative procedure can be facilitated by a number of simple additional surgical manoeuvres, such as enlarged or novel skin incisions or the division/resection of pectoralis muscles. In the era of sentinel lymph node biopsy as standard therapy for early breast therapy, palliative completion axillary dissection is an important surgical tool [18].

In palliative axillary surgery it is important to ensure that all options for systemic therapy to debulk extensive local disease have been explored and applied. Careful consideration needs to be given to use of local radiotherapy to control axillary disease. Prior irradiation considerably increases the technical challenge and threatens the success of palliative axillary surgery. Where possible all surgical options should have been completed or explored prior to employing local radiotherapy. In palliative axillary surgery, issues such as post-operative lymphoedema, sensory changes and upper-limb motor dysfunction must be anticipated and managed. They should not limit the extent of surgical excision, as the goal remains clear surgical margins [19].

The contraindications to resection of axillary disease are involvement of the axillary artery and brachial plexus. The axillary vein can usually be resected with relatively little morbidity, particularly if there is prior tumour-related venous thrombosis. The axillary artery, if resected, can be reconstructed with either a reverse vein graft or prosthetic (usually PTFE) graft. Axillary artery involvement is usually associated with brachial plexus involvement that is virtually impossible to resect with any hope of surgical clearance. Sacrifice of the axillary artery or brachial plexus without hope of complete tumour resection is not palliative and is not justifiable. Resection of the brachial plexus for neuropathic pain can be devastatingly disappointing. Forequarter amputation as an approach to uncontrolled local disease is not palliative in breast cancer. Attempts at axillary neurovascular bundle resection, with or without reconstruction, will lead to very high levels of morbidity and often mortality if complications arise. These procedures must be planned and undertaken with full specialist support. Patient selection is paramount [20].

20.3 Local Surgery in Metastatic Breast Cancer

It has become common practice to offer newly diagnosed breast cancer patients early radiological staging to exclude the presence of stage IV, metastatic breast cancer. Typically, an unstandardised combination of chest X-ray, liver ultrasound, CT chest and abdomen, whole-body isotope bone scan and more recently PET scan has been performed, prior to undertaking surgical resection of the primary breast tumour [21].

The rationale of this approach is to demonstrate those patients who were "incurable" by current therapy and to spare them the assault of local breast surgery, particularly mastectomy. It also allows systemic therapy to be commenced earlier and specific complications that might be associated with metastatic disease dealt with in a timely fashion. This approach has meant that for most women with metastatic breast cancer, the primary has remained in place with little local treatment. Local breast and axillary surgery was generally confined to those women with progressive symptomatic tumours. However, new effective therapies for advanced breast cancer, the ability to demonstrate with imaging low-volume metastatic disease and recognition of the potential for slow-tempo disease progression have changed the rationale of this approach [22].

Patients are often surviving considerable periods with stage IV breast cancer. In these patients, the majority of the tumour burden will often be the primary cancer in the breast or axilla. Recent publications have also cast the role of palliative local breast surgery in a new light. Noncontrolled retrospective studies have suggested an improved survival for patients who have the primary malignancy resected in the presence of confirmed metastatic disease [23].

The best results are seen in patients with complete primary tumour resection in the setting of low-volume, bone-predominant metastatic disease. The optimal timing of primary disease resection is unclear. Clearly the choice to delay primary disease resection until it is apparent that metastatic disease is low tempo and responsive to systemic therapy will bring biases to any reported survival benefits. What is therefore not clear is whether upfront resection of the primary disease will favourably influence survival from metastatic disease in breast cancer.

Prospective studies are in progress, with the intention of clarifying this issue [24].

What can be drawn from these results is that surgeons can offer primary resection of primary breast cancer in patients with metastatic disease (often highly desired by patients), confident that there will be no adverse effect on patient survival.

20.4 Metastectomy in Stage IV Breast Cancer

The key goals in metastectomy in breast cancer are to reduce disease-related morbidity and to improve quality of life. Secondary goals are improved disease-free survival and the elusive possibility of cure.

The common sites for metastasis resection in breast cancer are the bone, lung, liver and brain [25].

20.4.1 Bone

The bone is the most common site for breast cancer metastases. Low-volume, bone-only disease is relatively common and often responds well to systemic therapy, particularly endocrine agents. Bone lesions are relatively simple to diagnose and confirm radiologically. Bone tumours are associated with significant pain and loss of function. It is no surprise that these are the most commonly surgically resected breast cancer metastases [26].

Indications for surgery are lack of response to therapy, local pain, fracture or high potential of fracture in weight-bearing long bones. Long bones are the most frequently operated upon, but surgical decompression of vertebral metastases with the potential for spinal cord compression is perhaps the most dramatic and important metastectomy in breast cancer [27].

Sternal metastases may be considered a special case of bone disease. Many represent local relapse only, being solitary and relatively indolent. Local resection for isolated sternal metastases may be a curative procedure [28].

20.4.2 Lung

Pulmonary metastatic breast cancer is often associated with widespread disease in multiple sites. Even when the tumours are confined to the lungs, they are often multiple and associated with extensive pleural involvement.

When an isolated lung metastasis is encountered, it can be resected, both for confirmation of diagnosis and therapeutic control. Often the issue is whether a lung tumour represents a primary pulmonary lesion or secondary disease from breast cancer. PET isotope scanning can be helpful in excluding other disease sites [29].

Resection of metastases can be amenable to resection using video-assisted thoracoscopic techniques, which reduces operative morbidity considerably. Provided a complete resection of tumour can be achieved, formal pneumonectomy and lobectomy appear to have no advantage over a wedge resection, with considerable differences in operative morbidity and mortality, favouring the simpler procedure [30].

20.4.3 Liver

Isolated, solitary and localised hepatic metastases are rare in stage IV breast cancer. Liver metastases carry a poor prognosis, often requiring chemotherapy as the only applicable systemic therapy. Liver resection for metastatic breast cancer is rarely employed [31].

However, if the same criteria for resection of hepatic colorectal cancer metastases are applied to breast cancer patients (primary site free from recurrence, localised or solitary hepatic disease, exclusion of other sites of metastasis and the ability to resect the liver tumours with clear margins, retaining enough hepatic parenchyma for hepatic function/regeneration), similar outcomes to hepatic resections are seen in breast and colorectal cancer patients [32].

20.4.4 Brain

Cerebral metastases from breast cancer are relatively common, although rarely are they the first or an isolated site of disease. Breast cancer is the most common solid tumour that metastasises to the leptomeninges, but this disease is not considered surgically resectable [33].

MRI has increasingly made the diagnosis cerebral metastatic disease more rapid and reliable. Systemic therapies in breast cancer may not cross the blood–brain barrier, and so the brain can be a sanctuary site for breast cancer cells, when other sites have responded to treatment or remain clear. Certain factors—younger patients, oestrogen receptor-negative disease and Her2-positive disease—seem to increase the likelihood of cerebral metastases [34]. These patients may benefit from consideration of surgical resection. Seizures are a frequent presentation or symptom of cerebral disease in breast cancer patients. Surgery may represent the best palliation for this distressing complication.

Resection of cerebral metastases can be considered when few lesions are present, the location is favourable for resection and rapid symptom control is indicated. Surgical resection can be associated with considerable morbidity and needs to be carefully planned for in selected cases. Usually the procedure will be a debulking of tumour rather than complete resection. The alternative local therapy for cerebral metastases is whole-brain radiotherapy. Indeed, even when successful cerebral surgery has been performed, post-operative whole-brain radiotherapy is still indicated to reduce local recurrence rates [35].

References

1. Osborne MP. William Stewart Halsted: his life and contributions to surgery. Lancet Oncol. 2007;8(3):256–65.
2. Bleyer A, Welch HG. Effect of three decades of screening mammography on breast-cancer incidence. N Engl J Med. 2012;367(21).
3. Redig AJ, McAllister SS. Breast cancer as a systemic disease: a view of metastasis. J Intern Med. 2013; 274(2):113–26.
4. Ruiterkamp J, Ernst MF. The role of surgery in metastatic breast cancer. Eur J Cancer. 2011;47 Suppl 3:S6–22.
5. Lannin DR, Haffty BG. End results of salvage therapy after failure of breast-conservation surgery. Oncology (Williston Park). 2004;18(3):272–9.
6. Groheux D, Espié M, Giacchetti S, Hindié E. Performance of FDG PET/CT in the clinical management of breast cancer. Radiology. 2013;266(2):388–405.
7. Conte P, Guarneri V. The next generation of biologic agents: therapeutic role in relation to existing therapies in metastatic breast cancer. Clin Breast Cancer. 2012;12(3):157–66.
8. Alvarado M, Ewing CA, Elyassnia D, Foster RD, Shelley Hwang E. Surgery for palliation and treatment of advanced breast cancer. Surg Oncol. 2007;16(4):249–57.
9. Harris S. Radiotherapy for early and advanced breast cancer. Int J Clin Pract. 2001;55(9):609–12.
10. Newing RK, Pribaz JJ, Bennett RC, Buls J. Omental transposition and skin graft in the management of chest wall recurrence of carcinoma of the breast. Aust N Z J Surg. 1979;49(5):546–51.
11. Stoeckel WT, David L, Levine EA, Argenta AE, Perrier ND. Vacuum-assisted closure for the treatment of complex breast wounds. Breast. 2006;15(5):610–3.
12. Aukema TS, Russell NS, Wesseling J, Rutgers EJ. Extensive soft tissue resection with autologous tissue closure for locally recurrent breast cancer: lasting local control and acceptable morbidity. Eur J Surg Oncol. 2009;35(5):469–74.
13. Behnam AB, Nguyen D, Moran SL, Serletti JM. TRAM flap breast reconstruction for patients with advanced breast disease. Ann Plast Surg. 2003;50(6): 567–71.
14. Rand RP, Grant J, Moe RE. Anterior chest-wall reconstruction with the extended TRAM double-pedicle free flap. J Reconstr Microsurg. 1995;11(2):131–4.
15. Yu SC, Kleiber GM, Song DH. An algorithmic approach to total breast reconstruction with free tissue transfer. Arch Plast Surg. 2013;40(3):173–80.
16. Chang DW. Breast Reconstruction with Microvascular MS-TRAM and DIEP Flaps. Arch Plast Surg. 2012;39(1):3–10.
17. Levy Faber D, Fadel E, Kolb F, Delaloge S, Mercier O, Mussot S, Fabre D, Dartevelle P. Outcome of full-thickness chest wall resection for isolated breast cancer recurrence. Eur J Cardiothorac Surg. 2013;44(4):637–42.
18. Sikov WM. Locally advanced breast cancer. Curr Treat Options Oncol. 2000;1(3):228–38.
19. Veronesi G, Scanagatta P, Goldhirsch A, Rietjens M, Colleoni M, Pelosi G, Spaggiari L. Results of chest wall resection for recurrent or locally advanced breast malignancies. Breast. 2007;16(3):297–302.
20. Fadel E, Chapelier A, Bacha E, Leroy-Ladurie F, Cerrina J, Macchiarini P, Dartevelle P. Subclavian artery resection and reconstruction for thoracic inlet cancers. J Vasc Surg. 1999;29(4):581–8.
21. Xu G, Zhao L, He Z. Performance of whole-body PET/CT for the detection of distant malignancies in various cancers: a systematic review and meta-analysis. J Nucl Med. 2012;53(12):1847–54.
22. Smith NZ. Treating metastatic breast cancer with systemic chemotherapies: current trends and future perspectives. Clin J Oncol. 2012;16(2):E33–43.
23. Petrelli F, Barni S. Surgery of primary tumors in stage IV breast cancer: an updated meta-analysis of published studies with meta-regression. Med Oncol. 2012;29(5):3282–90.
24. Neuman HB, Morrogh M, Gonen M, Van Zee KJ, Morrow M, King TA. Stage IV breast cancer in the era

of targeted therapy: does surgery of the primary tumor matter? Cancer. 2010;116(5):1226–33.
25. Scully OJ, Bay BH, Yip G, Yu Y. Breast cancer metastasis. Cancer Genomics Proteomics. 2012;9(5):311–20.
26. Eastley N, Newey M, Ashford RU. Skeletal metastases – the role of the orthopaedic and spinal surgeon. Surg Oncol. 2012;21(3):216–22.
27. Tancioni F, Navarria P, Mancosu P, Pedrazzoli P, Morenghi E, Santoro A, Baena RR, Scorsetti M. Surgery followed by radiotherapy for the treatment of metastatic epidural spinal cord compression from breast cancer. Spine (Phila Pa 1976). 2011;36(20):E1352–9.
28. Singletary SE, Walsh G, Vauthey JN, Curley S, Sawaya R, Weber KL, Meric F, Hortobágyi GN. A role for curative surgery in the treatment of selected patients with metastatic breast cancer. Oncologist. 2003;8(3):241–51.
29. Nichols FC. Pulmonary metastasectomy. Thorac Surg Clin. 2012;22(1):91–9.
30. Solaini L, Prusciano F, Bagioni P, di Francesco F, Solaini L, Poddie DB. Video-assisted thoracic surgery (VATS) of the lung: analysis of intraoperative and postoperative complications over 15 years and review of the literature. Surg Endosc. 2008;22(2):298–310.
31. Dittmar Y, Altendorf-Hofmann A, Schüle S, Ardelt M, Dirsch O, Runnebaum IB, Settmacher U. Liver resection in selected patients with metastatic breast cancer: a single-centre analysis and review of literature. J Cancer Res Clin Oncol. 2013;139(8): 1317–25.
32. Howlader M, Heaton N, Rela M. Resection of liver metastases from breast cancer: towards a management guideline. Int J Surg. 2011;9(4):285–91.
33. Lin NU, Bellon JR, Winer EP. CNS metastases in breast cancer. J Clin Oncol. 2004;22(17):3608–17.
34. Stemmler HJ, Heinemann V. Central nervous system metastases in HER-2-overexpressing metastatic breast cancer: a treatment challenge. Oncologist. 2008;13(7):739–50.
35. van den Bent MJ. Management of metastatic (parenchymal, leptomeningeal, and epidural) lesions. Curr Opin Oncol. 2004;16(4):309–13.

21 Thyroid and Parathyroid

Nadine R. Caron and Laurie Simard

Contents

This chapter focuses on locally advanced and metastatic thyroid cancer as well as parathyroid cancer. Treatments for thyroid and parathyroid cancers are aimed at primary, regional, and distant sites for respective malignancies and their symptoms associated with tumor burden. In addition, both benign and malignant pathologies often have associated endocrine symptoms that are treated with addressing tumor burden and/or medical management. This chapter will discuss management options in various forms of local invasion from both diseases. Treatment of metastatic disease tailored to histologic subtypes as well as to metastatic site will be addressed. It is meant to focus on surgical management but the various roles of chemotherapy, radiation, and other medical modalities will also be discussed.

21.1 Thyroid

In its most common, well-differentiated form, thyroid cancer has an excellent prognosis. In rare cases, it presents as locally invasive and potentially non-resectable disease. Dealing with these invasive tumors and their metastatic disease can be challenging, balancing the aggressiveness and morbidity of the treatment with the morbidity and mortality associated with advanced papillary, follicular, medullary, or anaplastic thyroid cancer. Locoregional invasion of neck structures can lead to distressing symptoms and life-threatening conditions. Metastatic tumor growth can also

N.R. Caron, MD, MPH, FRCSC (✉)
Department of Surgery and Northern Medical Program, University of British Columbia, 3333 University Way, Prince George, BC V2N 4Z9, Canada
e-mail: caronn@unbc.ca

L. Simard, MD, FRCSC
Department of General Surgery, CHUS Hotel Dieu, 101-984 King Ouest, Sherbrooke, QC J1G 2E8, Canada
e-mail: laurie.simard@usherbrooke.ca

M. Wichmann, G. Maddern (eds.), *Palliative Surgery*, DOI 10.1007/978-3-642-53709-7_21, © Springer-Verlag Berlin Heidelberg 2014 cause regional symptoms and organ dysfunction. Palliation of locoregional and distant disease is equally important. Options may involve, either alone or in combination, surgery, external beam radiation therapy (EBRT), and chemotherapy, and in the well-differentiated thyroid cancers (papillary and follicular), additional options include radioactive iodine (RAI) therapy and L-thyroxine suppression therapy.

21.1.1 Well-Differentiated Thyroid Carcinomas (WDTC)

21.1.1.1 Local Invasion

Evolution of this disease is usually slow and an aggressive approach in the face of locoregional invasion can provide a survival advantage. As local tumors can compete with distant metastases for RAI uptake and reduce the efficacy of this treatment, surgical resection, when possible, is recommended.

Airway Obstruction/Invasion

Laryngotracheal involvement can lead to significant respiratory distress and airway compromise secondary to extrinsic compression, intraluminal tumor growth, vocal cord paralysis from recurrent laryngeal nerve involvement, or a combination of these. Although this is the most common site of locoregional invasion, no randomized controlled trials have compared shave resection followed by adjuvant treatment to the more radical laryngotracheal excision with reconstruction. Surgical approach is decided based on tumor characteristics, the implications of the surgery, the patient's comorbidities, and their subsequent choice after discussion of the options. Regardless of the surgical option chosen, adjuvant therapy in the form of RAI and/or EBRT should be considered [1]. Other treatment options are available in cases of inoperability. Minimally invasive therapies of Nd-YAG laser and/or tracheal stenting have been described. In a case series, they yielded immediate and long-term success in 92 % of patients and were well tolerated [2]. Tracheostomy becomes indicated in cases of impending airway obstruction and is rarely necessary in WDTC. If required, it should be performed in the operating room under general anesthesia to optimize challenging circumstances. Some tumor debulking and isthmusectomy may be necessary.

Great Vessels

Malignant carotid involvement is rare, and data on the subject are lacking [1]. In cases of hemorrhage, surgery or selective arterial embolization may be considered. Venous involvement commonly presents as an incidental finding or superior vena cava (SVC) syndrome. With internal jugular vein involvement, surgery is the primary treatment option and, as the obstruction is often compensated, resection is generally well tolerated [3]. Complete surgical excision of the primary lesion, with jugular resection and/or thrombectomy, can palliate impending SVC syndrome [3]. Adjuvant treatment in the form of RAI and EBRT should be considered. In inoperable cases, venous stenting is an interesting alternative.

Esophagus

Available data are limited. When surgery or esophageal stenting is not feasible, gastrostomy tubes are the alternative. Total parenteral nutrition is rarely required.

21.1.1.2 Regional and Distant Metastasis

Survival in the presence of distant metastatic disease is highly variable, depending on location and extent of disease and presence of RAI uptake (ranges from greater than 50 % at 10 years to less than 50 % at 3 years) [4]. The most common distant metastatic sites are the lung, bone, liver, and brain. Treatment planning depends on the patient's performance status and other disease sites; 5–20 % of patients with distant lesions will eventually die from progressive locoregional disease [1]. Surgery is considered the best option in selected cases of limited distant disease while the most common alternative is RAI ablation. Survival improvement related to complete surgical excision was described in a retrospective study (5-year disease-specific survival of 78 % vs. 46 %, $p = .03$) [5]. When secondary disease is confirmed at time of initial diagnosis, resection of the primary and regional disease optimizes success of RAI treatment of metastasis, especially those which are not amenable to surgical intervention. EBRT may be useful in controlling inoperable, persistent, or recurrent locoregional disease that is not RAI avid [1]. Chemotherapy options are limited but may be considered, preferably in a clinical trial setting in non-iodine avid, symptomatic lesions or in lesions that progress despite RAI therapy. Table 21.1 describes the characteristics of each metastatic site and associated available treatment options.

21.1.2 Medullary Thyroid Carcinoma (MTC)

MTC does not concentrate RAI and responds less to EBRT than WDTC. The clinical course of patients with metastatic MTC is highly variable, ranging from indolent disease with survival for decades to aggressive, rapidly fatal outcomes [7]. Patients with advanced disease may suffer from flushing and diarrhea related to tumor secretion of bioactive substances (calcitonin and others). Debulking the tumor burden often controls these symptoms [7]. Table 21.2 depicts the role of the different treatment options available in MTC.

21.1.3 Anaplastic Thyroid Carcinoma (ATC)

ATC is one of the most aggressive solid neoplasms with a median survival of 6 months after diagnosis [9]. It most commonly presents as a large, firm thyroid mass causing hoarseness, vocal cord paralysis, dysphagia, cervical pain, and dyspnea. Diagnosis is available via fine-needle aspiration or core biopsy and, if necessary, open surgical biopsy [10]. Routine intraoperative frozen sections are not recommended but may be helpful either to ensure adequate sampling or to confirm diagnosis if it will change surgical procedure [10]. Initial staging includes appropriate locoregional imaging with computerized tomography (CT) scan or magnetic resonance imaging (MRI) as well as distant disease assessment with positron emission tomography (PET)-CT scan or, if not available, cross-sectional imaging of the brain, chest, abdomen, and pelvis [10]. Direct laryngoscopy will assess vocal cord mobility and for any disease extension into the laryngotracheal area [10]. Most cancer-related deaths are due to rapid locoregional growth so therapeutic efforts should be concentrated here. A multidisciplinary team with therapeutic decisions individualized based on patient and disease factors is needed. These patients are often best managed by multimodal therapy, including surgery and EBRT ± chemotherapy [10]. Due to its poor prognosis, aggressive approaches in metastatic ATC should be used sparingly. See Fig. 21.1.

21.1.4 Surgery

Complete surgical excision, not including major structures such as the larynx and esophagus, should be performed [10]. Unfortunately, this is rarely possible. There is currently no known survival advantage of achieving microscopically negative margins compared to grossly negative margins. Therefore, an en bloc resection should be considered whenever all gross disease can be resected, but tumor debulking with grossly positive margins should not be attempted [10]. The definition of "unresectable" may vary among institutions, depending on tumor extent and expertise. In cases of inoperability, neoadjuvant EBRT and/or chemotherapy should be considered, possibly rendering the tumor suitable for surgery [10]. As there is a high risk of relapse after response to EBRT ± chemotherapy, surgery should be performed when feasible in these cases.

Tracheostomy for airway compromise is technically challenging and has a high rate of healing complications, which can delay EBRT. It should be considered in cases of impending airway obstruction, not prophylactically [10]. If performed, this must be undertaken in the operating room under general anesthesia and should not be performed in the emergency department or on the

Table 21.1 Characteristics and treatment options available in the different metastatic sites of well-differentiated thyroid cancers: papillary and follicular

Metastatic site	Presentation/particularity[a]	Role of surgery	RAI therapy	EBRT	Others
Lung	Often multicentric or "miliary" in distribution Often asymptomatic Possible dyspnea, obstructive pneumonia, hemoptysis, and respiratory failure	In resectable and limited disease	Mainstay of treatment in RAI-avid lesions [1]	Palliative role in obstructive lesions [1]	Endobronchial laser therapy in case of hemorrhage Thyroid suppression only in asymptomatic, non-RAI-avid, stable lesions
Bone	Often multicentric Common sites include the vertebrae, ribs, and pelvis May present with pain, fracture, or neurologic deficit No data support treatment of stable, asymptomatic, unresectable, or non-RAI-avid thyroid lesions	Indicated in symptomatic lesions and in selected cases of asymptomatic lesions in weight-bearing areas [5]	Often shows lesser response than lung lesions but may improve survival in avid lesions	Palliation of symptomatic inoperable lesions	Radio-frequency ablation, cryoablation, and selective arterial embolization as a last resort in selected cases [1] Bisphosphonates proven in other primaries to prevent, inhibit, and delay cancer-associated skeletal complications
Brain	Typically older patients with a higher tumor burden and less differentiated disease with poor prognosis	Mainstay of treatment with possible survival improvement [6]	May be used in avid disease but with variable results	Palliation of inoperable disease, either as whole-brain radiation or stereotactic guided	Corticosteroids in symptomatic disease and during radiation/RAI treatment No recommendation for prophylactic antiseizure treatment [1]
Liver	Options derived from data on other primaries	In resectable and limited disease	In RAI-avid lesions	Stereotactic-guided therapy may be used	Radio-frequency ablation in amenable lesions

[a]Metastatic disease identified via clinical, radiologic, and biochemical monitoring (thyroglobulin, anti-thyroglobulin antibody)

Table 21.2 Role of the treatment options available in medullary thyroid cancer (MTC)

	Surgery	EBRT	Chemotherapy	Others
Role and indication	Aggressive surgical treatment of locoregional, recurrent, and distant disease is the mainstay of treatment	Maintains a role primarily in palliation of symptomatic bony and cerebral metastasis May be used for symptomatic locoregional disease but often less responsive	Limited role, reserved to rapidly progressive and symptomatic cases, may achieve symptom control but without survival improvement	Radiolabeled octreotide and metaiodobenzylguanidine (MIBG) show encouraging results for short-term disease stabilization, pain control, and quality of life improvement [8] Immunotherapy seems promising but not yet clinically applicable

Data from: Greenblatt and Chen [7]

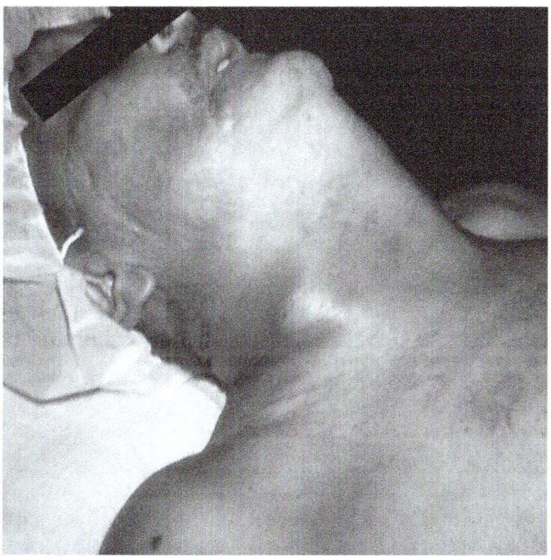

Fig. 21.1 Clinical features of anaplastic thyroid cancer (Used with permission from Surks and Korenman [17])

ward [10]. Pretracheal tumor debulking or isthmusectomy may be necessary. Most patients requiring a tracheostomy have aggressive disease with a poor prognosis. It may relieve airway distress but provides minimal prolongation of life with potential prolonged suffering, so it should be a fully informed decision made by the patient and their healthcare team.

21.1.5 Adjuvant and Palliative Treatment Options

Table 21.3 summarizes the role of the different adjuvant and palliative treatment options available for ATC.

21.2 Parathyroid

Palliation is relevant in two clinical scenarios: parathyroid carcinoma and persistent or recurrent benign hyperparathyroidism with symptomatic hypercalcemia.

21.2.1 Parathyroid Carcinoma (PTC)

PTC is found in less than 1 % of cases of primary hyperparathyroidism (HPT) [12]. Its etiology is still poorly understood, and most of the data on its molecular pathogenesis come from studies of the rare HPT-jaw tumor syndrome [12] as 15 % of these patients develop PTC [13]. A mutation highly specific to PTC (tumor suppressor gene CDC73) could be used as a diagnostic tool in equivocal cases [12]. PTC has also rarely been reported in cases of familial isolated HPT and multiple endocrine neoplasia type 1 and 2A [13].

21.2.1.1 Presentation

Although rare, PTC is vital to diagnose. Table 21.4 depicts useful characteristics in differentiating benign from malignant disease. In addition, laryngeal nerve involvement and lymphadenopathy should be considered suspicious [12]. The rare nonfunctional carcinomas commonly present as locally advanced disease [12].

21.2.1.2 Diagnosis

Investigations

First-line preoperative localizing studies are ultrasound scan (US) and sestamibi scan. In

Table 21.3 Role of the treatment options available in anaplastic thyroid carcinoma (ATC)

	Surgery	EBRT	Chemotherapy	Others
Role and indication	Preferred approach when at least grossly negative margins can be achieved without major morbidity [10]	Neoadjuvant setting: may render inoperable cases operable [10]	Usually combined with radiation as a radiosensitizer [11]	Endobronchial techniques (Nd-YAG laser coagulation and stenting) may be used in selective cases
	No indication for tumor debulking with gross positive margins [10]	Adjuvant setting: shown, in case series [11], to improve survival in the presence of positive margins	Chemotherapy alone is disappointing [9]	Selective embolization of the thyroid arteries (SETA) may alleviate local symptoms and control hemorrhage if needed
	Tracheostomy performed in cases of impending airway obstruction [10]	Palliative setting (inoperable primary): as a definitive, high-dose regimen or as a palliative, low-dose regimen depending on performance status [10]	Preferred option in diffusely threatening metastatic disease [10] as it may lead to disease stability or regression but without survival improvement	
	May be indicated in metastatic disease if it is the only way to preserve function (i.e., spinal compression, pathological fractures) [10]			

Table 21.4 Characteristics differentiating benign from malignant parathyroid disease

	Benign disease	Parathyroid carcinoma
Women to men ratio	3–4:1	1:1
Average age at presentation	55 years old	48 years old
Serum calcium	<11.2 mg/dl (2.8 mmol/l)	>14 mg/dl (3.5 mmol/l)
Hypercalcemic crisis (shortened QT interval on ECG and apathy that if left untreated can lead to coma and death)	Rare	Possible
Serum PTH	Mild elevation	3–10-fold elevation
Renal involvement (renal colic, nephrocalcinosis)	<20 %	55–85 %
Radiological skeletal features (osteitis fibrosa cystica, osteoporosis, pathological fractures)	<5 %	44–90 %
Palpable neck mass	Rare	30–70 %

Data from: Fang and Lal [12] and Shane [14]

addition, CT scan and MRI may reveal local invasion and pathologic lymphadenopathy [13]. When clinically relevant and in cases of reoperation for recurrence, laryngoscopy is used to assess vocal cord mobility. Invasive studies, such as selective venous catheterization, are mainly indicated for recurrent disease when other modalities are nondiagnostic [13]. Fine-needle aspiration (FNA) of masses suspicious for PTC is contraindicate due to the high risk of tumor seeding and low diagnostic rate [12]. Cross-sectional imaging is indicated in the presence of symptoms suggestive of metastasis and when postoperative calcium and parathyroid hormone (PTH) fail to normalize [12]. While disease-related lytic bone lesions might appear positive on 18-fluorodeoxyglucose (FDG)-PET, its role in PTC is unclear [13].

Pathology

Intraoperative diagnosis of PTC is clinical with no proven benefit of frozen section of the parathyroid lesion [12]. Morphologic features of PTC include a larger tumor (median diameter 3.3 cm) and an irregular, firmer mass with a whitish-gray color [12]. PTC is commonly adherent to or invading surrounding structures, namely, the strap muscles, thyroid gland, trachea, esophagus, and recurrent laryngeal nerve [14]. Some histologic criteria, including capsular or vascular invasion, fibrous trabeculae, and numerous mitotic figures, have been suggested for diagnosis but none are sensitive or specific enough [12]. Immunohistochemical staining for Ki-67 and parafibromin has been studied, but they also lack sensitivity and specificity [12, 13]. A combination of the clinical, morphologic, and histologic criteria should be used.

Prognosis

PTC is an indolent disease with survival rates estimated at up to 90 % at 5 years and 67 % at 10 years [13]. Morbidity and mortality are rarely due to tumor burden but commonly result from consequences of chronic hypercalcemia. Prognostic factors include initial margin status, lymph node involvement, and distant metastasis [13]. Nonfunctional tumors at diagnosis are associated with a worse prognosis [12].

21.2.1.3 Treatment

Surgery (Fig. 21.2)

Primary Tumor

Complete resection is the only chance for cure so PTC should be resected en bloc with any adjacent invaded structure. This commonly includes a hemithyroidectomy, the adjacent lymphatic tissue, the strap muscles, the thymus, and rarely the recurrent laryngeal nerve [12]. Tumor spillage should be avoided to decrease tumor seeding. Some recommend prophylactic ipsilateral central lymph node dissection (LND), but modified radical lateral LND should be carried out only in the presence of confirmed disease [12] via FNA biopsy of abnormal lymph node(s). Since PTC has been reported to coexist with either benign parathyroid adenoma or hyperplasia, a bilateral neck exploration should be performed [14]. The use of intraoperative rapid intact PTH assay (IOPTH) may be useful to assure that most, if not all, of the disease has been resected. If the IOPTH does not normalize, the options are further neck exploration with its associated potential complications or to complete the planned surgery for the primary disease and search for distant metastases postoperatively [13]. Cases of postoperative diagnosis of PTC are more complex. Patients with negative resection margins, with equivocal lesions, or with postoperative calcium and PTH normalization may be observed [12, 14]. However, re-excision with ipsilateral hemithyroidectomy and central lymph nodes is recommended in the presence of tumor aggressiveness and capsular or vascular invasion and if calcium and PTH fail to normalize after the initial surgery in the absence of distant disease on further imaging [13]. Close postoperative monitoring of calcium levels is mandatory as large doses of intravenous calcium and oral calcitriol may be required [13].

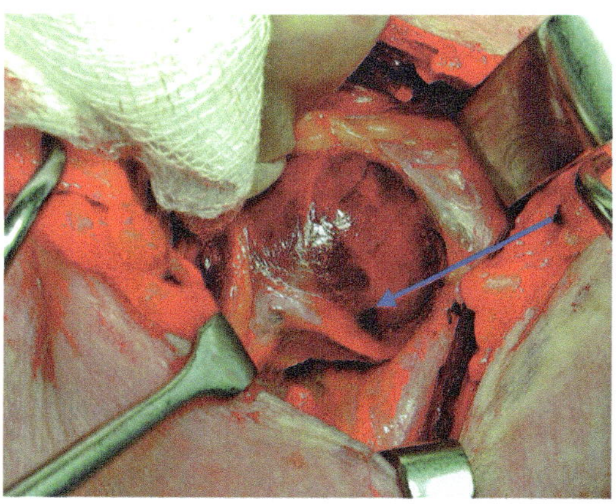

Fig. 21.2 Demonstrates the attachment of recurrent laryngeal nerve to large parathyroid tumor (Used with permission from Lynn and Lynn [18])

Recurrent and Metastatic Disease

Recurrence rate after surgery ranges from 20 to 60 % and is lower with en bloc ipsilateral thyroid resection [12]. Although rarely curative, surgery is considered the mainstay of treatment of recurrent and metastatic disease [12]. It often renders patients normocalcemic for a period, facilitates medical management, and may improve survival [14]. The major drawback is possible increased morbidity associated with repeat surgeries [15]. EBRT may be considered in cases of unresectable, recurrent neck diseaseor to palliate bone metastases [12]. The lung, bone, and liver are the most common sites of distant disease [12]. Preoperative imaging, including venous catheterization in equivocal cases, should be performed to confirm the location and extent of these local-regional recurrences and metastatic sites [15].

Table 21.5 Characteristics of the different drugs used in the management of hypercalcemia

	Mechanism of action	Onset of action	Duration of effect	Doses	Particularities
Loop diuretic	Increases renal calcium excretion	Hours	Used in the short term until acute-phase controlled	Adjusted based on the patient's volume status	Used only when diuresis is established Monitor for fluid or electrolyte imbalance
Bisphosphonates	Inhibits osteoclast activity	2–4 days	Long term	Intravenous administration, agent dependent	Introduced early in clinical course and maintained for long-term control
Calcitonin	Inhibits osteoclast activity and increases renal calcium excretion	12–24 h	48 h	Intramuscular or subcutaneous administration, 4 IU/kg each 12 h up to 6–8 IU/kg every 6 h	Used in severe symptomatic cases (serum calcium at >14 mg/l (3.5 mmil/l)) as a bridge for the delayed onset of action of bisphosphonates
Cinacalcet	Calcimimetic, increases sensitivity of the calcium sensing receptors thus decreasing PTH secretion	1–4 weeks	Long term	Dose titration, from 30 mg daily to maximum 90 mg four times daily	Does not alter the disease course but is recommended for palliation of symptomatic hypercalcemia in inoperable patients

Data from Fang and Lal [12] and Givi and Shah [13]

21.2.1.4 Adjuvant Therapies

Data on chemotherapy use in PTC are scarce and disappointing with short-lived responses. It is primarily considered in refractory hypercalcemia [12]. In retrospective studies, EBRT has led to decreased recurrence rates and improved survival [16] and may be considered in patients at high risk of locoregional recurrence (i.e., gross capsular invasion, positive margins, and intra-operative capsule rupture) [12].

21.2.2 Medical Management of Hypercalcemia

Acute, symptomatic hypercalcemia is initially treated with volume correction using isotonic saline, followed by a range of medical options (Table 21.5). Volume restoration is performed at an initial rate based on severity of hypercalcemia and then adjusted to maintain a urine output around 100 ml/h [12].

21.3 Summary

In the thyroid and parathyroid conditions discussed, treatments are aimed at primary, regional, and distant sites for respective malignancies and their symptoms associated with tumor burden. In addition, both benign and malignant pathologies often have associated endocrine symptoms that are treated with addressing tumor burden and/or medical management.

References

1. Cooper DS, Doherty GM, Haugen BR, Kloos RT, Lee SL, Mandel SJ, Mazzaferri EL, McIver B, Pacini F, Schlumberger M, Sherman SI, Steward DL, Tuttle RM. Revised American Thyroid Association management guidelines for patients with thyroid nodules and differentiated thyroid cancer. Thyroid. 2009;19(11):1167–214.
2. Noppen M, Poppe K, D'Haese J, Meysman M, Velkeniers B, Vincken W. Interventional bronchoscopy for treatment of tracheal obstruction secondary

to benign or malignant thyroid disease. Chest. 2004;125:723–30.
3. Hyer SL, Dandekar P, Newbold K, Haq M, Wechalakar K, Harmer C. Thyroid cancer causing obstruction of the great veins in the neck. World J Surg Oncol. 2008;6:36.
4. Robbins RJ, Wan Q, Grewal RK, Reibke R, Gonen M, Strauss HW, Tuttle RM, Drucker W, Larson SM. Real-time prognosis for metastatic thyroid carcinoma based on 2-[18F]fluoro-2-deoxy-D-glucose-positron emission tomography scanning. J Clin Endocrinol Metab. 2006;91(2):498.
5. Stojadinovic A, Shoup M, Ghossein RA, Nissan A, Brennan MF, Shah JP, Shaha AR. The role of operations for distantly metastatic well-differentiated thyroid carcinoma. Surgery. 2002;131:636–43.
6. Chiu AC, Delpassand ES, Sherman SI. Prognosis and treatment of brain metastases in thyroid carcinoma. J Clin Endocrinol Metabol. 1997;82:3637–42.
7. Greenblatt DH, Chen H. Palliation of advanced thyroid malignancies. Surg Oncol. 2007;16:237–47.
8. Pasieka JL, McEwan AJ, Rorstad O. The palliative role of 131I-MIBG and 111In-octreotide therapy in patients with metastatic progressive neuroendocrine neoplasms. Surgery. 2004;136:1218–26.
9. Giuffrida D, Gharib H. Anaplastic thyroid carcinoma: current diagnosis and treatment, review article. Ann Oncol. 2000;11:1083–9.
10. Smallridge R, Ain KB, Asa SL, Bible KC, Brierley JD, Burman KD, Kebebew E, Lee NY, Nikiforov YE, Rosenthal MS, Shah MH, Shaha AR, Tuttle M. American Thyroid Association guidelines for management of patients with anaplastic thyroid cancer. Thyroid. 2012;22(11):1104–39.
11. Haigh PI, Ituarte PH, Wu HS, et al. Completely resected anaplastic thyroid carcinoma combined with adjuvant chemotherapy and irradiation is associated with prolonged survival. Cancer. 2001;91:2335–42.
12. Fang SH, Lal G. Parathyroid cancer : review article. Endocr Pract. 2011;17 Suppl 1:36–43.
13. Givi B, Shah JP. Overview parathyroid carcinoma. Clin Oncol. 2010;22:498–507.
14. Shane E. Clinical review: parathyroid carcinoma. J Clin Endocrinol Metab. 2001;86(2):485–93.
15. Kebebew E, Arici C, Duh QY, Clark OH. Localization and reoperation results for persistent and recurrent parathyroid carcinoma. Arch Surg. 2001;136:878–85.
16. Busaidy NL, Jimenez C, Habra MA, Schultz PN, El-Naggar AK, Clayman GL, Asper JA, Diaz Jr EM, Evans DB, Gagel RF, Garden A, Hoff AO, Lee JE, Morrison WH, Rosenthal DI, Sherman SI, Sturgis EM, Waguespack SG, Weber RS, Wirfel K, Vassilopoulou-Sellin R. Parathyroid carcinoma: a 22-year experience. Head Neck. 2004;26(8):716.
17. Surks M, Korenman S. Atlas of clinical endocrinology, Thyroid disease, vol. 1. Philadelphia: Current Medicine; 1999.
18. Lynn WR, Lynn JA. How to perform a successful exploration of the neck for primary hyperparathyroidism. In: Talati JJ, Tiselius H-G, Albala DM, Ye Z, editors. Urolithiasis. London: Springer Science; 2012.

Adrenal Gland

22

Nadine R. Caron and Laurie Simard

Contents

Adrenal lesions may present as an incidental finding, with locoregional symptoms or with symptoms related to hormonal secretion. They should be investigated for possible hormonal secretion, and the risk of malignancy, either primary or secondary, should be assessed. This chapter concentrates on adrenocortical carcinoma and pheochromocytoma since they represent the most common malignant adrenal lesions. The focus is made on surgical resection, which is the mainstay of treatment for locoregional and isolated metastatic disease. Other palliative options, such as radiation, chemotherapy, and other modalities may alleviate symptoms related to the mass effect and control hormonal secretion in inoperable cases. These options, as well as possible medical therapies, will also be reviewed.

22.1 The Adrenal Incidentaloma and Associated Risk of Malignancy

Adrenal incidentalomas may be found in 4–7 % of abdominal CT scans. Up to 5 % of these will be adrenocortical carcinomas (ACC), and 2.5 % will be metastatic cancers [1]. Figure 22.1 presents a suggested management algorithm for such incidentally discovered adrenal masses. Malignancy is suspected by combination of clinical, biochemical, and radiological characteristics. An endocrine syndrome can be found in 60 % of ACC, most commonly Cushing syndrome (50 %), virilization (<10 %), or a combination

N.R. Caron, MD, MPH, FRCSC (✉)
Department of Surgery and Northern Medical Program, University of British Columbia, Prince George, BC V2N 4Z9, Canada
e-mail: caronn@unbc.ca

L. Simard, MD, FRCSC
Department of General Surgery, CHUS Hotel Dieu, Sherbrooke, QC J1G 2E8, Canada
e-mail: laurie.simard@usherbrooke.ca

M. Wichmann, G. Maddern (eds.), *Palliative Surgery*,
DOI 10.1007/978-3-642-53709-7_22, © Springer-Verlag Berlin Heidelberg 2014

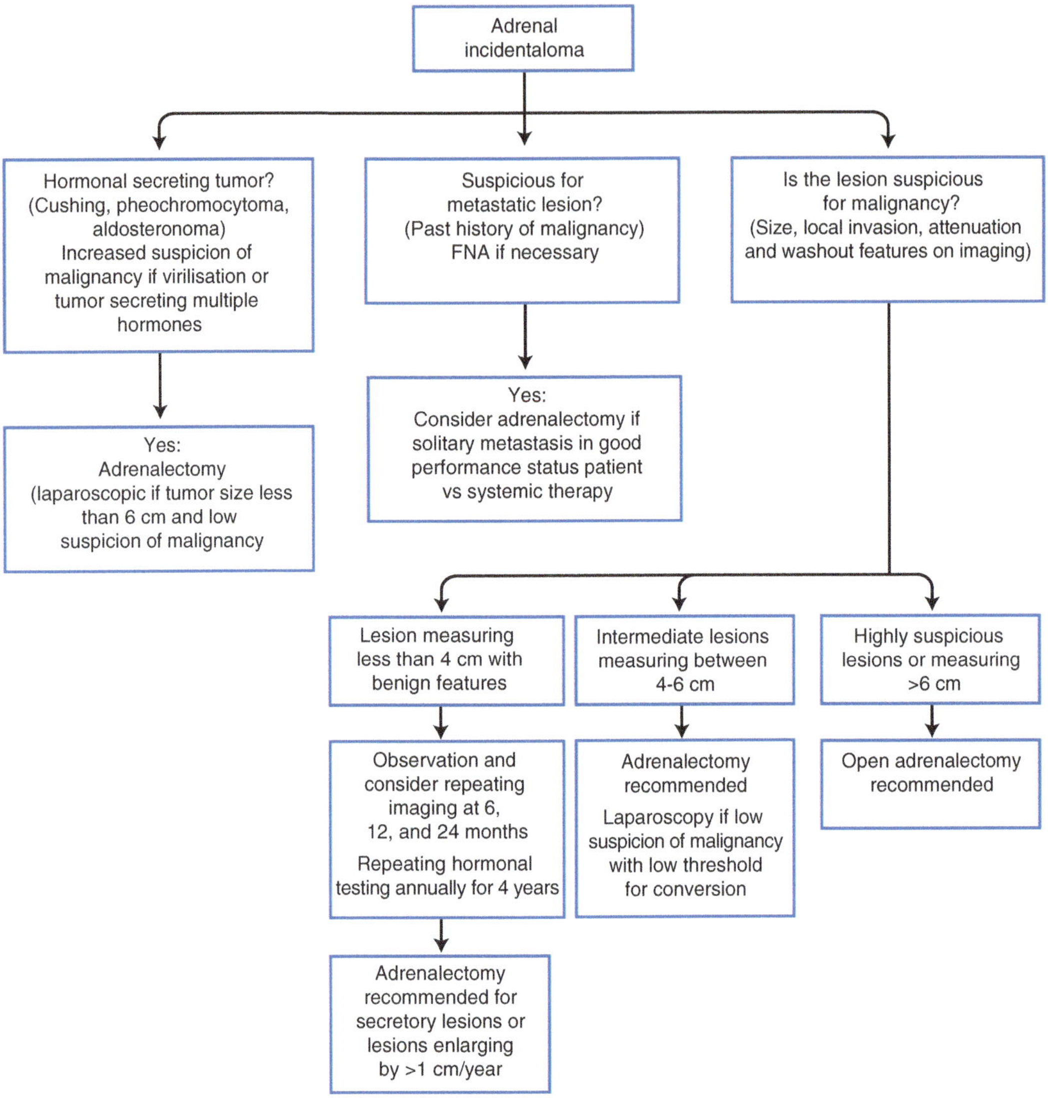

Fig. 22.1 Management algorithm for incidentally diagnosed adrenal masses

of both (25 %) [2]. On imaging, both size and appearance (attenuation and washout) are important. Ninety-five percent of ACC are greater than 5 cm at diagnosis [2]. Resection is recommended for incidentalomas >4 cm [1] since ACC is estimated to represent only 2 % of smaller lesions [3]. Tumor growth on serial radiologic imaging is also vital to consider. Other suspicious characteristics on imaging are an attenuation value of >10 Hounsfield units (HU) on unenhanced computerized tomography (CT) and >30 HU on enhanced scans as well as a delayed washout (less than 60 % at 15 min). CT scan and magnetic resonance imaging (MRI) are considered equivalent, but MRI may allow better assessment of extra-adrenal extension. Use of 18-Fluorodeoxyglucose (FDG)-PET may increase sensitivity and specificity, but due to limited experience and high costs, it is not routinely recommended [3]. Fine needle aspiration (FNA) biopsy can differentiate adrenal and non-adrenal tissue and is therefore indicated in suspicion of metastatic disease (once pheochromocytoma ruled out via biochemical testing) [1]. The idea that laparoscopy leads to increased recurrence is now controversial, and some series suggest comparable outcomes, particularly for lesions <10 cm in diameter and when the surgery is performed by an experienced surgeon [4]. Current consensus with resection of *likely* ACC (local invasion, diameter of >6 cm or suspicious imaging features) is still via open surgery in order to avoid tumor rupture [3].

22.2 Adrenocortical Carcinoma (ACC)

ACC are very rare malignant tumors (1–2 per million per year) [2]. Randomized clinical trials are lacking, and thus, the majority of the data on its management comes from small published series. The malignancy of an adrenal lesion is determined on histology with Weiss score, graded from zero to nine with each of the following criteria administered one point if confirmed on pathology: high mitotic rate, atypical mitoses, high nuclear grade, low percentage of clear cells, necrosis, diffuse architecture of tumor, capsular invasion, sinusoidal invasion, and venous invasion. A score of three or greater is associated with malignancy. Ki67 immunohistochemical staining has been found to be helpful in confirming malignancy and correlating with prognosis [5].

22.2.1 Prognosis

The two major prognostic factors are disease stage and margin status on pathology from initial surgery. In presence of metastatic lesions, the 5-year survival drops from 58–66 % to 0–24 %, and survival is usually less than 13 months [5]. The most common sites for distant disease are the lungs, liver, and bones. Significant prognostic factors include a Weiss score of >3, a mitotic index of >6/10 HPF, and a large tumor burden (>12 cm) [3]. Survival is improved by complete tumor resection, but even in presence of radical resection, relapse is seen in 75–85 % of patients [6]. This supports the need for adequate surgery and adjuvant treatments.

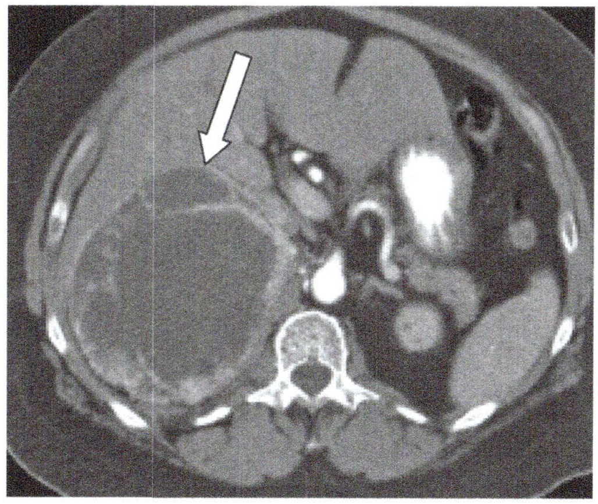

Fig. 22.2 A 38-year-old male presenting with an abdominal mass. Contrast-enhanced CT demonstrates a 10-cm right adrenal complex mass (*arrow*), proven to be adrenal carcinoma at histology (Used with permission from Boland [14])

22.2.2 Treatment

Treatment for ACC should consider patient factors and the oncology and potential endocrinology aspects of the tumor.

22.2.2.1 Surgery

Whenever feasible and safe, complete en bloc resection of the primary tumor and distant or recurrent disease should be performed [3, 7]. In particular, the threshold to perform nephrectomy should be low if invasion is suspected, providing preoperative confirmation of bilateral kidneys and good renal function is obtained. Direct invasion of the vena cava or intracaval tumor thrombus does not contraindicate surgery [3]. Surgical debulking may be considered in certain selected cases, but this approach has not demonstrated improvement in survival, and data are lacking to support it. Decision-making factors include the presence of symptomatic hormone hypersecretion, rate of progression, tumor grade, and patient performance status [3]. Debulking mainly serves to control tumor-related endocrine syndromes and possibly to increase the efficacy of other therapies although these patients, due to their reserved prognosis, may be better palliated medically. There is currently no role for neoadjuvant therapy in unresectable tumors. See Fig. 22.2.

22.2.2.2 Chemotherapy

The data on the use of adjuvant mitotane come from retrospective studies and the benefit on survival of these data is unclear. A published report [6] has shown that adjuvant mitotane, compared to surgery alone, led to prolonged disease-free survival (42 months vs. 10–25 months) and improved median overall survival (110 months vs. 52–67 months) in completely resected ACC. However, other series [7] have failed to demonstrate the same result. Mitotane should be considered for patients with the highest risk of recurrence, including high-grade disease, intraoperative tumor spillage, and presence of vascular or capsular invasion [6]. When used, a minimal duration of 2 years under the guidance of a medical oncologist is recommended [3]. While receiving mitotane, monitoring includes measurement of ACTH, urinary free cortisol, thyroid function, serum testosterone, lipids, and electrolytes [3]. Adrenal insufficiency must be supplemented, most commonly consisting of glucocorticoid and fludrocortisone. Other side effects include gastrointestinal (nausea, vomiting, diarrhea) and neurologic symptoms (lethargy, confusion, dizziness, ataxia). At this time, no other chemotherapy regimen, alone or in combination with mitotane, has been proven to be more effective than mitotane alone, but some centers do have combination protocols that are considered on a case-by-case basis. In the face of acknowledged palliative setting (locally advanced or metastatic disease), there is no survival benefit demonstrated with mitotane alone or in combination [8].

22.2.2.3 Radiation

ACC was previously thought to be radioresistant. Though not prospectively proven, some studies have shown a reduced local recurrence rate with adjuvant external beam radiation therapy (EBRT) [3]. Possible indications for EBRT include incomplete resection, uncertain resection status, intraoperative tumor violation, positive lymph nodes, diameter of >8 cm with evidence of vascular invasion, and a Ki67 of >10 %. Clear indications include palliation of metastatic disease to the brain and bone and with documented spinal cord compression or superior vena cava syndrome [3]. Radiation may also be considered in the presence of non-resectable persistent or recurrent local disease [3], but preferably administered in symptomatic cases only. It is generally well tolerated with mostly mild to moderate nausea, anorexia, and liver and kidney function impairment.

22.2.2.4 Additional Potential Palliative Treatment Options

Radiofrequency ablation (RFA) can be considered in inoperable patients or in the presence of metastatic disease, where the benefits of surgery are slim and do not outweigh the risks [3]. Its long-term efficacy and effect on survival remain unconfirmed. It is best considered in primary tumors that are <5 cm in diameter, located away from vital structures and large blood vessels [3], and in the treatment of liver metastasis. For arterial embolization, there is limited information, but it may provide adequate palliation of pain and a decrease in hormone production without major side effects [9]. Embolic agents include alcohol foam, stainless steel coils, ethanol, and gelfoam.

22.2.2.5 New Therapies/Under Investigation

Different immunotherapies are being studied in ACC, including the use of dendritic cells and DNA vaccination [3] and cytotoxic adenoviral gene therapy. Many growth factors have been found to be overexpressed in ACC (i.e., vascular endothelial growth factor, epidermal growth factor receptor, and insulin-like growth factor type 2) and may be promising targets as the field of oncogenomics develops.

22.3 Medical Management of Adrenal Hypersecretion

Palliative control of hypercortisolism is usually achieved with metyrapone and/or ketoconazole [2]. Their effect is apparent within a few days and is assessed by measuring the 24-h urine cortisol. If control is not achieved, mitotane and/or mifepristone (glucocorticoid receptor antagonist) can be added [2].

22.4 Pheochromocytoma (PCC) and Paraganglioma

Pheochromocytomas are part of the neuroendocrine tumor family. They commonly present with episodic hypertension, headache, diaphoresis, and tachycardia but can also be found incidentally. To diagnose a malignant PCC, the presence of local invasion and distant metastasis is needed, and such lesions are not curable. Up to 25 % are part of a hereditary syndrome, most commonly multiple endocrine neoplasia and von Hippel-Lindau. Initial management targets control of hypertension and prevention of hypertensive crisis. This starts with an alpha-adrenergic blocker and may then include beta-adrenergic and calcium channel blockade. Metyrosine, a catecholamine synthesis inhibitor, can also be used. Patients with malignant disease have an average 5-year survival of approximately 50 % [10]. Common sites for distant disease are the bones, liver, and lungs. Treatment options for malignant PCC include surgery (the mainstay of treatment), metaiodobenzylguanidine (MIBG) radiotherapy, and systemic antineoplastic therapy. There are no randomized control trials to determine which nonsurgical treatment is more effective. Therapies targeted at the adrenal bed, including EBRT, RFA, cryoablation, and arterial embolization, have been described in case series, and they should be used selectively [10]. As for other metastatic tumors, these modalities can also be considered for treatment of symptomatic metastatic lesions (e.g., EBRT to bone metastasis, RFA for liver lesions). See Fig. 22.3.

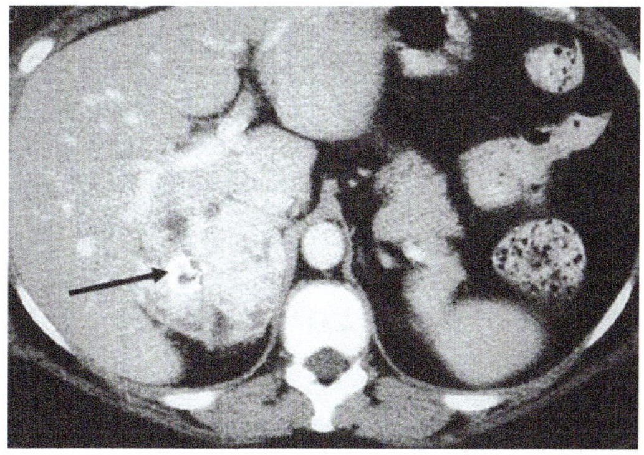

Fig. 22.3 A 56-year-old female with a pheochromocytoma. Contrast-enhanced CT image demonstrates a 5-cm hypervascular mass containing calcification (*arrow*) in the right adrenal gland. Although its imaging appearance is nonspecific, the patient had a history of "panic attacks" and laboratory evidence to support the diagnosis of pheochromocytoma. At surgical pathology, a pheochromocytoma was diagnosed (Used with permission from Hindman and Israel [15])

22.4.1 Surgery

Surgical resection after medical preparation for elevated catecholamine secretion should be considered in all cases of localized and isolated metastatic disease. Laparoscopy is the preferred approach for PCC with a low risk of malignancy [11]. However, in case of doubt, conversion to an open procedure should be performed. In a series of 176 operated patients, PCC had a 15 % rate of recurrence, and of those recurrences, 52 % were malignant. Risk factors for recurrent disease were familial cases of PCC, extra-adrenal tumors (paragangliomas), right-sided tumor, and operative capsule breach [12]. Although there are no firm data to support resection of metastasis, it appears to improve symptoms from abnormal hormone secretion and possibly increase survival [10]. Tumor debulking is considered a mainstay of treatment, palliating the hypersecretory state and possibly improving the efficacy of MIBG radiotherapy on residual lesions. However, its role is unclear in asymptomatic low-secreting tumors [10].

22.4.2 Chemotherapy

Systemic treatment, with a combination of cyclophosphamide, vincristine, and dacarbazine, is considered in patients with rapidly progressive and symptomatic disease and in cases negative for MIBG uptake or refractory to this treatment [10]. Tyrosine kinase inhibitors, such as sunitinib, appear promising but unproven.

22.4.3 MIBG Radiotherapy

MIBG is a selective treatment option when coupled with radioactive iodine. A retrospective study of 116 patients [13] demonstrated partial tumor response in 24–45 % of patients. It is generally well tolerated with possible mild myelosuppression. This treatment option is considered in slow-growing disease with positive uptake on MIBG scintigraphy. The benefit of a high-dose regimen does not outweigh the risks of increased toxicity and is not recommended [10].

22.4.4 Combination Therapy

Overall, MIBG radiotherapy and systemic chemotherapy have approximately the same tumor response rate and toxicity profile. Superiority of one over the other has not been demonstrated regarding their effect on overall survival. A combination of both treatments has not been demonstrated beneficial in small series [10].

22.5 Summary

Adrenal lesions may present (1) as an incidental finding on imaging study performed for unrelated reason, (2) as clinical presentation with risk factors for or symptoms suspicious for adrenal mass, and (3) in evaluation for endocrinopathies. They are concerning for possible endocrine syndromes or malignancies (primary and secondary) and are best investigated and treated within multidisciplinary teams. Surgical resection is the mainstay of treatment for locoregional and isolated metastatic disease, but other palliative options may alleviate symptoms related to the mass effect and control hormonal secretion in inoperable cases.

References

1. Young Jr WF. The incidentally discovered adrenal mass. N Engl J Med. 2007;356:601–10.
2. Allolio B, Fassnacht M. Clinical review: adrenocortical carcinoma: clinical update. J Clin Endocrinol Metab. 2006;91:2027–37.
3. Schteingart DE, Doherty GM, Gauger PG, Giordano TJ, Hammer GD, Korobkin M, Worden FP. Management of patients with adrenal cancer: recommendations of an international consensus conference. Endocr Relat Cancer. 2005;12:667–80.
4. Brix D, Allolio B, Fenske W, Agha A, Dralle H, Jurowich C, Langer P, Mussack T, Nies C, Riedmiller H, Spahn M, Weismann D, Hahner S, Fassnacht M. German Adrenocortical Carcinoma Registry Group, Laparoscopic versus open adrenalectomy for adrenocortical carcinoma: surgical and oncologic outcome in 152 patients. Eur Urol. 2010;58(4):609.
5. Assié G, Antoni G, Tissier F, Caillou B, Abiven G, Gicquel C, Leboulleux S, Travagli JP, Dromain C, Bertagna X, Bertherat J, Schlumberger M, Baudin E. Prognostic parameters of metastatic adrenocortical carcinoma. J Clin Endocrinol Metab. 2007;92:148–54.
6. Terzolo M, Angeli A, Fassnacht M, Daffara F, Tauchmanova L, Conton PA, Rossetto R, Buci L, Sperone P, Grossrubatscher E, Reimondo G, Bollito E, Papotti M, Saeger W, Hahner S, Koschker AC, Arvat E, Ambrosi B, Loli P, Lombardi G, Mannelli M, Bruzzi P, Mantero F, Allolio B, Dogliotti L, Berruti A. Adjuvant mitotane treatment for adrenocortical carcinoma. N Engl J Med. 2007;356:2372–80.
7. Crucitti F, Bellantone R, Ferrante A, Boscherini M, Crucitti P. The Italian Registry for Adrenal Cortical Carcinoma: analysis of a multiinstitutional series of 129 patients. The ACC Italian Registry Study Group. Surgery. 1996;119(2):161.
8. Fassnacht M, Terzolo M, Allolio B, Baudin E, Haak H, Berruti A, Welin S, Schade-Brittinger C, Lacroix A, Jarzab B, Sorbye H, Torpy DJ, Stepan V, Schteingart DE, Arlt W, Kroiss M, Leboulleux S, Sperone P, Sundin A, Hermsen I, Hahner S, Willenberg HS, Tabarin A, Quinkler M, de la Fouchardière C, Schlumberger M, Mantero F, Weismann D, Beuschlein F, Gelderblom H, Wilmink H, Sender M, Edgerly M, Kenn W, Fojo T, Müller HH, Skogseid B, FIRM-ACT Study Group. Combination chemotherapy in advanced adrenocortical carcinoma. N Engl J Med. 2012; 366(23):2189.
9. O'Keeffe FN, Carrasco CH, Chamsangavej C, Richli WR, Wallace S. Arterial embolization of adrenal tumors: results in nine cases. AJR Am J Roentgenol. 1988;151:819–22.
10. Scholz T, Eisenhofer G, Pacak K, Dralle H, Lehnert H. Clinical review: current treatment of malignant pheochromocytoma. J Clin Endocrinol Metab. 2007; 92:1217–25.
11. Shen WT, Sturgeon C, Clark OH, Duh QY, Kebebew E. Should pheochromocytoma size influence surgical approach? A comparison of 90 malignant and 60 benign pheochromocytomas. Surgery. 2004;136(6):1129.
12. Amar L, Servais A, Gimenez-Roqueplo AP, Zinzindohoue F, Chatellier G, Plouin PF. Year of diagnosis, features at presentation, and risk of recurrence in patients with pheochromocytoma or secreting paraganglioma. J Clin Endocrinol Metab. 2005;90(4): 2110.
13. Loh KC, Fitzgerald PA, Matthay KK, Yeo PP, Price DC. The treatment of malignant pheochromocytoma with iodine-131 metaiodobenzylguanidine (131I-MIBG): a comprehensive review of 116 reported patients. J Endocrinol Invest. 1997;20:648–58.
14. Boland GWL. Adrenal imaging. Abdom Imaging. 2011;36(4):472–82.
15. Hindman N, Israel GM. Adrenal gland and adrenal mass calcification. Eur Radiol. 2005;15(6):1163–7.

Urology

23

Dan Spernat

Contents

D. Spernat, MBBS, MPH, MEd, AFRACMA, FRACS
Department of Urology,
The Queen Elizabeth Hospital,
Woodville Road, Woodville 5011, SA, Australia
e-mail: daniel.spernat@health.sa.gov.au

Primary and secondary malignancies can affect the urological system. The intention of palliative surgery is to improve the patient's quality of life. However, urological intervention may also increase life expectancy. The most commonly performed palliative urological procedures are ureteric stenting and fulguration of bleeding bladder and prostate tumours. Ureteric stents or nephrostomy tubes may reverse obstructive renal failure. The improved renal function may increase life expectancy and allow for palliative chemotherapy to be considered. However, ureteric stents may not be able to overcome the compressive forces of malignancy. Therefore, nephrostomy tubes may be required to alleviate the obstruction. One must bear in mind the quality of life implications of nephrostomy tubes. Nephrostomy tubes require regular changes and have an increased risk of infection and the potential for dislodgement. There is also a role for palliative resection of the primary tumour in some metastatic solid organ malignancies. This may be to reduce bleeding and pain such as in metastatic bladder cancer. Additionally resection of the primary lesion has been shown to improve survival, despite metastases, in renal cell carcinoma.

23.1 Kidney

The triad of symptoms that renal cell carcinoma (RCC) historically presented with were mass, hematuria and pain. Due to the increased use of CT scanning, many renal masses are now

M. Wichmann, G. Maddern (eds.), *Palliative Surgery*,
DOI 10.1007/978-3-642-53709-7_23, © Springer-Verlag Berlin Heidelberg 2014

incidentally discovered. Importantly this has led to an increased proportion of organ-confined masses being detected [1]. Regardless up to one-third of cases will present with synchronous metastatic disease [2].

Cytoreductive nephrectomy has potential quality of life benefits as it may reduce bleeding, pain from clot colic as well as paraneoplastic symptoms [3]. Approximately 1–2 % of patients also demonstrate regression of metastases [4]. Furthermore patients who underwent cytoreductive nephrectomy followed by systemic interferon alpha treatment enjoyed a 30–50 % survival advantage over patients who were treated with systemic interferon alpha alone [5]. Nevertheless, mean survival amongst this group remains poor with median survival improving from 7.8 months to 13.6 months [5].

Since 2005 tyrosine kinase inhibitors (TKIs) have become the first-line systemic therapy for metastatic RCC. The available data suggest that cytoreductive nephrectomy remains an integral part of treatment of these patients [6]. This recommendation is only valid for patients with good performance status [7]. Several factors have been identified on multivariate analysis to determine a patient's appropriateness for cytoreductive nephrectomy. Patients with four or more of the risk factors listed next did not benefit from cytoreductive nephrectomy compared to patients treated with medical therapy alone [6]. Poor prognostic factors are:

1. Serum albumin below normal
2. Lactate dehydrogenase above normal
3. Tumour stage T3 or T4
4. Symptomatic metastatic disease
5. Liver metastases
6. Retroperitoneal or supradiaphragmatic lymphadenopathy

Moreover, the percentage of tumour burden removed at the time of cytoreductive nephrectomy predicts progression-free survival on univariate and multivariate analysis [6]. Timing of cytoreductive nephrectomy is controversial. Presurgical therapy followed by nephrectomy has the potential advantages of down staging irresectable disease, reducing time to systemic therapy and assessing the tumours' response to targeted therapy. However, there are no randomised controlled trials comparing pre- to postsurgical-targeted therapy [6].

Cytoreductive nephrectomy is a challenging operation due to loss of tissue planes, local invasion and tumour neovascularisation. Therefore, these operations should be undertaken in a centre of excellence and may require a multidisciplinary approach with vascular surgery input. Due to the potential impact on wound healing, haemorrhage and intraoperative adhesions, it is recommended that the TKIs be ceased for at least 2 weeks prior to surgery [8].

The gold standard treatment for organ-confined ureteric or renal pelvis transitional cell carcinoma (TCC) is nephroureterectomy [9]. Patients with synchronous or asynchronous metastatic disease have a universally poor outcome [9]. Chemotherapy regimens are based on the chemosensitive properties of bladder TCC and are therefore extrapolated for upper tract TCC [9].

Patients presenting with advanced upper tract TCC that are symptomatic from bleeding or pain from clot colic may benefit from palliative nephroureterectomy. These advantages must be balanced against the negative impact that nephrectomy has on renal function as this may preclude palliative chemotherapy or result in dose reduction [10]. There is no evidence that removal of the primary tumour improves chemotherapy response [10]. Moreover, by avoiding dose modification chemotherapeutic response may be improved [10]. A ureteric stent may resolve the renal colic by disobstructing the ureter and therefore improve renal function sufficiently for the patient to be able to tolerate chemotherapy.

Palliative nephroureterectomy for advanced upper tract TCC may be technically difficult. Laparoscopic surgery may be possible depending on the site of the lesion and which surrounding structures are involved. In the event of a non-resectable symptomatic upper tract TCC, radiotherapy may improve local control [11]. Radiotherapy combined with cisplatin-gemcitabine chemotherapy may provide increased disease-free survival and an overall survival advantage [12].

23.2 Bladder

Cystectomy has traditionally been reserved for patients without evidence of metastatic disease [13]. However, patients with metastatic bladder cancer may require treatment to control local disease and the distant metastases. For metastatic bladder TCC the current standard of care involves a transvesical debulking of the bladder tumour (TURBT) with adjuvant chemotherapy and radiotherapy [14]. Current chemotherapeutic regimes include cisplatin and gemcitabine, and this may provide a survival advantage [15].

However, palliative cystoprostatectomy (men) or anterior pelvic exenteration (women) remains an option for patients with significant local symptoms such as refractory haemorrhage. Muscle-invasive bladder tumours may also result in ureteric obstruction. Ureteric stenting may be insufficient to disobstruct the ureters. Ureteric obstruction occurs secondary to direct blockage of the ureter by tumour and invasion of the ureteric wall interrupting peristalsis [13]. Furthermore, non-urothelial carcinomas of the bladder respond poorly to chemo- and radiotherapy, and therefore palliative cystectomy may be required to control local symptoms.

As cystectomy carries greater morbidity than radiotherapy, it should be considered only if there are no other options [13]. Moreover, perioperative morbidity and mortality is greater in those over 75 years of age [16]. Palliative cystectomy may be a technically challenging operation, especially in T4b tumours [13]. Therefore, palliative diversion with nephrostomy tubes or via an ileal conduit may provide adequate symptom relief.

23.3 Ureteric Obstruction

Malignancy may cause ureteric obstruction and renal failure. The obstruction may be due to direct invasion or external compression from lymph node masses. Disobstructing the ureters may resolve renal failure and thus increase the life expectancy of the patient. Additionally, this may improve the renal function sufficiently for the patient to be able to tolerate chemotherapy. However, ureteric stents may not be able to overcome the compressive forces, and nephrostomy tubes may be a palliative option.

There are many different ureteric stents that are commercially available. Broadly, these stents may be made from polymers or metal alloys. The polymer stents are the standard JJ stents with one pig tail placed in the renal pelvis and the other in the bladder. The alloy stents are either semipermanent short stents (Memokath™ 051, PNN Medical A/S, Denmark) which are placed across the occluded segment or long stents that run from the renal pelvis to the bladder (Resonance®, Cook Medical, USA).

Resonance® stents are reported to have longer dwell times than polymer stents [17]. Moreover, Blaschko et al. have reported that Resonance® stents are more resistant to extrinsic compression than polymer JJ stents and have superior flow characteristics [18]. However, this experience is not universal, and some authors have reported poorer flow characteristics with Resonance® stents compared with polymer JJ stents [19]. Stent symptoms are likely to be similar to polymer JJ stents as the Resonance® stent also projects in to the bladder and renal pelvis where it may cause irritation.

The Memokath™ 051 stent is a semipermanent, thermo-expandable nickel-titanium ureteral stent. It has been designed for long-term use in patients with benign or malignant ureteral strictures [20]. Memokath™ ureteral stents may be more resistant to external compression than the JJ stent in patients with malignant strictures [21, 22]. The stent is designed to cover only the strictured section of the ureter reducing symptoms compared to a standard JJ stent [23]. Furthermore, the stent should not extend into the patient's bladder or into the renal pelvis.

23.4 Prostate

There has been a trend towards a lower stage of disease at diagnosis due to screening [24]. Regardless patients who present with cT3b-T4N0 or N1 disease present specific challenges – there is a need for local and micrometastatic disease control. Most patients with lymph node-positive disease will ultimately fail treatment [24]. Whilst many urologists are reluctant to perform radical prostatectomy (RP) in patients who are lymph node positive, there is evidence of improved cancer-specific and overall survival in those who undergo RP [25].

Thus RP is an important component of multimodal strategies of lymph node-positive prostate cancer [24]. Early adjuvant hormone therapy has been shown to improve cancer-specific and overall survival significantly [24]. There also appears to be a benefit from maximal multimodal therapy where RP is followed by adjuvant radiotherapy to the prostatic fossa and combined androgen blockade in lymph node-positive patients [24].

Nevertheless, many patients will not be fit enough for radical prostatectomy, and T4b tumours can be a technically challenging operation. RP is especially challenging where the prostate is adherent to the pelvic side wall. Therefore, many patients will be palliated with radiotherapy and neoadjuvant androgen deprivation. These patients may suffer recurrent hematuria or outflow obstruction and may require palliative TURP or fulguration of the prostate fossa. Suprapubic catheter placement, hyperbaric oxygen, or conjugated oestrogens may also be of benefit in this situation [26, 27]. Ureteric obstruction may also complicate locally advanced prostate cancer.

23.5 Testicular Cancer

Radical orchidectomy is important for the staging and treatment of testicular malignancy. However, patients with disseminated disease and life-threatening metastases should be stabilised with chemotherapy and orchidectomy delayed until medically safe [28]. Orchidectomy remains important in this group as the pathological subtype impacts on prognosis. Moreover, the testis is a sanctuary site that may not respond to systemic chemotherapy.

Patients with primary seminoma and a stable residual retroperitoneal mass after chemotherapy should be monitored [28]. However, should the mass increase in size or the HCG level increase, further treatment is warranted. Further treatment may involve salvage chemotherapy, surgery or radiotherapy [28].

Patients with non-seminoma who have a residual retroperitoneal mass and normal tumour markers post-chemotherapy require surgical resection [28]. Whilst only 10 % of residual masses contain viable tumour, 50 % contain teratoma that may dedifferentiate [28]. Moreover, there are no reliable imaging modalities to distinguish between these lesions. Should viable tumour be identified, salvage chemotherapy is indicated. Similarly, patients with residual retroperitoneal mass and elevated tumour markers should be treated with salvage chemotherapy [28].

A retroperitoneal mass that persists despite salvage chemotherapy should be resected. Similarly, if there is marker progression and no further chemotherapeutic options, then resection is appropriate if complete resection of the mass is feasible [28]. Post-chemotherapy retroperitoneal lymph node dissection (RPLND) is technically challenging and should be carried out by an experienced surgeon with ICU backup. Vascular surgery input may be necessary as portions of the aorta or vena cava may need to be resected en bloc.

23.6 Penile and Scrotal Malignancies

Many patients with potentially curable penile cancers refuse penectomy. Therefore there is a very limited role in patients with metastatic disease. However, penile and scrotal lesions which are ulcerated, painful and with or without fistulae may benefit from palliative resection [29]. In addition metastases to inguinal lymph nodes may erode through surrounding structures including skin and vessels. Therefore, palliative resection should be considered for enlarging metastatic lymph nodes.

As the surgery can be extensive and destructive, neoadjuvant chemotherapy may be of benefit [30]. To minimise potential complications surgery should be carried out by a surgeon with experience in malignant groin exploration. Additionally complex flaps may be required to close the defect, and therefore involvement of a plastic surgeon or a melanoma expert may be helpful. Lymph nodes that are not resectable may benefit from palliative radiotherapy [29].

Locally advanced penile lesions may also involve the urethra leading to obstruction. Therefore, even if penectomy is refused, palliative perineal urethrostomy may be of benefit. Should the patient consent to penectomy, the decision to perform a partial vs. radical penectomy should be made on the basis of being able to achieve clear margins whilst also leaving the patient with sufficient penile length to hold the penis for urination. Generally 2 cm of residual length is considered adequate [29].

23.7 Adrenal

Adrenocortical carcinoma is a rare condition with an overall 5-year survival rate of approximately 35 % [31]. These tumours often metastasise and invade local structures. Management is surgical as these tumours are generally not sensitive to chemo- and radiotherapy. Complete surgical resection results in a higher 5-year survival [31]. Moreover, as some of these tumours are functional, resection may reduce symptoms [32]. Due to the close proximity of the adrenal to the kidney, direct invasion is common [31]. Recalcitrant hematuria may also necessitate en bloc resection. Surgical excision via a thoracoabdominal incision provides excellent access for these complex masses [32].

References

1. Parsons JK, Schoenberg MS, Carter HB. Incidental renal tumours: casting doubt on the efficacy of early intervention. Urology. 2001;57:1013–5.
2. Bukowski RM. Natural history and therapy of metastatic renal cell carcinoma: the role of interleukin-2. Cancer. 1997;80:1198–220.
3. Wein AJ. Campbell-Walsh urology: ninth edition review. Elsevier Saunders: Philadelphia, Edinburgh; 2007, p. 1567–637.
4. Walther MM, Yan JC, Pass HI, Linehan WM, Rosenberg SA. Cytoreductive surgery before high dose interleukin-2 based therapy in patients with metastatic renal cell carcinoma. J Urol. 1997;158: 1675.
5. Flanign RC, Mickisch G, Sylvester R, Tangen C, Van Poppel H, Crawford ED. Cytoreductive nephrectomy in patients with metastatic renal cancer: a combined analysis. J Urol. 2004;171:1071–6.
6. Crispen PL, Blute ML. Role of cytoreductive nephrectomy in the era of targeted therapy for renal cell carcinoma. Curr Urol Rep. 2012;13(1):38–46.
7. Ljungberg B, Cowan NC, Hanbury DC, Hora M, Kuczyk MA, Merseburger AS, et al. EAU guidelines on renal cell carcinoma: the 2010 update. Eur Urol. 2010;53(3):398–406.
8. Harshman LC, Yu RJ, Allen GI, Srinivas S, Gill HS, Chung BI. Surgical outcomes and complications associated with presurgical tyrosine kinase inhibition for advanced renal cell carcinoma (RCC). Urol Oncol. 2013;31(3):379–85.
9. Wein AJ. Campbell-Walsh urology: ninth edition review. Elsevier Saunders: Philadelphia, Edinburgh; 2007, p. 1638–52.
10. Lerner SE, Blute ML, Richardson RL, Zincke H. Platinum based chemotherapy for advanced transitional cell carcinoma of the upper urinary tract. Mayo Clin Proc. 1996;71(10):945–50.
11. Hall MC, Womack JS, Roerborn CG, Carmody T, Sagalowsky AI. Advanced transitional cell carcinoma of the upper urinary tract: patterns of failure, survival and impact of postoperative adjuvant radiotherapy. J Urol. 1998;160(3 Pt 1):703–6.
12. Czito B, Zietman A, Kaufman D, Skowronski U, Shipley W. Adjuvant radiotherapy with and without concurrent chemotherapy for locally advanced transitional cell carcinoma of the renal pelvis and ureter. J Urol. 2004;172(4 Pt 1):1271–5.
13. Stenzl A, Witjes JA, Comerat E, Cowan NC, De Santis M, Kuczyk M, et al. Treatment of muscle-invasive and metastatic bladder cancer: update of the EAU Guidelines. Eur Urol. 2011;59(6):1009–18.
14. Wein AJ. Campbell-Walsh urology: ninth edition review. Elsevier Saunders: Philadelphia, Edinburgh; 2007, p. 2468–78.
15. Dimopoulos MA, Deliveliotis C, Moulopoulos LA, Papadimitriou C, Mitropoulos D, Anagnostopoulos A, et al. Treatment of patients with metastatic urothelial carcinoma and impaired renal function with single agent docetaxel. Urology. 1998;52(1):56–60.
16. Zebic N, Weinknecht S, Kroepfl D. Radical cystectomy in patients aged>or=75 years: an updated review of patients treated with curative and palliative intent. BJU Int. 2005;95(9):1211–4.
17. Rao MV, Polcari AJ, Turk TMT. Updates on the use of ureteral stents: focus on the Resonance® stent. Med Devices (Auckl). 2011;4:11–5.
18. Blaschko SD, Deane LA, Krebs A, Abdelshehid CS, Khan F, Borin J, et al. In-vivo evaluation of flow characteristics of novel metal ureteral stent. J Endourol. 2007;21(7):780–3.
19. Spernat D, Chopra S, King Q. In Vivo comparison of pressure/flow characteristics of novel

long-dwell alloy ureteral stent (Resonance) vs. standard polyurethane double pigtail stent (Sof-flex, Cook) – implications in established renal dysfunction. BJU Int 2010;105(S1):39–41.
20. Staios D, Shergill I, Thwaini A, Junaid I, Buchholz NP. The Memokath stent. Expert Rev Med Devices. 2007;4(2):99–101.
21. Zaman F, Poullis C, Back C, Moraitis K, Junaid I, Buchholz N, et al. Use of a segmental thermoexpandable metal alloy stent in the management of malignant ureteric obstruction: a single centre experience in the UK. Urol Int. 2011;87(4):405–10.
22. Maan Z, Patel D, Moraitis K, El-Husseiny T, Papatsoris AG, Buchholz NP, et al. Comparison of stent-related symptoms between conventional Double-J stents and a new-generation thermoexpandable segmental metallic stent: a validated-questionnaire-based study. J Urol. 2010;24(4):589–93.
23. Maan Z, Patel D, Moraitis K, El-Husseiny T, Papatsoris AG, Buchholz NP, et al. Comparison of stent-related symptoms between conventional Double-J stents and a new-generation thermoexpandable segmental metallic stent: a validated-questionnaire-based study. J Endourol. 2010;24(4):589–93.
24. Heidenreich A, Bolla M, Joniau S. EAU guidelines on prostate cancer. Eur Urol. 2012. Access from http://www.uroweb.org/gls/pdf/08%20Prostate%20Cancer_LR%20March%2013th%202012.pdf
25. Steuber T, Budaus L, Walz J, Zorn KC, Schlomm T, Chun F, et al. Radical prostatectomy improves progression free and cancer specific survival in men with lymph node positive prostate cancer in the prostate-specific antigen era: a confirmatory study. BJU Int. 2011;107(11):1755–61.
26. Spernat D, Aw H, Eapen R, Appu S. The use of hyperbaric oxygen therapy in radiation-induced haemorrhagic cystitis. Internet J Urol. 2011;8(2).
27. Miller J, Burfield GD, Moretti KL. Oral conjugated estrogen therapy for treatment of hemorrhagic cystitis. J Urol. 1994;151(5):1348–50.
28. Albers P, Albrecht W, Algaba F, Bokemeyer C, Cohn-Cedermark G, Fizazi K, et al. Guidelines on testicular cancer. Eur Urol. 2005;48(6):885–94.
29. Wein AJ. Campbell-Walsh urology: ninth edition review. Elsevier Saunders: Philadelphia, Edinburgh; 2007, p. 959–92.
30. Pizzocaro G, Algaba F, Solsona E, Tana S, Van Der Poel H, Watkin N, et al. EAU penile cancer guidelines 2009. Eur Urol. 2010;57(6):1002–12.
31. Wein AJ. Campbell-Walsh urology: ninth edition review. Elsevier Saunders: Philadelphia, Edinburgh; 2007, p. 1821–67.
32. Niaz WA, Alvi S. Metastatic malignant pheochromocytoma of adrenal gland. J Coll Physicians Surg Pak. 2008;18(5):305–7.

Gynaecology

24

John Miller

Contents

J. Miller, MBBS, FRANZCOG, CGO
Department of Gynaecology,
The Queen Elizabeth Hospital,
Woodville Road, Woodville, SA 5011, Australia
e-mail: j.miller@naonc.com.au

Palliative surgery in gynaecology is primarily concerned with patients suffering from gynaecological cancers. The aim is to aid symptom control and improve quality of life, not necessarily prolonging survival. Its main indication in gynaecology is the treatment of bowel obstruction in patients with recurrent ovarian cancer.

24.1 Introduction

The role of palliative surgery in gynaecology is primarily concerned with patients suffering from malignancies of the gynaecological tract. These involve the ovary (primary or secondary), primary peritoneal cancer, fallopian tube, uterus, cervix, vulva and vagina. The role of colpocleisis for benign severe prolapse is beyond the scope of this chapter which will focus on gynaecological oncologic conditions.

Palliative surgery can be defined as surgery performed to control the cancer, reduce symptoms and improve quality of life for those whose cancer is not able to be entirely removed. Palliative surgery may increase the patient's life expectancy as well, particularly if it allows for the reintroduction of cancer-specific therapies such as chemotherapy. Palliative care is aimed towards symptom control and improved quality of life, not necessarily prolonging survival. Surgery may provide the best symptom control, but its indication must be individualised taking into account life expectancy, risk of surgical morbidity and mortality and the patient's level of

M. Wichmann, G. Maddern (eds.), *Palliative Surgery*,
DOI 10.1007/978-3-642-53709-7_24,

functioning. Palliative surgery focussing on the patient's quality of life and comfort requires recognition of their autonomy and potential for personal rehabilitation and development whilst still maintaining realistic expectations.

Effective anti-disease therapy offers the best chance of good symptom relief, and treatment of symptoms must be directed at the underlying cause if possible. Remember symptoms can be due to the cancer or the therapy or have a completely unrelated aetiology. Therefore thorough evaluation of the patient with advanced gynaecological cancer must be undertaken. Once palliative treatment is initiated, there must be ongoing evaluation of its effectiveness and outcome. Factors to consider when evaluating therapy include stage of disease and rate of progression, natural history, burden of investigations and therapy versus patient gains, potential to prevent future symptoms and the potential for patient rehabilitation (physical, psychological, social and spiritual).

24.2 Ovarian Cancer

Epithelial ovarian cancer which accounts for >90 % of all ovarian malignancies is advanced at diagnosis in ~70 % of cases. The tumour is usually spread throughout the peritoneal cavity, often with associated ascites and possible pleural effusions. Primary peritoneal and tubal cancers tend to behave in a similar fashion, and their treatment is comparable to that for ovarian cancer. Metastatic ovarian cancer can therefore have physiological effects, mass effects (including those tumours metastatic to the ovary from other primary sites), gynaecological effects and particularly in advanced disease effect on gastrointestinal function.

Primary cytoreductive surgery is still the mainstay of therapy for its assumed benefit in three main areas [1]. Physiological benefits of removing bulky tumour masses, particularly ovarian and omental disease, in regard to improving gut function and decreasing ascites. Improved tumour perfusion and increased growth fraction increasing the likelihood of response to chemotherapy and decreasing the potential for developing drug resistance. Immunologic benefits as large tumour masses appear to have an immunosuppressive function. Optimal cytoreduction also leads to superior survival [2]. Prognosis is affected by the maximum diameter residual disease, with survival best in those who have all their disease resected. Patients whose largest residual lesion is no greater than 5 mm fare better than those with nodules up to 15 mm, who in turn do better than those with less than optimal cytoreduction and bulky residual disease. If optimal primary cytoreduction is not thought possible, or the patient has a poor performance status or significant comorbidities, there is a role for neoadjuvant chemotherapy with a view to interval debulking surgery if chemosensitive. Greater than 70 % of patients with ovarian cancer respond to chemotherapy. However, most recur intraperitoneally and become resistant to chemotherapy. There is now thought to potentially be a role for repeat surgical cytoreduction in patients with recurrent disease [3]. Selected patients with disease thought to be operable showed a survival benefit after repeat cytoreductive surgery compared to chemotherapy alone.

24.3 Uterine Cancer

Cancer of the endometrium is the most common gynaecological cancer with 1 in 49 women in Australia being affected by age 85 [4]. Its main symptom is abnormal vaginal bleeding (especially postmenopausal bleeding), but it may also exhibit symptoms from local mass effect or symptoms secondary to metastatic spread. Spread is more likely in certain histological subtypes such as sarcomas and clear cell or serous papillary carcinomas.

Advanced uterine cancer can cause problems with bleeding, pain or fistulae possibly necessitating the use of palliative surgical procedures.

24.4 Cervical Cancer

Cancer of the cervix is the most common gynaecological cancer worldwide, with the incidence being much higher in third world countries without a screening programme. Unfortunately patients in developing countries often present with advanced disease that may be locally invasive into adjacent structures or organs. It is hoped that in the future the incidence of invasive cervical cancer will decrease due to the introduction of the human papillomavirus (HPV) vaccine.

Locally advanced or metastatic cervical cancer is usually primarily treated with chemoradiation rather than radical hysterectomy. When cervical cancer recurs centrally in a radiated field, pelvic exenteration may offer the only hope of cure. However, there may also be a role for palliative exenteration in certain cases of cervical cancer complicated by vesico- or colovaginal fistulae. Less morbid urinary or gastrointestinal diversions may be more appropriate if pure symptom control is the aim.

Recurrent cervical cancer may also present with ureteric obstruction. Retrograde stenting is often appropriate, but if this is not technically feasible, strong consideration must be given to the appropriateness of percutaneous nephrostomy in patients whose poor prognosis or symptoms from pelvic tumour may make a less traumatic demise from renal failure a kinder option.

24.5 Vaginal Cancer

Primary vaginal cancer is rare, accounting for only 1–2 % of gynaecological malignancies. By far the majority of vaginal carcinomas are secondary from other primary sites, particularly the cervix, uterus and colon. Chemoradiation is the usual primary therapy for vaginal cancers. In patients with central recurrence after radiation therapy, surgery, often in the form of pelvic exenteration, may be the only treatment available. Vaginal cancer can also be complicated by rectovaginal or vesicovaginal fistulae which may also make exenteration a suitable treatment option, or if not feasible necessitate diversion procedures.

24.6 Vulvar Cancer

Cancer of the vulva accounts for ~4 % of female genital tract malignancies. By far the majority are squamous cell carcinomas, but there are other aggressive histological subtypes including melanoma and sarcoma. Vulvar cancer can cause pain and bleeding and surgical excision is usually the best form of symptom control. Plastic surgical reconstruction may be required to cover the defect following removal of large vulvar cancers, especially if it is recurrent cancer in a radiotherapy field. Involvement of the anus, rectum or urethra is often initially treated with chemoradiation with a view to shrinking the tumour in the hope a less radical surgical procedure may be required.

24.7 Gynaecological Cancer Symptoms

Gynaecological malignancies can cause a number of symptoms, with surgery having a potential role in the treatment of many of these symptoms.

24.7.1 Psychosocial

Surgery to remove the tumour can have a positive psychological affect on the patient. Even if it is not curative, it may prolong survival sufficiently for the patient to get their affairs in order or attend important events.

24.7.2 Pain

Pain can be due to a number of causes including local effects or ulceration as well as infiltration of nerves. There are a number of procedures that can be of potential benefit in controlling pain. These include nerve blocks or ablation, dorsal rhizotomy (ablation of dorsal root fibres) for unilateral perineal lesions and cordotomy (interruption of spinothalamic tracts) for nociceptive pain.

24.7.3 Bleeding

Uterine cancers in particular may cause significant and distressing vaginal bleeding. Even if the tumour is metastatic, there is often a role for the so-called simple toilet hysterectomy to remove the uterus to control the bleeding. The hysterectomy will also prevent further local spread of the disease.

24.7.4 Mass Effect

Large ovarian tumours, either primary or secondary from other sites, (particularly GIT and breast), may cause local pressure effects resulting in pain, bloating, abdominal distension and problems with gut function. There is a role for tumour markers to help determine if an ovarian tumour is primary or metastatic. However, it must be remembered that tumour markers are just a guide and the definitive answer needs a tissue diagnosis. Raised CA125 suggests a primary serous ovarian tumour. CEA may be elevated in colorectal tumours as well as mucinous ovarian lesions, and consideration must be given to a colonoscopy in patients with a raised CEA in association with an ovarian mass. CA19.9 can be raised in hepatobiliary and pancreatic lesions as well as mucinous ovarian tumours and indicate the need for upper abdominal imaging. If a patient has a past history of breast cancer, their CA15.3 should be checked as ovarian tumours may represent a recurrence of breast cancer (even if their primary breast tumour was a long time previously because of the risk of late recurrence). Even if the removal of the ovarian tumour does not prolong survival, there is a role to debulk them to improve the patient's quality of life for the time they have left.

There is some suggestion that ovaries can behave as a sanctuary site resistant to chemotherapy, and their removal, particularly if it is a large tumour, may help improve response to treatment and prolong survival.

24.7.5 Bowel

Gynaecological cancers can cause a number of gastrointestinal symptoms including nausea and vomiting, constipation, anorexia and diarrhoea. However, it is intestinal obstruction which is the main indicator for palliative surgery in gynaecology. Intestinal obstruction is the most frequent cause of death in advanced ovarian cancer. Obstruction may be present at multiple sites and can be mechanical or due to decreased motility. Mechanical obstruction is usually via extrinsic compression of the small intestine by tumour or lymph nodes, whilst dysmotility is usually secondary to infiltration of the myenteric plexus. Patients who have received pelvic radiotherapy may also be complicated by obstructive symptoms caused by radiation strictures.

Palliative surgery for gastrointestinal tract obstruction must be individualised with careful selection of those who may benefit. The decision between surgery and conservative therapy is based on the extent of disease, operability, life expectancy, chances of response to further antineoplastic therapy, general condition and patient preference. If surgery is contemplated the procedure must be feasible with acceptable morbidity to the patient who is often in poor condition with limited life expectancy. The procedure must be likely to improve the patient's symptoms and quality of life [5].

A Cochrane review in 2010 [6] looked at palliative surgery versus medical therapy for bowel obstruction in ovarian cancer. Only one study by Mangili et al. [7] met the inclusion criteria. This was a retrospective review of 47 women with advanced ovarian cancer. Twenty-seven underwent palliative surgery and 20 were treated conservatively with octreotide. The outcomes looked at were reported overall survival and perioperative mortality and morbidity.

Six (22 %) patients undergoing surgery had serious complications, and three (11 %) died as a result of these complications. However, surgery had a significantly ($p<.001$) better survival than conservative therapy.

The incidence of bowel obstruction in patients with ovarian cancer is 25–50 % [8], and the life expectancy of patients with bowel obstruction in ovarian cancer is 4 months [9]. There are no definite prognostic factors to predict the outcome of surgery in patients with malignant bowel obstruction, and the management of these patients remains controversial. Krebs and Gopleruds [10] score patients with bowel obstruction based on age, nutrition, tumour, ascites, chemotherapy and radiotherapy. This score has been reported to offer eligibility criteria for those who can benefit from surgery.

In another study [11] looking at surgery versus chemotherapy for intestinal obstruction in advanced ovarian cancer, the only significant factor predicting a greater than 6 months disease-free period was prior response to platinum-based chemotherapy. Mangili [7] reported survival was superior for surgery compared to octreotide and that surgical palliation should be considered in patients with a good performance status.

If palliative surgery is considered in patients with bowel obstruction, there are various options to consider. These include laparotomy and surgical resection or bypass of the obstructed segment or segments, a diverting stoma proximal to the obstruction, colorectal stents or a venting gastrostomy (percutaneous endoscopic gastrostomy or PEG). Flexible self-expanding metallic stents to bypass a localised obstruction, either proximal small bowel or colon (especially distal to the splenic flexure), have been shown to have a role in palliation of bowel obstruction in patients with recurrent gynaecological malignancies [12]. Palliative laparoscopic end colostomy formation is feasible in some patients with malignant obstruction or fistulae [13] and provides good symptom relief with a less morbid surgical procedure.

Decompressive percutaneous endoscopic gastrostomy (PEG) can be used to control nausea and vomiting in patients with gynaecological cancers [14]. It is used for patients with small bowel obstruction who have a limited lifespan or are poor surgical candidates, or who have recurrent small bowel obstructions.

Leitdo et al. [3] looked at the outcome of palliative procedures for malignant bowel obstruction due to recurrent ovarian cancer. Twenty-six patients were reviewed, 14 with small intestinal obstruction and 12 with large intestinal obstruction. Fourteen patients (54 %) underwent operative procedures, and 12 patients (46 %) underwent endoscopic procedures. Symptom improvement or resolution within 30 days occurred in 23 patients (88 %); 71 % of operative and 50 % of endoscopic patients still had symptom control at 60 days. The median survival of patients who were operated on was 191 and 78 days for those who underwent endoscopic procedures. Recurrence of symptoms or death by 90 days occurred in ~50 % of patients.

24.7.6 Fistulae

Fistulae between the urinary or gastrointestinal tracts and the vagina can be a distressing complication of patients with gynaecological malignancies, especially those with locally advanced cervical cancer. Surgical correction is the treatment of choice if feasible, but this may not be possible especially if the tissue has received a radical dose of radiotherapy. If this is the case, diverting colostomy for rectovaginal or ileal loop diversion for vesicovaginal fistulae may be considered.

24.7.7 Central Recurrence

Central recurrence of cervical cancer may be treated via a pelvic exenteration with a curative intent if there is no evidence of distant disease. Exenteration is not usually considered in patients with distant metastases or unresectable pelvic wall disease. However, if these patients have significant symptoms from local disease such as bleeding, discharge, pain or fistulae, then palliative pelvic exenteration can be a therapeutic option. A study looking at palliative exenteration [15] reported a significant complication rate of 38.4 % and 2-year overall survival of 15.4 %. However all of the patients undergoing palliative pelvic exenteration achieved symptom control and reported improved quality of life.

24.7.8 Ureteric

Patients with advanced cervical cancer can get ureteric blockage leading to an obstructive uropathy. A study looking a palliative urinary diversion by percutaneous nephrostomy and stenting [16] reported increased short-term survival but no significant difference in quality of life. Therefore percutaneous nephrostomy should only be undertaken if months of relative symptom-free survival is anticipated and not performed in patients with locally advanced disease causing severe symptoms significantly affecting their quality of life.

24.7.9 Ascites

Recurrent ascites is a common complication in patients with advanced gynaecological malignancies, especially recurrent ovarian cancer. Repeated paracentesis may be required, and this can be a great inconvenience to patients, necessitating numerous hospital admissions and invasive procedures. The PleurX peritoneal catheter drainage system, which is tunnelled in under radiological guidance, can be used for repeated drainage of ascitic fluid in the community setting. Its safety and effectiveness were confirmed in a study by Tapping et al. [17], and it can be used as a first-line approach in patients with refractory malignant ascites.

Peritoneovenous shunts for the management of malignant ascites have tended to be utilised less frequently due to their reported complication rate of ~40 %, particularly risk of occlusion or DIC.

24.8 Summary and Key Points

The primary intention of palliative surgical procedures is to relieve symptoms and improve quality of life in patients with advanced disease. Its effectiveness is judged by the presence and durability of patient-acknowledged symptom resolution [18]. Surgery to remove the tumour and treat the disease may often offer the best chance at symptom control. It may also offer the possibility of reintroduction of other therapies which may help improve the patient's quality of life. Gynaecological malignancies can have an effect on a number of other systems, especially gastrointestinal and urinary. Management of bowel and urinary symptoms is very well covered in the colorectal and urology chapters of this book, and the same principles apply in patients with gynaecological cancer. Gynaecological surgeons must develop a very good multidisciplinary approach to the care of their patients to optimise their quality of life once they are in the palliative stage of their disease.

References

1. Berek JS, Hacker NF. Practical gynecologic oncology. 3rd ed. Philadelphia: Lippincott Williams and Wilkins; 2000.
2. Hoskins WJ, McGuire WP, Brady MF, Homesley HD, Creasman WT, Berman M, et al. The effect of diameter of largest residual disease on survival after primary cytoreductive surgery in patients with suboptimal residual epithelial ovarian carcinoma. Am J Obstet Gynecol. 1994;170:974–9.
3. Leitdo Jr MM, Chi DS. Surgical management of recurrent ovarian cancer. Semin Oncol. 2009;36(2):106–11.
4. Report to the nation uterine cancer. 2012. Cancer Australia.
5. Rezk Y, Timmins PF, Smith HS. Palliative care in gynecologic oncology. Am J Hosp Palliat Med. 2011;28(5):356–74.
6. Kueukmetin A, Naik R, Galaal K, Bryant A, Dickinson H. Palliative surgery versus medical management for bowel obstruction in ovarian cancer. Cochrane Database Syst Rev. 2010;(7):CD007792.
7. Mangili G, Aletti G, Frigerio L, Franchi M, Panacci N, Vigano R, et al. Palliative care for intestinal obstruction in recurrent ovarian cancer: a multivariate analysis. Int J Gynaecol Cancer. 2005;15:830–5.
8. Caprotti R. Palliative surgery for recurrent bowel obstruction due to advanced ovarian cancer. Minerva Gineologica. 2006;58(3):239–44.
9. Pothuri B. Palliative surgery for bowel obstruction in recurrent ovarian cancer: an updated series. Gynecol Oncol. 2003;89(2):306–13.
10. Gadducci A, Cosio S, Fanuchi A, Genazzani AR. Malnutrition and cachexia in ovarian cancer patients: pathophysiology and management. Anticancer Res. 2001;21(4B):2941–7.
11. Bryan DN, Radbod R, Beck JS. An analysis of surgical versus chemotherapeutic intervention for the management of intestinal obstruction in advanced ovarian cancer. Int J Gynaecol Cancer. 2006;16(1):125–34.
12. Caceres A, Zhou Q, Iasonos A, Gerdes H, Chi DS, Barakat RR. Colorectal stents for palliation of large bowel obstructions in recurrent gynaecologic cancer: an updated series. Gynecol Oncol. 2008;108(3):482–5.
13. Dos Santos LA, Schomoritz BM, Huang M, Holcomb K, Ramirez PT, Caputo TA. Palliative laparoscopic end colostomy in a nonagenarian. JSLS. 2008;12(4):410–3.

14. Meyer L, Pothuri B. Decompressive percutaneous gastrostomy tube use in gynaecologic malignancies. Curr Treat Options Oncol. 2006;7(2):111–20.
15. Guimaraes GC, Baiocchi G, Ferreira FO, Kumagai LY, Fallopa CC, Aguiar S, Rossi BM, Soares FA, Lopes A. Palliative pelvic exenteration for patients with gynaecological malignancies. Arch Gynecol Obstet. 2011;283(5):1107–12.
16. Lapita MC, Buckley BS. Impact of palliative urinary diversion by percutaneous nephrostomy drainage and ureteral stenting among patients with advanced cervical cancer and obstructive uropathy: a prospective cohort. J Obstet Gynecol Res. 2011;37(8):1061–70.
17. Tapping CR, Ling L, Razack A. PleurX drainage in the management of malignant ascites: safety, complications, long term patency and factors predictive of success. Br J Radiol. 2011;10:1259.
18. Dunn GA. Surgical palliative care: recent trends and developments. Surg Clin North Am. 2011;91(2):277–92. vii.

Orthopaedics

25

Samuel Young and René Zellweger

Contents

The authors would like to acknowledge the assistance of Dr. Richard Beaver, Consultant, Orthopaedic Surgeon, Royal Perth Hospital, for the clinical cases and radiographs used in this chapter.

S. Young, MBBS(Hons)
R. Zellweger, FRACS, FACS (✉)
Department of Orthopaedic Surgery,
Royal Perth Hospital,
Wellington Street, Perth, WA 6000, Australia
e-mail: s_e_young@optusnet.com.au;
rene.zellweger@health.wa.gov.au

Metastatic disease is the number one cause of morbidity to cancer patients. The bone is a frequent site of metastatic disease. Surgery has the potential to improve function and quality of life through stabilisation or reconstruction. Communication between the treating surgeon and subspecialist colleagues is essential to optimise outcomes for patient care. The aim of palliative orthopaedic treatment is to alleviate pain and restore mobility and dignity to patients suffering with terminal cancer.

Key Messages to Surgeons

1. Metastatic bone disease is a common and significant cause of morbidity in cancer patients.
2. Surgery can offer improvements in function and quality of life and can often be performed in general orthopaedic centres.
3. Local biology in pathological fractures is altered and union is unpredictable. More aggressive surgical techniques may be required.
4. Arthroplasty is evolving as a more reliable option for these patients compared to standard internal fixation techniques.
5. Communication between the treating surgeon and radiation oncologists, medical oncologists and specialist orthopaedic oncologists should be encouraged and is essential in most situations.

M. Wichmann, G. Maddern (eds.), *Palliative Surgery*,
DOI 10.1007/978-3-642-53709-7_25, © Springer-Verlag Berlin Heidelberg 2014

25.1 Introduction

Metastatic disease is the primary cause of morbidity and mortality to cancer sufferers. The bone is the third most commonly encountered site of metastasis after the liver and lung. It is the most common site amongst breast and prostate primary carcinoma. Overall it is estimated that up to 84 % of all patients with metastatic disease will suffer bony lesions. The most common primary solid tumours that exhibit this pattern originate in the breast, lung, thyroid, prostate and kidney. Haematological malignancies such as lymphoma and myeloma also share this propensity.

Morbidity from metastatic bone disease (MBD) is significant. Up to 70 % of patients will develop bone pain. Pathological fracture, spinal compression and associated immobility are all burdens that may be experienced. There is evidence that on average, a patient with MBD will undergo a skeletal-related event (pain, fracture, radiotherapy, surgery) every 3–6 months [1].

With an ageing population and improvements in modern chemotherapeutic regimens, we can assume the number of patients afflicted will only continue to rise. For some tumour types, notably breast and prostate tumours, bony metastasis is not necessarily associated with a reduction in life span compared to visceral metastasis.

In addition to the individual, MBD carries a burden to society. In the US alone, it is estimated that 13 billion US dollars were spent managing metastatic disease in 2005 [2].

The aim of palliative care is improvement in the quality of life of patients and families who face life-threatening illness, by providing pain and symptom relief and spiritual and psychosocial support from diagnosis to the end of life. The goals of palliative orthopaedic treatment are relief of pain and restoration of mobility and function to generate improved quality of life. Orthopaedic surgeons are well equipped to facilitate these goals.

Whilst a large volume of research has been conducted in this field in the last half century, many patients who may benefit from orthopaedic surgery are not recognised and referred for consideration of stabilisation. Orthopaedic surgeons should understand the principles of managing patients with MBD. This involves being able to recognise these patients, investigate appropriately and stabilise surgically when appropriate. The treating surgeon needs to be able to work effectively in a multidisciplinary environment recognising the need to involve oncologists, radiation physicians and, potentially, referral to subspecialist units when complicated reconstruction is required.

In this chapter, the authors will provide the reader with the principles of treatment in the hope that they feel comfortable managing patients with MBD in their own practice. Whilst many cases will require subspecialist involvement, the majority can be managed locally. This helps to alleviate some of the psychological burden associated with this life-threatening diagnosis.

25.2 Basic Science

It has been noted for many years that the bone is a common site for metastatic disease. We now recognise that the viscera and the spine are interconnected through the valveless channels of Batson's plexus. This helps to explain the propensity for metastasis to occur in the spine and pelvis. In addition it helps to explain the observation that whilst any malignancy may metastasise to the bone, over 80 % of MBD is caused by five primary tumours, namely breast, prostate, lung, thyroid and renal tumours, all of which have access to this system. Long bone lesions are seen most commonly in the proximal segments, thought to be due to increased blood flow. Two thirds of long bone lesions are encountered in the femur, and the majority of the remainder are in the humerus.

The bone is also a significant host of growth factors. It has been postulated that tumour cells expressing appropriate adhesion molecules can bind and cause the destruction of bone releasing these growth factors, which can potentiate growth of metastatic foci [3].

The majority of metastatic lesions encountered are lytic in nature. Lysis is not due to direct tumour destruction. It occurs via the release of cytokines, causing recruitment of osteoclasts. This is thought to occur as part of the metastatic cell binding. It is critical that the surgeon appreciates the alteration to local biology [3]. It should not be assumed that fractures will progress to healing as most will not [4]. Fixation needs to be selected that will withstand a lack of load sharing.

25.3 Clinical Presentation

Skeletal lesions are the major cause of pain in cancer patients and the main reason they will present to the orthopaedic surgeon. Metastases to the liver and lung may be asymptomatic for long periods, whilst MBD may cause pain early in the disease.

In patients with metastatic carcinoma, a low threshold of suspicion should be maintained that pain may be musculoskeletal in nature. Typically the pain is deep, unrelenting and progressive, and night pain is a concern. That said, many patients will present with more non-specific symptoms. Vague headache can be a sign of skull base involvement, and backache may be related to spinal metastasis.

Spinal cord compression or cauda equina syndrome is seen less commonly than long bone fracture. However, it needs to be appreciated due to the potential for permanent loss of function. There may be a history of back pain exacerbated by activities which increase visceral pressure (i.e. coughing, sneezing). Neurological deficits can be reported. Motor weakness is the most common, followed by pain, sensory disturbance and sphincter loss.

Patients may also present with the sequelae of hypercalcaemia. Classical presentations of hypercalcaemia, such as nephrolithiasis, bone pain and psychiatric effects, are less frequent, and patients may simply report fatigue, anorexia and constipation.

25.4 Investigation

Patients with MBD can present at different stages of their disease. Some will present with a diagnosed primary tumour with a documented lesion that has progressed and is causing symptoms. In this population we can proceed directly to surgical planning. Extensive investigation is not required.

In those patients not known to have metastatic disease or malignancy, a more careful approach should be undertaken. Whilst lytic skeletal lesions are 500 times more likely to be metastasis than primary sarcoma, primary lesions do exist [2]. The "rodded sarcoma" or "whoops procedure" creates a very difficult reconstructive problem for the orthopaedic oncologist. In cases where the diagnosis is in doubt, the authors recommend discussion with an experienced orthopaedic oncologist. This will help to prevent adverse outcomes to patients [5].

25.4.1 Clinical Assessment

Appropriate assessment begins with history and physical examination. Determining a history of carcinoma or a family history is important. A systems review and an assessment of risk factors (i.e. smoking, obesity, alcohol) should also be undertaken. The severity of the pain helps to guide management. It should be noted if pain is present at rest, or only with use, as this alters quality of life. Current medical condition is relevant as is chemotherapy which may be ongoing. It is important to enquire about previous surgery or radiotherapy to the site as this may dictate surgical planning.

Physical examination is mandatory. The soft tissues overlying the lesions and planned surgical sites must be assessed as should distal neurological function. All findings should be carefully documented. In cases of metastasis with unknown primary, examination of the breast, thyroid and prostate may lead to the diagnosis. Metastatic renal cell and thyroid carcinoma are highly vascular and bruits may be detected.

25.4.2 Laboratory Assessment

Essential tests vary depending on clinical scenario. In cases where diagnosis needs to be made, the following are considered mandatory:

1. Full blood count: The film may show changes consistent with marrow packing disorders such as myeloma. Anaemia is also common amongst cancer patients and should be detected preoperatively.

2. Erythrocyte sedimentation rate (ESR) and C-reactive protein (CRP) are markers for infection, a potential differential diagnosis in MBD. ESR is also elevated in myeloma.
3. Urea and electrolytes: Renal function can be impaired and potassium metabolism is often altered in this population.
4. Liver function tests: This can indicate poor synthetic function and is an independent predictor of a poor outcome and alerts the surgeon to potential healing problems and coagulopathy. Elevated enzymes may be due to hepatic metastasis.
5. Coagulation profile can be altered by poor liver function and should be documented prior to invasive procedures.
6. Serum calcium: Whilst not common, it must be diagnosed as it can be lethal if untreated. More common in lung carcinoma and haematological malignancies.
7. Serum and urine quantitative electrophoresis are diagnostic in myeloma.
8. Prostate specific antigen is often elevated with prostatic metastatic disease.

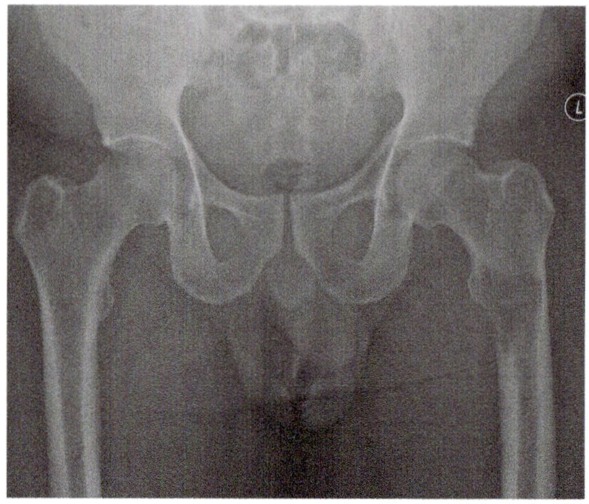

Fig. 25.1 Lytic lesion in the left proximal femur of a 40-year-old male. Note the bony destruction and lack of blastic response

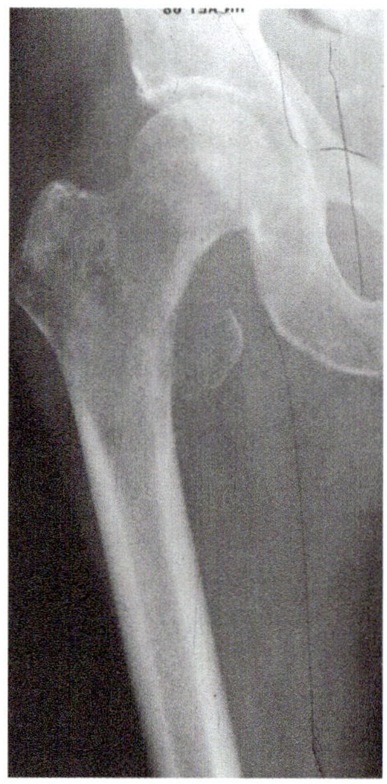

Fig. 25.2 Proximal femoral metastatic deposit secondary to transitional cell carcinoma. The isolated lesser trochanter fracture is considered pathognomonic of a sinister cause

25.4.3 Imaging

Plain x-rays yield the greatest volume of information for diagnosis and surgical planning. X-rays must be of high quality and include the full length of the bone. Orthogonal views must be obtained. A chest x-ray is routine to look for both primary tumour and visceral metastasis as well as for other co-morbidities relevant to the anaesthetic assessment.

Metastatic lesions can mimic other pathologies but tend to affect medullary and cortical bone and have a narrow zone of transition and minimal periosteal reaction (Figs. 25.1 and 25.2). Blastic lesions are frequently seen in prostate carcinoma. In women they can be seen in breast carcinoma although, overall, lytic lesions are more common. Acral metastasis (distal to the elbow or knee) is classically associated with lung carcinoma although renal cell cancer may also exhibit this behaviour. Isolated cortical metastasis is associated with lung carcinoma.

New presentations are advised to have a Technetium-99 bone scan. It will not necessarily determine primary lesions but can assist in identifying if a lesion is monostotic or polyostotic

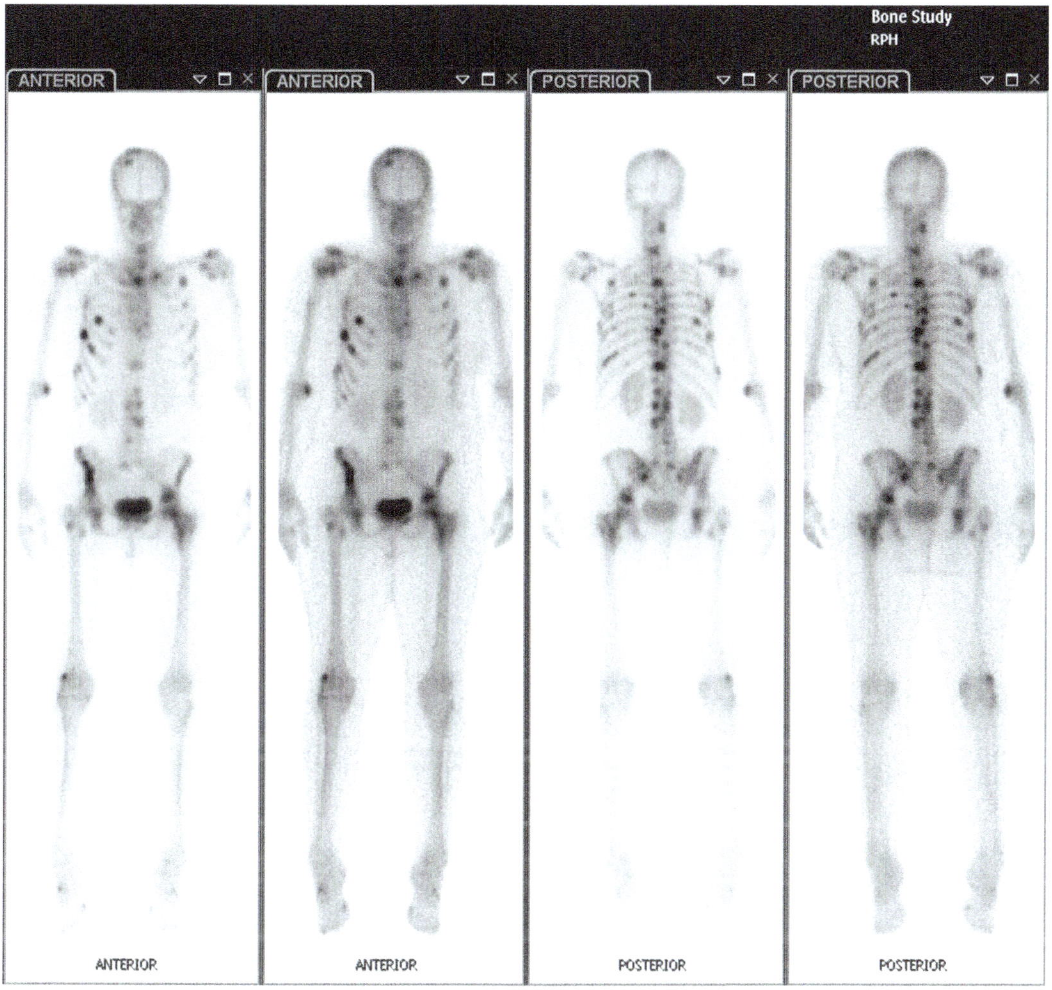

Fig. 25.3 Technetium-99 bone scan of a patient with breast cancer. The disease has metastasised throughout the skeleton

(Fig. 25.3). This can help look for other sites of potential disease and delineate those patients for whom curative resection may be intended. It also acts as a baseline for response to treatment. Surgeons must note that bone scans are only hot if osteoblastic activity is present. Some cancers can cause lysis without osteoblastic growth and will be cold. The classic example is myeloma. Renal cell tumours may also exhibit this behaviour.

CT scanning of lesions is generally of little use in diagnosis, although it may help in surgical planning. Scanning of the viscera, however, is probably the single most high-yield investigation for determining primary lesions. CT scan of the chest, abdomen and pelvis can detect the primary tumour in 85 % of cases [6] (Fig. 25.4). Importantly, if it fails to do so, then it is unlikely that further invasive investigation will assist.

Positron emission tomogram (PET) scanning has been examined recently to aid in this situation. It possesses greater diagnostic accuracy in locating small (5 mm) lesions. As such it is increasingly being used in lesions with unknown primary tumours. Its other use is determining patients for whom curative resection may be considered. It is generally only available in tertiary referral hospitals, limiting its use.

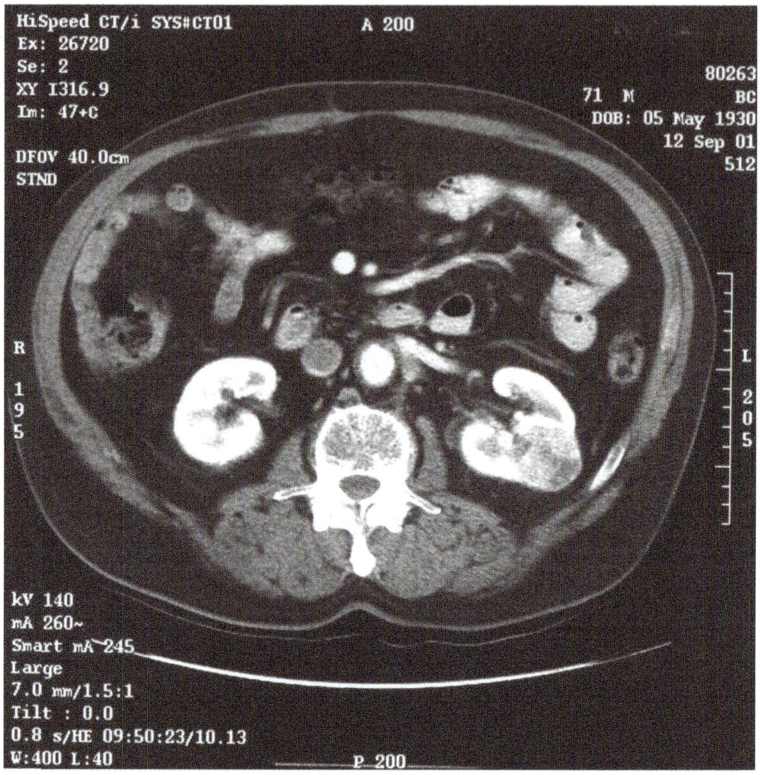

Fig. 25.4 Selected CT slice of a patient who presented with a lesion in the proximal humerus. Investigation revealed a mass in the left kidney. Subsequent biopsy demonstrated a renal cell carcinoma

25.4.4 Biopsy

In cases where the diagnosis is unclear, a biopsy is the next step. Even if the diagnosis is clear, it is common practice to send operative material for histopathology to confirm the clinical suspicion.

We recommend discussion with an orthopaedic oncologist if the diagnosis is in doubt prior to performing a biopsy. It may not be necessary for the patient to be transferred but can prevent problems with subsequent treatment. Certain centres have radiology staff capable of performing biopsies under CT or US guidance.

The biopsy can be as simple as sending reamings from intramedullary (IM) nailing or as a separate procedure prior to planned reconstruction. When performing open biopsy the principles are based on the need to cause minimal contamination. If wide resection is subsequently needed, the biopsy tract must be excised with the lesion as it is considered contaminated with malignant cells.

Longitudinal incisions should be used violating as few compartments as possible. Neurovascular structures should be avoided and meticulous haemostasis is required. Drains should be placed at the inferior apex of the wound, if required.

Material should be sent for both histological analysis and bacterial culture and sensitivity. Prior discussion with a pathologist can aid in deciding what samples the medium should be transported in (i.e. fresh or formalin).

25.5 Management

Treatment for patients with MBD is primarily palliative, with the goals of limiting pain and rapidly restoring function. The aims for each patient will vary depending on the situation. Some patients will require surgery to facilitate community ambulation, whilst others simply need stability to allow nursing care.

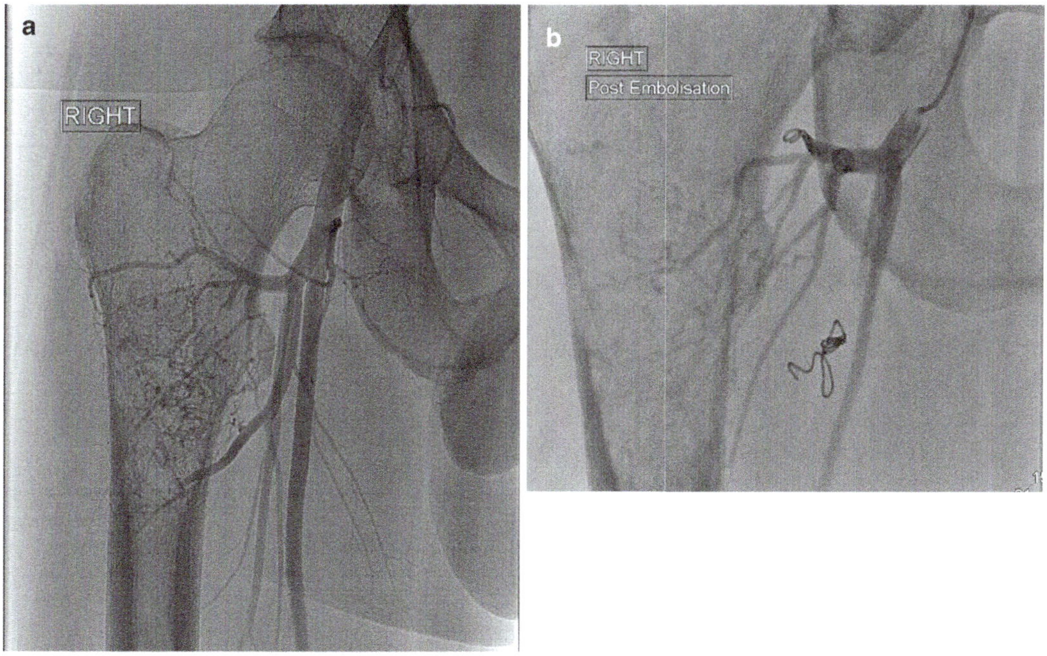

Fig. 25.5 (**a**, **b**) Pre- and post-angiography and coiling of a highly vascular renal cell carcinoma deposit in the right proximal femur. The coils and decreased flow can be seen

The likely outcome and risks involved need to be clearly communicated to the patient and family.

Management of these patients can be divided into the preoperative optimisation, operative planning and intervention followed by postoperative rehabilitation and adjuvant treatment.

25.5.1 Preoperative Assessment

25.5.1.1 Medical Optimisation

Patients with MBD often suffer from other medical co-morbidities and the sequelae of their cancer. Malnourishment, anaemia, coagulopathy and hypercalcaemia can be present. The clinician should be alert to these possibilities. Early involvement of other medical disciplines and the anaesthetist may be required. Spinal anaesthesia may be favoured if lung function is compromised, though it is contraindicated if central metastases are present due to the risk of coning. Malignancy increases the risk of thromboembolic disease, and we recommend routine use of mechanical prophylactic devices, specifically intermittent pneumatic compression pumps. Chemical prophylaxis is indicated if it does not interfere with planned surgery or anaesthesia. Hypercalcaemia, whilst rare, increases the risk of adverse outcomes in the perioperative period. Correction can usually be achieved with intravenous fluid and bisphosphonate infusions.

25.5.1.2 Embolisation

Renal and thyroid carcinoma lesions may be highly vascular. Embolisation is advisable to decrease the risk of bleeding. This should be performed even if closed techniques such as intramedullary nailing are to be employed. CT angiography can provide an idea of the vascularity of the lesion. Embolisation should be performed within 48 h and preferably 24 h prior to surgery to provide optimal effect (Fig. 25.5a, b).

25.5.1.3 Adjuvant Treatment

The treating surgeon should be aware of the principles of adjuvant therapies. These include radiotherapy and chemotherapy including bisphosphonates. Radiation therapy is virtually always used postoperatively. It helps alleviate pain and "mops up" tumour cells dispersed through operation. The entire bone is included. A single course is usually all that is required. When operating through the skin that has previously been irradiated, it is important to know the dosage. Wound healing complications can be expected if cumulative dose was over 50 Gy; 60 or more Gy will almost guarantee wound breakdown.

Chemotherapy can impair wound healing. Surgery should be delayed until after the effects on neutrophils have ceased. Because of the variability between agents, surgeons should consult their oncology colleagues preoperatively.

25.5.2 Operative Planning and Surgery

There are several important principles in the surgical treatment of MBD. It is established that surgical stabilisation increases patients' ability to ambulate, be discharged home and achieve pain relief. Decision-making needs to be individualised. The period of recovery or protected rehabilitation should not be longer than the anticipated life expectancy. Paradoxically, this often requires the use of more invasive surgical techniques to facilitate stability and early pain-free function. Surgeons should aim to undertake only one operation to stabilise a lesion.

Broad principles are outlined below [4]:

1. Prognosis guides treatment. Patients with life expectancy less than 6 weeks should be treated with analgesia and radiotherapy. For a prognosis of 6 weeks to 6 months, internal fixation using osteosynthesis is recommended. If the patient is likely to live longer than 6 months, arthroplasty or endoprosthetic reconstruction should be strongly considered.
2. All affected areas of the bone should be considered in the proposed reconstruction.
3. Mechanical stability that allows immediate use and weight bearing must be obtained.
4. Radiotherapy is administered post surgery. This reduces pain and helps to clear cancer cells disseminated locally by the surgery.

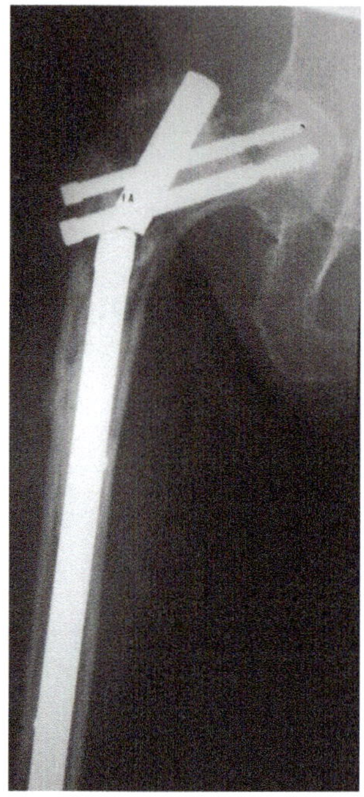

Fig. 25.6 Example of fatigue failure of osteosynthesis. The patient had myeloma affecting the right proximal femur. Intramedullary nail with cement augmentation was used. The patient outlived the implant

Determining the prognosis is one of the most difficult aspects of managing these patients, yet it is critical to outcome. Typically, clinicians have a tendency to underestimate the patients' life expectancy. This has the potential to under-treat and place patients at risk for failure of fixation and further surgery (Fig. 25.6). Scoring systems are available to help, but often consultation with the patients' oncologist or general practitioner may provide the most useful assessment. The following features are associated with a better prognosis:

1. Primary tumour breast, prostate, myeloma or lymphoma
2. Solitary skeletal metastasis
3. Absence of visceral metastasis
4. Absence of pathological fracture

Renal cell carcinoma is a tumour that is difficult to predict. Its biological activity can be highly variable as is the prognosis. We encourage surgeons to seek expert opinion when dealing with this tumour.

Management of long bone lesions varies with the anatomical site. The femur and the humerus are the most commonly affected bones. In the lower limb IM nailing is the treatment of choice. It carries the advantages of whole bone protection, minimally invasive insertion and resistance to axial loading. The decreased soft tissue insult and improved mechanical strength facilitate early weight bearing and rehabilitation. In the femur we advocate the use of long cephalo-medullary nails. These maximise the amount of bone protected and reduce the need for re-operation [7, 8].

The main disadvantage with IM nailing is the embolisation of tumour, fat and thrombus to the lungs with resulting potential cardiopulmonary compromise. This phenomenon is also seen in trauma surgery. However, the mortality rates are increased in the MBD population. It is thought to be due to increased permeability of the bone coupled with increased vascularity. The effect is magnified in bilateral disease and in the intact bone.

Multiple techniques have been suggested to reduce the incidence of embolic load. These include drilling decompressive vents distally, use of unreamed nails and, more recently, the use of the reamer-irrigator-aspirator (RIA) device.

Femoral venting has only been shown to be of benefit in reducing peak pressure in animal studies. The main problem is the generation of a stress riser, and it is currently not routinely performed in our institution. Other methods include removal of the guide wire prior to nail insertion allowing decompression on marrow contents through the nail. However, this can only be done if the reduction is maintained.

Unreamed solid nails have the theoretical advantages of decreased embolic load, shorter operating time and less trauma to endosteal blood supply. However, the available literature from the trauma setting has not demonstrated a clinical advantage. This may stem from the fact that the highest pressures are generated by the femoral opening broach rather than during the reaming process. The disadvantage of unreamed nails is the decreased diameter. This reduces bending rigidity and increases unsupported length.

The reamer-irrigator-aspirator (DePuy-Synthes™, Switzerland) device has been developed for use in the multitrauma patient to reduce the embolic load from multiple long bone nails. It has found alternative uses in bone graft harvesting and also in treatment of metastatic deposits. The principle is a high-speed (900 rpm) sharp single-use reamer. This is attached to an irrigation tube providing continuous fluid and suction to remove debris. Currently, no literature exists to support its routine use in the management of MBD.

In the majority of patients, the development of pulmonary complications probably relates more to preoperative global condition and haemodynamic stability rather than any of the variables listed previously. Therefore, we advocate preoperative optimisation and intraoperative attention to haemodynamic status. We recommend using standard reamed statically locked nailing of long bone lesions without venting, removing the guide wire prior to insertion if possible. Reaming is gentle, progressing slowly, and the anaesthetist is advised at the time of the potential for embolic effects.

Bilateral femoral nailing for MBD increases the risk to the patient for cardiopulmonary compromise. Where possible, the second surgical procedure should be delayed until the patient has recovered from the surgical insult.

Controversy exists in the surgical management of diaphyseal lesions in the humerus. The surgical options are either IM nailing or plate stabilisation, usually in conjunction with polymethylmethacrylate (PMMA) augmentation. Nailing in the humerus carries the disadvantages of rotator cuff violation and poor rotational rigidity to a bone subjected to, predominantly, rotational loads. For these reasons some surgeons advocate an open approach with plate fixation, often with PMMA augmentation (Fig. 25.7a, b). This is a more rigid construct but requires greater surgical dissection and limited ability to protect the entire bone. There is no consensus within the literature, and we suggest surgeons use the technique they feel most comfortable with.

The increasing use of arthroplasty or endoprosthetic reconstruction (EPR) for MBD is important to note. This has been driven by the improved understanding of altered local biology in metastasis and by failures of osteosynthesis. In metastatic deposits proliferation of osteoclasts leads to unpredictable fracture healing. Union

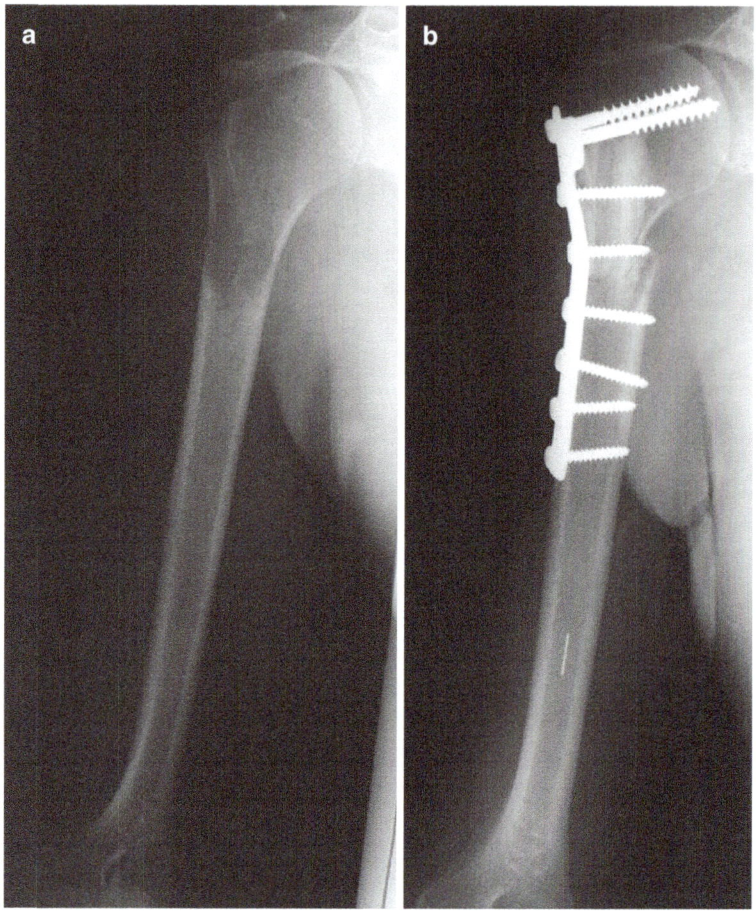

Fig. 25.7 (**a**, **b**) A 71-year-old male with disseminated renal cell carcinoma. This has been treated with osteosynthesis augmented with PMMA bone cement

rates vary from 67 % in myeloma to virtually 0 % in lung carcinoma [2]. Even after radiotherapy, tumours can continue to grow and destroy the bone (Fig. 25.8a, b). This can cause implant fatigue/failure and ongoing pain as well as limiting reconstructive options. EPR has become the treatment of choice for periarticular disease.

The femur and specifically the hip are disproportionately over-represented in the frequency of long bone MBD locations. Up to 75 % of all surgery for MBD is performed in the hip. Arthroplasty has an increasing role due to its reliability and familiarity to most orthopaedic surgeons. Immediate weight bearing can be allowed, and ongoing follow-up can be minimised to decrease the social burden to the patient and family.

In the proximal femur, lesions that cross the intertrochanteric line proximally should be treated with arthroplasty. Osteosynthesis in this region for MBD and related fractures has an unacceptably high revision rate [8]. Planning is essential. A CT may be required to assess local bone stock and to detect lesions distally in the femur and acetabulum. These will all need to be dealt with in the planned reconstruction. Surgical approach is dictated by the surgeons' preference.

Cemented components should be used in femoral reconstruction. Cemented stems allow immediate weight bearing, and radiation can be administered with no concerns over stem ingrowth. Choice of prosthesis is dictated by the surgeons' preference. However, the use of calcar-replacing prostheses may be needed if the bone is deficient in this region. Involvement of the greater trochanter is a difficult problem. It can be curetted safely and packed with cement but as much as possible should be retained to aid in implant stability.

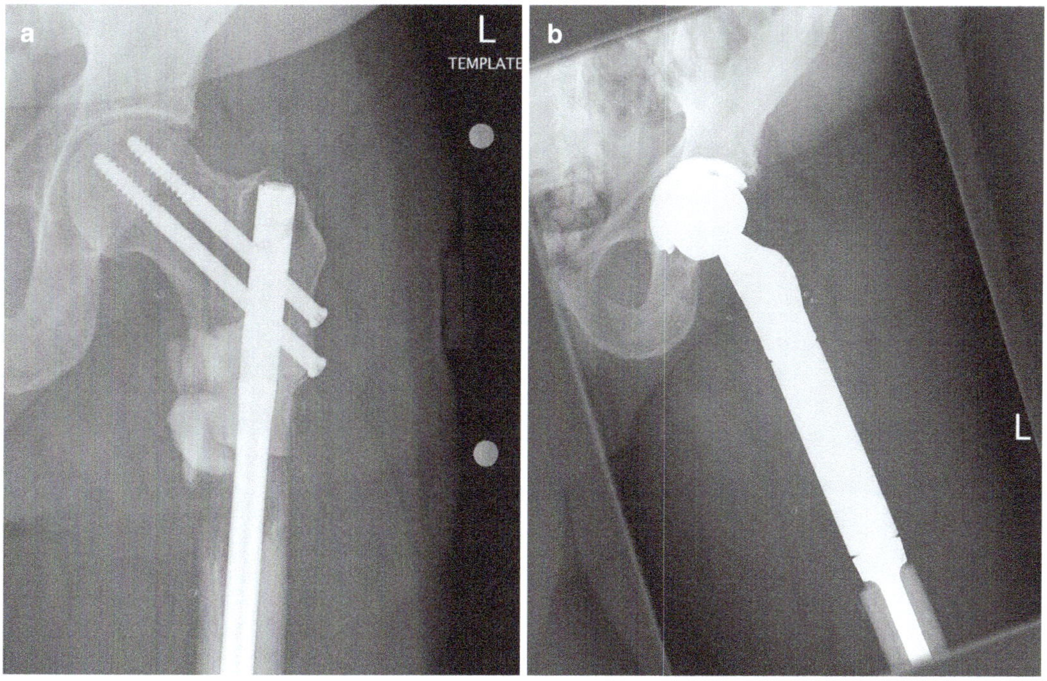

Fig. 25.8 (**a**) Patient from Fig. 25.1 several weeks after internal fixation with PMMA augmentation. The disease has progressed distally. Note the coils from preoperative embolisation. (**b**) Patient from Figs. 25.1 and 25.8a showing revision to a tumour prosthesis

Stem length is important. The tip of the stem must bypass the distal extent of the lesion by two cortical diameters in order to minimise the stress riser effect. This will often require the use of long stem implants. We prefer low viscosity cement and slow introduction of the stem to minimise pressure changes and embolisation. Distal cement restrictors are not necessary when using long stems. The addition of antibiotics to the cement is encouraged, and the dose can be increased safely. We accept that increased antibiotic adversely affects the cement quality. However, infection is of greater concern in deconditioned patients with a terminal illness. For patients with a poorer prognosis, a unipolar head can be used. The decision to use a total hip arthroplasty is based on patient function, life expectancy and the presence of concurrent osteoarthritis or acetabular metastasis.

Massive metaphyseal bone loss may necessitate the use of a proximal femoral replacement or tumour prosthesis. These operations are technically challenging with a high complication rate, and referral to a specialist centre is advised.

Acetabular reconstruction principles follow those found in revision hip arthroplasty. These techniques are complex and should only be undertaken by surgeons experienced in revision hip arthroplasty. Areas of MBD are akin to defects seen from polyethylene wear and should be defined with CT (Fig. 25.9a, b). The difference is the lack of a favourable local biological environment. Bone graft cannot be expected to integrate. If the disease is isolated to the acetabulum, curettage and cementation to the lesion with use of a modified Harrington technique can be employed [9]. More commonly, the joint is affected, or there is disease on the femoral side making arthroplasty a more appropriate choice. Currently, cemented acetabular components are considered "gold standard". Uncemented ultraporous metal cups have recently been used for the management of these lesions, and whilst their use is appealing, more work must be done before routine use can be recommended. Large areas of lysis should be curetted, and the defects can be filled with cement. A cup can be subsequently

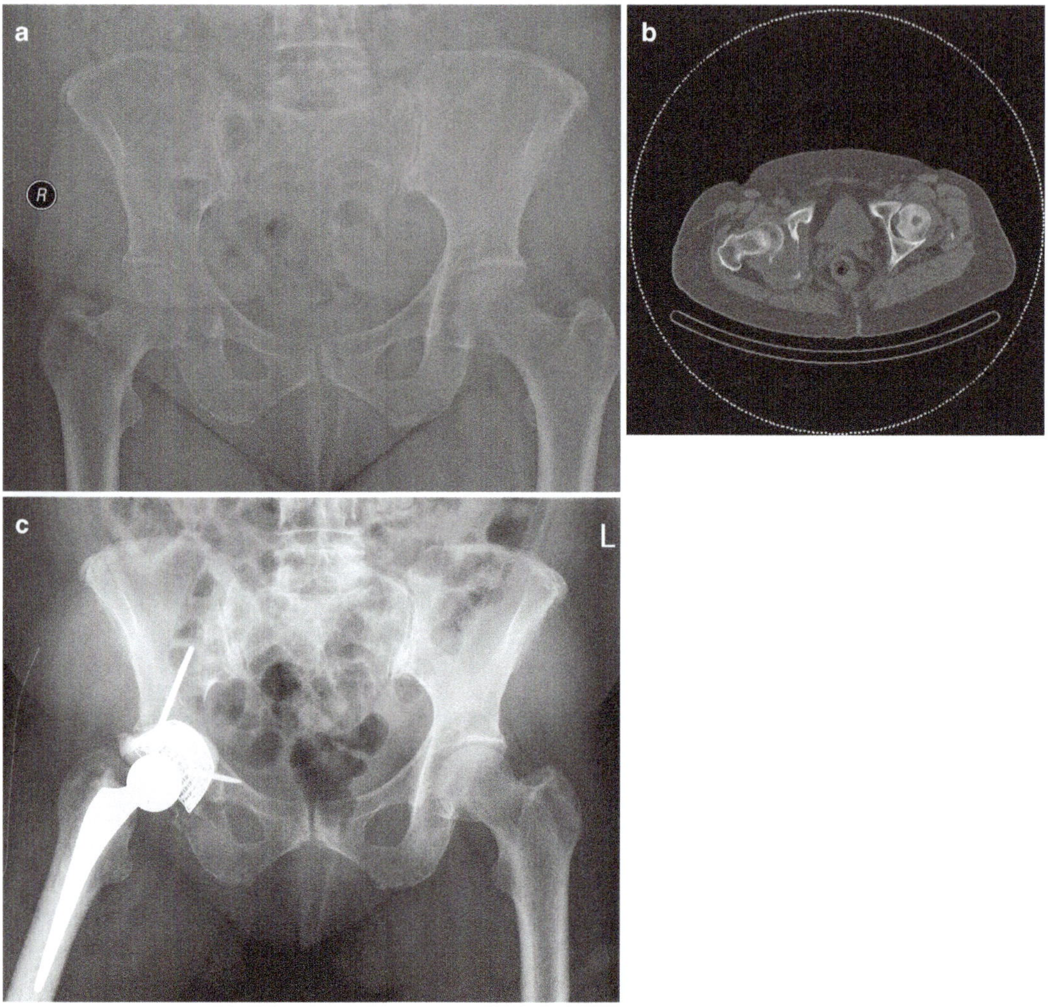

Fig. 25.9 (**a**, **b**) Patient with MBD affecting the right hip secondary to lung cancer. Plain x-ray does not demonstrate the extent of the process. The CT better defines the deficiency of the posterior bone and joint penetration (**c**) Reconstruction for the patient seen in **a**, **b**. After curettage of the acetabular defect, a cemented cup is placed. This is protected using a combination of mesh and a modified Harrington rod technique

cemented into this. Additional techniques are available if the support for the cement is poor. A modified Harrington rod technique can be used where threaded pins can be driven into the ilium, cut short and the cemented cup rested on this (Fig. 25.9c). Alternatively a cage may be used. Metal on polyethylene articulations are preferred, and where possible, large heads should be employed to improve stability. Intercalary resection (Fig. 25.10a–c) and endoprosthetic replacement are being used increasingly for patients with metastatic disease. Immediate and reliable weight bearing and pain control are strong incentives. This is offset by the increased surgical dissection, blood loss and infection risk. We recommend that the use of these implants and megaprostheses in general be confined to subspecialist surgeons.

MBD around the knee is far less common. The principles of management are the same as elsewhere. If internal fixation is utilised, then it must be robust enough to allow early weight bearing. Often destruction of local bone stock will preclude this, and an arthroplasty will be required.

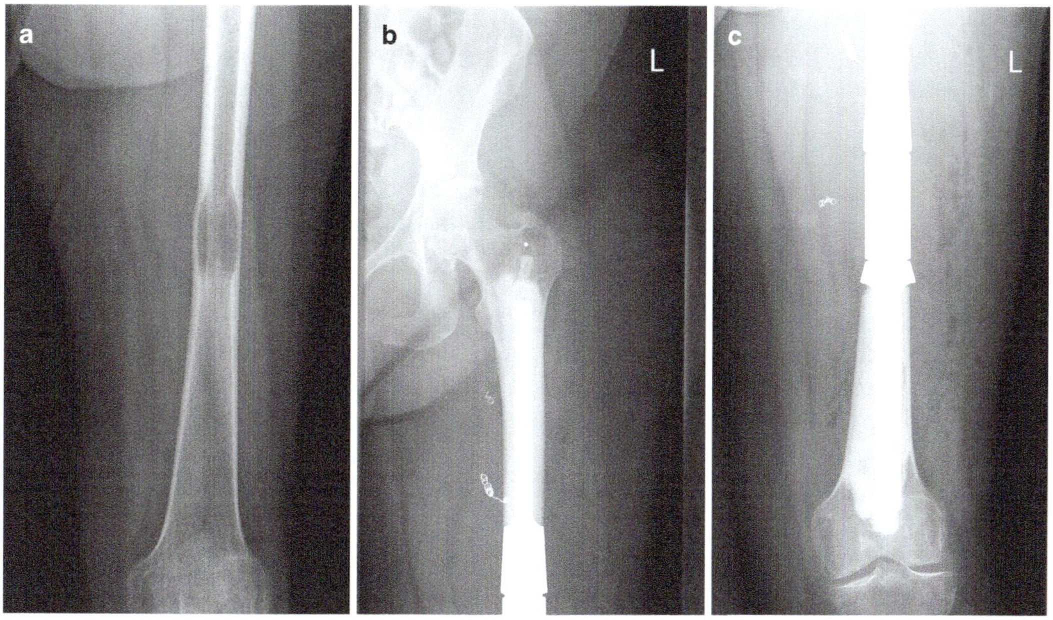

Fig. 25.10 (**a–c**) A 67-year-old female with MBD secondary to renal cell carcinoma. Due to good prognosis and high functional status, the patient underwent excision and reconstruction using an intercalary prosthesis. Excellent result was obtained in terms of pain relief and function. Note the coils from preoperative embolisation

Planning is critical and attention to common arthroplasty decision-making should be employed. Cemented stems should bypass lesions. A rotating hinge design should be used if collateral ligament insertion sites are involved. Care should be taken with soft tissue dissection. The preservation of the tibial tuberosity is essential. This may compromise tumour debulking, but in the palliative setting maintaining the extensor function is of greater importance.

In the humerus, endoprosthetic replacement has a well-defined role in trauma management, and this has been extended to deal with MBD. Resection and hemiarthroplasty offer reliable pain relief in the shoulder. Function is dependent on the condition and reconstructive capacity of the tuberosities. The patient must be counselled as to the likely diminished functional outcome. Reverse total shoulder arthroplasty has been suggested as an alternative to improve function. Currently, complication rates related to instability and unclear long-term outcomes limit its wide-spread use. Therefore, we cannot recommend it at this time except by recommendation of sub-specialists. In the elbow, arthroplasty for MBD has been utilised with success. Care should be taken to define the extent of the disease. In a series of 20 cases, a high rate (25 %) of local recurrence was seen [10]. Importantly, in this series, routine radio and chemotherapy did not alter wound healing or infection rates.

25.5.2.1 Impending Fracture

Patients may present with disease prior to fracture. The decision on when to intervene, and when to observe, is often difficult. Intervening prior to fracture improves patient outcomes, returns function sooner and decreases hospital stays. If the surgeon feels a patient is at risk of impending fracture in the lower limb, weight bearing should immediately be ceased and the patient admitted to hospital.

There are multiple reported methods for determining if a lesion is likely to progress to fracture. Both radiographic and clinical measures have been suggested. In our institution Mirels' scoring system is used to aid in prediction [11].

It is summarised in Table 25.1. The lesion site is predictive with the highest risk seen in peritrochanteric lesions. The size is determined by

Table 25.1 Mirels' scoring system

	Score = 1	Score = 2	Score = 3
Site	Upper limb	Lower limb	Trochanteric
Size	<1/3	1/3–2/3	>2/3
Pain	Mild	Moderate	Severe
Nature	Blastic	Mixed	Lytic

proportion of the bones total diameter affected by the metastasis. Blastic lesions (common in prostate) have a lower risk of fracture. Pain is difficult to define; mild and severe are relative terms. We prefer to consider pain as (1) not an issue to the patient, (2) pain with mechanical loading and (3) rest pain.

The patient is given a score out of 12. Seven or less is associated with a 4 % risk of fracture after irradiation. Eight is associated with 15 % and nine or greater with 33 % risk of fracture. The value of eight or greater is generally accepted as an indication for prophylactic intervention. In practical terms, the decision is made after discussion and counselling the patient. Realistically, pain in the lower limb, especially around the hip, will generally require stabilisation as the risk of progression is high.

Intervention in intact long bones, whilst advantageous, carries its own risks. A fracture allows decompression of the medullary canal. Embolic material will disperse through this gap rather than enter the vascular system. Instrumentation of an intact long bone increases peak intramedullary pressures beyond that seen after fracture. Patients should be counselled about the increased risk. Despite this, there is still no evidence that prophylactic measures to reduce pressures alter clinical outcome. We do not routinely recommend such measures and suggest surgeons use techniques familiar to them.

25.5.3 Postoperative Care

Early mobilisation should be encouraged as soon as practical with the use of aids and physical therapy. We recommend routine use of mechanical thromboembolic prophylaxis with calf pumps. Chemical prophylaxis can be used as appropriate. The use of drains is at the discretion of the surgeon though we find them rarely necessary. A single dose of a broad-spectrum cephalosporin on induction should be given though we do not routinely administer antibiotics beyond this time. Mobilisation of the shoulder may need to be limited for up to 6 weeks allowing time for soft tissue recovery. In the hip, flexion should be limited to 90° for 6 weeks to prevent dislocation.

25.5.4 Amputation

Amputation is rarely performed for MBD. Improvements in surgical reconstruction techniques and the relative rarity of distal metastases (which may be more feasibly dealt with by amputation) have decreased the need for such radical surgery.

Practically, amputation should be reserved for cases in which reconstruction is not possible and pain cannot be controlled by non-surgical means. The patients' prognosis must be considered as the period of rehabilitation in this debilitated cohort may be longer than in others. Patients should be counselled that even below-knee amputations may leave them wheelchair dependent based on the prognosis and on their general health condition. It will be advantageous for the patient to meet preoperatively with rehabilitation specialists and possibly other patients who have experienced an amputation. The psychological effects of such surgery to the terminally ill patient and their family can be severe and must be anticipated.

Very little literature exists on this subject, in keeping with its infrequent use. Palliative amputation has been used in the upper limb for soft tissue metastasis invading the brachial plexus [12]. In the foot and ankle, reconstruction that allows early weight bearing is difficult making amputation a feasible alternative.

Surgical technique must be meticulous and shall be performed by a surgeon who is familiar with the procedure to avoid further unnecessary suffering of the already compromised patient. Wound healing problems are commonly encountered, and chemotherapy must often be ceased until healing is assured. Haemostasis is critical, and the use of drains prevents haematoma with possible detrimental consequences for the patient. Careful follow-up is advised to ensure wound healing, properly fitted prosthesis and mental health.

Conclusion

The aims of palliative orthopaedic treatment are to alleviate pain and restore function, mobility and dignity to patients suffering with terminal cancer. Treating surgeons will often find themselves to be team leaders in the patients' management. A multidisciplinary approach involving other staff in the decision-making process is important. It is critical that the patients and their family are involved in this process from diagnosis, through treatment and to bereavement. Clear, straightforward communication is essential to a good outcome.

This chapter provides the treating surgeon with an understanding of the principles of orthopaedic management in patients with metastatic bone disease. This includes appropriate clinical assessment and investigation as well as the technical management of these lesions. It is hoped the reader will feel confident managing appropriately in peripheral practices as well as knowing when to seek the assistance of a specialist centre.

References

1. Coleman R. Clinical features of metastatic bone disease and risk of skeletal morbidity. Clin Cancer Res. 2006;12(20 Suppl):6243–9.
2. Biermann J, Holt G, Valerae O, Schwartz H, Yaszemski M. Metastatic bone disease: diagnosis, evaluation, and treatment. Instr Course Lect J Bone Joint Surg. 2009;91-A:1518–30.
3. Coghlin C, Murray G. Current and emerging concepts in tumour metastasis. J Pathol. 2010;222:1–15.
4. Damron T, Sim F. Operative treatment for metastatic disease of the pelvis and proximal end of the femur. Instr Course Lect J Bone Joint Surg. 2000;82-A(1):114–26.
5. Mankin H, Mankin C, Simon M. The hazards of the biopsy, revisited. J Bone Joint Surg. 1996;78-A(5):656–63.
6. Simon M, Bartucci E. The search for the primary tumor in patients with skeletal metastasis of unknown origin. Cancer. 1986;58(5):1088–95.
7. Van der Hulst R, Van den Wildenburg F, Vroemen J, Greve J. Intramedullary nailing of (impending) pathological fractures. J Trauma. 1994;36(2):211–5.
8. Wedin R, Bauer H, Wersäll P. Failures after operation for skeletal metastatic lesions of long bones. Clin Orthop Relat Res. 1999;358:128–39.
9. Harrington K, Sim H, Enis J, Johnston J, Diok H, Gristina A. Methylmethacrylate as an adjunct in internal fixation of pathological fractures: experience with three hundred and seventy five cases. J Bone Joint Surg Am. 1976;58A:1047–55.
10. Athwal G, Chin P, Adams R, Morrey B. Coonrad-Morrey total elbow arthroplasty for tumours of the distal humerus and elbow. J Bone Joint Surg Br. 2005;87B(10):1369–74.
11. Mirels H. Metastatic disease in long bones. A proposed scoring system for diagnosing impending pathological fractures. Clin Orthop Relat Res. 1989;249:256–64.
12. Wittig J, Bickels J, Kollender Y, Kellar-Graney K, Meller I, Malawer M. Palliative forequarter amputation for metastatic carcinoma to the shoulder girdle region: indications, preoperative evaluation, surgical technique, and results. J Surg Oncol. 2001;77(2):105–13.

Index

M. Wichmann, G. Maddern (eds.), *Palliative Surgery*,
DOI 10.1007/978-3-642-53709-7, © Springer-Verlag Berlin Heidelberg 2014

R

S

GPSR Compliance

The European Union's (EU) General Product Safety Regulation (GPSR) is a set of rules that requires consumer products to be safe and our obligations to ensure this.

If you have any concerns about our products, you can contact us on ProductSafety@springernature.com

In case Publisher is established outside the EU, the EU authorized representative is:

Springer Nature Customer Service Center GmbH
Europaplatz 3
69115 Heidelberg, Germany

Batch number: 10166043

Printed by Printforce, the Netherlands